Health Equity, Diversity, and Inclusion

SECOND EDITION

Context, Controversies, and Solutions

Patti R. Rose, MPH, EdD

President and Founder
Rose Consulting Inc.
Miami, Florida

JONES & BARTLETT
LEARNING

D0905842

World Headquarters
Jones & Bartlett Learning
25 Mall Road
Burlington, MA 01803
978-443-5000
info@jblearning.com
www.jblearning.com

Jones & Bartlett Learning books and products are available through most bookstores and online booksellers. To contact Jones & Bartlett Learning directly, call 800-832-0034, fax 978-443-8000, or visit our website, www .jblearning.com.

Production Credits

VP, Product Management: Amanda Martin
Director of Product Management: Laura Pagluica
Product Manager: Sophie Fleck Teague
Product Specialist: Sara Bempkins
Project Specialist: Kelly Sylvester
Digital Project Specialist: Rachel DiMaggio
Senior Marketing Manager: Susanne Walker
Manufacturing and Inventory Control Supervisor: Amy Bacus
VP, Manufacturing and Inventory Control: Therese Connell
Composition: Exela Technologies
Project Management: Exela Technologies
Cover Design: Scott Moden
Senior Media Development Editor: Troy Liston
Rights Specialist: Maria Leon Maimone
Cover Image (Title Page, Chapter Opener): © schab/Shutterstock
Printing and Binding: Gasch Printing
Cover Printing: Gasch Printing

Library of Congress Cataloging-in-Publication Data

Names: Rose, Patti Renee, author.
Title: Health equity, diversity, and inclusion: context, controversies, and solutions / Patti R. Rose.
Other titles: Health disparities, diversity, and inclusion: context, controversies, and solutions
Description: Second edition. | Burlington, MA : Jones & Bartlett Learning, [2021] | Preceded by Health disparities, diversity and inclusion / Patti R. Rose. 2018. | Includes bibliographical references and index.
Identifiers: LCCN 2019048756 | ISBN 9781284197792 (paperback)
Subjects: MESH: Health Status Disparities | Social Determinants of Health | Cultural Diversity | Cultural Competency | United States
Classification: LCC RA563.M56 | NLM WA 300 AA1 | DDC 362.1089–dc23
LC record available at https://lccn.loc.gov/2019048756

6048

Printed in the United States of America
25 24 23   10 9 8 7 6 5 4

I lovingly devote this book to my beloved family—my husband Jeffrey Rose and our two beautiful children, Courtney and Brandon. With these individuals in my life, I have given and received unconditional love, experienced the true meaning of family, enjoyed amazing, intelligent conversation regularly, and experienced global travel with them, which is a true gift.

I also dedicate this book to all people who are suffering in the midst of social injustice, health and educational inequities, and health disparities. It is my hope that my words will continue to serve to inform on solutions to these ongoing problems and that health disparities, also known as "the gap", will be closed.

Contents

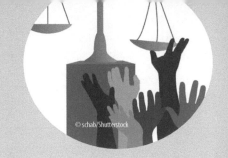

Chapter 12 Case Studies and Health Disparities . . .171

Chapter 13 What Is Diversity and Who Defines It? 185

Chapter 14 Diversity in Health Care: Making It Happen and Sustaining It 205

Chapter 15 Cultural Competence Versus Diversity: Why Cultural Competence Also Matters 219

Preface

As a young graduate student at Yale University pursuing a master of public health degree in the mid-1980s, I stumbled upon a topic that I was unfamiliar with—namely, health disparities in terms of race and ethnicity. I was taking a number of core courses, and within most, there was mention of a gap between the health statuses of Black and White people in the United States. I reflected upon this issue and decided that it would be a key area of interest for me, and indeed it has been to this day. I took pride in the fact that I was studying in a field, public health, in which I could make a real difference. I would be able to help close the health status gap. Not only did I take courses that emphasized health disparities, but I also attended "Closing the Gap" conferences, read books about it, and fiercely debated with classmates, and ultimately colleagues, about the causes.

Some argued that the primary reason for the gap was genetics, which I disagreed with, because I understood clearly that the illnesses that Black people were suffering from in the United States were not the same as those of Black people in Africa, for the most part. There were some genetic commonalities, such as disposition to sickle cell disease, but that served as a clear indicator that Black people in America were descendants of people in West Africa, primarily as a result of the slave trade.

Ultimately, after working in the field of public health for a couple of years, I decided to return to my studies to pursue a doctorate in community health education at Teachers College, Columbia University. Still, the health disparity existed, without much change, and I continued taking courses and learning more about the proverbial gap and its impact on other emerging majorities beyond Black people; further, I studied the importance of racial and ethnic diversity in the workforce, in terms of health, as it was touted as one of the many potential solutions to the problem. Many years later, in my role as an academic, I taught about health disparities and diversity, noting that the problems were the same as when I was a young student and that not only was the matter unresolved, in many ways it was worse.

The key aspects of this book are the discussions of health disparities, with an emphasis on solutions, and the ongoing need for diversity in the field of health. The issues of health disparities and diversity are framed by racial and ethnic considerations. This focus does not preclude the understanding that the term *diversity* is very broad, encompassing, beyond race and ethnicity, gender; the lesbian, gay, bisexual, transgender, queer or questioning, and intersex (LGBTQI) community; the disabled; and religious groups. However, this book seeks to identify health disparities along racial and ethnic lines.

The other area of focus is health equity. Although there are efforts to reach consensus around this definition, the Robert Wood Johnson Foundation defines it as follows:

"Health equity means that everyone has a fair and just opportunity to be as healthy as possible. This requires removing obstacles to health such as poverty, discrimination, and their consequences, including powerlessness and lack of access to good jobs with fair pay, quality education and housing, safe environments, and health care."

Health equity for all in the United States is a lofty goal, particularly given that health disparities are widening. It was felt by some that the Affordable Care Act (ACA), also known as Obamacare, would resolve these issues, leading to greater health equity, but it appears, thus far, that instead, the gap has widened, which is very unfortunate. Nevertheless, it is clear that the ACA is not universal health coverage, as private health corporations remain at the helm of health care in the United States. If we consider the history of the country, perhaps there is some insight, open for debate as to why security of health equity for all remains unachievable. 2019 commemorated the 400th anniversary of the transatlantic slave trade. Some argue that slaves arrived earlier. As pointed out by Torres Spellcy (2019):

There is a tendency of many people who write the history of America to have a view of the world centered on Jamestown and the Anglo American experience. When history fixates on the 13 original American colonies, the rest of the map, including Florida, seems to fall away. But it's worth expanding that picture to include Spanish-occupied territory in what is now the United States. When we consider those lands, we see that slavery actually dates back a full century before 1619. Slavery in Florida reveals how a multinational slave trade built on personal greed and white supremacy forced Africans and African Americans to build North American wealth in which they would not be able to share. Then, adding insult to injury, these early black slaves were erased from the standard narrative of American history.

The timeframe and dates as to when slavery began are important to clarify and remember, not only to ensure that no one forgets that this tragedy occurred, but also in terms of health disparities. Health inequity and the consideration of universal health coverage, points worthy of consideration, emerged from the 1619 Project, launched by *The New York Times* to explore slavery within the context of American History and to clarify existing historical understanding/teaching of the atrocity of slavery on American soil. In a PBS interview, the lead reporter of this body of work, Nikole Hannah-Jones, states the following:

…what we know is that white support for universal programs declines if they think that large numbers of black people are going to benefit from it. And this is a sentiment that goes all the way back to right after the end of the Civil War when the Freedmen's Bureau starts to offer universal health care for people who had literally just come out of bondage… And white people immediately pushed back against that believing that even people who had just come out of slavery should not get anything "for free," even though their labor clearly had built the entire, most of the economy of the country. And so that sentiment continues to this day.

This is a straightforward argument regarding universal health coverage and its relationship to lack of equity across the board, including health, for Black people, which also extends to certain other emerging majority groups. Whether one agrees with the argument made by Hannah-Jones or not, what is certain is that in terms of Black, Native American, and the ethnic group of Latino/Hispanic people, health equity in the United States is not the case. To achieve health equity moving forward, there must be less energy spent discussing the cause, resulting in total emphasis and focus on the solution. In general, the causes have been studied, researched, argued, and in many instances, established. Therefore, as this text explores causality, the aim is to highlight and explore solutions.

Additionally, throughout the book, use of the term *minority* is minimized in recognition of this term's obsolescence. The term is replaced by *emerging majority*, as it is clear that the United States has become more diverse than ever before. Emerging majority is used in this book to refer to the various racial groups and the Hispanic/Latino ethnic group. The terms Hispanic and Latino are used interchangeably when appropriate.

Cultural competence is highlighted as one of the many solutions to health disparities, as there is a need within the field of health to value and appreciate the diversity of all people as well as to continue learning about other cultures to ensure optimal provision of services. In this edition, a brief explanation of cultural proficiency is discussed along with the components of a related framework. Cultural proficiency is the ultimate goal, per the cultural competency continuum, and therefore is worthy of consideration toward health equity for all. The importance of science, technology, engineering, art, and math (STEAM) will also be discussed to explain why members of the emerging majority groups must venture into these areas of study and work in an effort to close the health status gap. This edition includes a new chapter, which focuses on the history of education in the United States and the relationship of education to health. This intersection between education and health in the United States and the parallel injustices within each are enlightening. Understanding these injustices is important as solutions toward health equity are considered. Another new chapter in this edition pertains to the elderly and health care. Topics such as chronic illnesses, mass incarceration of the elderly, the over-use of pharmaceuticals (as prescribed), and other relevant issues are explored. The purpose is to interrogate why and how the problems of the elderly impact health disparities and to further discuss the need for elder Americans to also experience health equity, which must be the case for people of all ages, throughout the continuum of their lives.

This second edition is aptly titled *Health Equity, Diversity, and Inclusion: Context, Controversies, and Solutions*, as all of these areas will be covered. The title change is not to de-emphasize health disparities but rather to highlight a forward thinking approach toward solutions regarding health equity, rather than dwelling in the gap with a sole focus on health disparities. The controversies highlighted throughout the text are mainly those associated with topics such as social injustice,

ACA, and immigration, with limited discussion about current politics around the latter issue, although concerns regarding those matters contribute to the issue of lack of health equity for all. Rather than simply reiterating and identifying problems related to health disparities and diversity, solutions toward health equity are given great emphasis in order to continue the dialogue related to solving the myriad problems that are gravely affecting the lives of many.

▶ References

Braveman, P., Arkin, E., Orleans, T., Proctor, D., & Plough, A. (2019). What is health equity? The Robert Wood Johnson Foundation. Retrieved from https://www.rwjf.org/en/library/research/2017/05/what-is-health-equity-.html.

PBS (2019). Transcript. The 1619 Project details the legacy of slavery in America. Retrieved from: https://www.pbs.org/newshour/show/the-1619-project-details-the-legacy-of-slavery-in-america

Torres-Spellcy, C. (2019). Everyone is talking about 1619. But that's not actually when slavery in America started. *The Washington Post*. Retrieved from https://www.washingtonpost.com/outlook/2019/08/23/everyone-is-talking-about-thats-not-actually-when-slavery-america-started/?fbclid=IwAR2XY5mJZOn97oa8MiLjcMF65FlvHKoD7PiUqfe-qOD4vHpmJak7Y7ba5Y4&noredirect=on

Acknowledgments

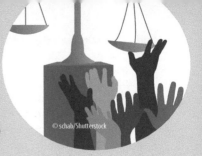

Opportunities to express gratitude are often missed as we embark on the complex day-to-day journey of life. Writing a book is an endeavor that involves many in the accomplishment of a goal that is worthy, as a book lasts in perpetuity with the potential to reach the hands of many. In this case, the book may impact lives, with hopes that words will turn into deeds toward necessary and positive change. To that end, I do not take lightly this opportunity to express my gratitude to some key, significant people in terms of my writing this *Second Edition* and beyond. I begin by thanking my husband, Jeffrey Rose, for his loving commitment to me, always, and to seeing this project through, by my side with never-ending support. He assisted by preparing tables of information, which was of great help in organizing this work and it was a delight to include his work in this project. I appreciate his attention to detail so much and his love and willingness to share his time from his busy schedule to give me his intelligent, honest feedback, time, and skills.

I also thank my children, Courtney and Brandon Rose. I am profoundly moved by my children and the wonderful young adults they are. They both inspire me and provoke me to think based upon new realities in the midst of social media, their generation, and their personal experiences as intelligent, young adults learning to navigate this challenging world. Courtney now holds an Ed.D from Teachers College, Columbia University, one of my alma maters, and she is one of the contributing authors for this text, along with one of her former classmates, Dr. Edmund Adjapong. Their contribution to this work, in the form of a chapter, is as wonderful as their understanding of the history of education; and the intersection between health and educational disparities is profound. There are parallels that should not be missed and they clarify this with great skill. I am filled with pride to watch Dr. Courtney Rose walk in my footsteps, as she was two-years-old when I achieved my doctorate at the same school. Now she is teaching in college classrooms, consulting, writing, and creating her own path. We are also co-hosts of our own podcast, the Ivy Roses, which is an added enjoyment as we continue the journey of educating together. Brandon is an accomplished young attorney. Watching him serve as a professional with such skill and adeptness motivates me to move forward with enthusiasm and tremendous energy in all that I do. I am most proud of how he serves in the community as a Guardian Ad Litem, assisting young people in need, and volunteering on boards to ensure that organizations that need assistance receive the help that he is able to provide. As he continues his journey through the legal and professional world in general, I am impressed with how he navigates, figures things out, and remains in the constant quest of determining how he can serve given his legal acumen and other skill sets. The words of encouragement and support from my husband and our children, as I take on the arduous task of writing, are thoroughly rewarding, as I know that my book will be in their hands upon completion. This gives me the energy and enthusiasm to complete the work with pride, knowing that the subject matter—health disparities, social justice, and solutions to inequities in the United States—represents meaningful, important work.

Additionally, I offer gratitude to Ms. Heather Aaron for responding to my interview questions regarding nursing homes with significant expertise in my chapter about the elderly and health disparities. She is an important voice to this book and clearly an expert on the subject matter.

Finally, and above all, I thank God. There is definitely a force in my life that is greater than my mind can imagine that leads, guides, and protects my beloved family and me and inspires my work through an intuitive voice that is forever present. For this blessing, mere words of gratitude are insufficient, but I express them humbly. I always lean on the strength and courage of God, and doing so has never failed me.

About the Author

© schab/Shutterstock

Dr. Patti Rose acquired her Master's Degree from Yale University, followed by her Doctorate (Ed.D) from Teachers College, Columbia University. She has served as a Faculty member (from Adjunct Professor, Instructor, to the Associate Professor Level) at the University of Miami, Florida Atlantic University, Florida International University, Springfield College, Worcester State College, Nova Southeastern University, and Barry University. In recent years, courses that she has developed and taught include Black Women in Medicine and Healing; Psychosocial Health and Healing and Women (online course); Race and Healthcare in America; Culture, Race, and Diversity Issues in the United States; Mass Incarceration and the Impact on the Black Community; and Black Women in Medicine and Healing. In the summer of 2013, she taught Chinese college students as a Visiting Professor at Jiaotong University in Shanghai, China for 6 weeks, and during the summers of 2014, 2015, and 2016 for 5 weeks in Guangzhou, China at Jinan University. She also taught at Feng Chia University in Taichung, Taiwain in 2017, at Jinan University in Shenzhen, China in 2018, and at Chengdu Polytechnic University in Chengdu, China in 2019. She will teach at Chengdu Polytechnic University in Chengdu, China again during the summer of 2020. She also serves as the Educational Consultant and Liaison for the Essex County College of New Jersey and the JNC International Summer School Program of China Partnership.

Dr. Rose has given keynote addresses, conference presentations, and workshops for many national colleges and universities and other venues, including the Louisiana State University (LSU) School of Veterinary Medicine; Yale University; Teachers College, Columbia University; LeMoyne College; Ross University; Des Moines University Medical School; Miami Dade College; the American Public Health Association; the National Association of Healthcare Executives; The National Association of Black Veterinarians; and beyond. Her international presentations have included conferences in Nairobi, Kenya; Barcelona, Spain; Paris, France; Aruba, St. Thomas; and Puerto Rico (a United States territory). Her administrative roles include serving as Director and Founder of her own firm, Rose Consulting, her current role, and prior service as President and CEO of Plainfield Health Center in Plainfield, New Jersey, and as Vice President of Behavioral Health Services at The Jessie Trice Center for Community Health, one of the largest community health centers in the nation, in Miami, Florida.

She is the author of several books, including *Cultural Competency for Health Administration and Public Health*, published in 2011, *Cultural Competency for the Health Professions*, published in 2013, and *Health Equity, Diversity, and Inclusion: Context, Controversies and Solutions, Second Edition*, publishing in 2020, all by the same publisher, Jones & Bartlett Learning. She also has many published articles, including a piece in the *Harvard Journal of Minority Public Health*, which focused on teenage pregnancy in the Black community. Her work currently includes serving as administrator and sole writer for her blog, Natural Is Cool Enough (N.I.C.E.), which has a national and international following, a *Huffington Post* blogger, and being the co-creator and co-host of a podcast, *The Ivy Roses*, which can be found on numerous podcast platforms including iTunes, iHeartRadio, Sound Cloud, and beyond. She developed a DVD, *Cultural Competency: A Public Health Imperative*, through her consultation for a project directed by the Alumni Office of the Yale University School of Public Health, where she also received the Public Health Service Award (2004) for her commitment to community health service.

Dr. Rose has language skills in both Spanish and Mandarin based on her travels and intense study and speaking practice in both languages. Dr. Rose's passion is to travel the globe to understand the world and to share her knowledge of various cultures, history, health education and health promotion, health equity, social injustice (including health disparities), globalism, and diversity through her writing, teaching, and speaking engagements. Her current research is focused on health disparities and health equity, particularly in the United States, from a social justice vantage point, utilizing a cultural lens, and through comparative analysis, from a national and global perspective. Her cultural travel, work, and research have included journeys to Puerto Rico, Mexico, Fiji, Turkey, Africa (South Africa, Kenya, Senegal, Ghana, Tanzania, Egypt, Zanzibar, and the Cape Verde Islands), Sri Lanka, Dubai, Australia, New Zealand, Europe (Spain, Italy, Ireland, France, Portugal, Iceland, the United Kingdom, Greece, and the Netherlands), the Caribbean (Jamaica, Tortola, St. Lucia, St. Thomas, Barbados), Latin and Central America (Cuba, Honduras, Nicaragua, Costa Rica, Panama, the Dominican Republic, and Guatemala), and Asia (Japan, China, Vietnam, Singapore, Bali, South Korea, India, The Maldives, and Thailand).

Her professional affiliations have included the American College of Healthcare Executives, the American Public Health Association, the Black Executive Forum, and the National Association of Health Services Executives. She was appointed by the U.S. Department of Commerce, National Institute of Standards and Technology, to serve in the capacity of Examiner on the 2004 Board of Examiners of the Malcolm Baldrige National Quality Award. She is currently the President of the South Florida Chapter of the Yale Black Alumni Association and a frequent Yale Alumni Schools Committee college applicant evaluative interviewer. Dr. Rose has been married for 34 years and is the mother of two.

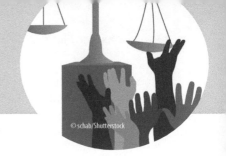

CHAPTER 1

Introduction

Health is a state of complete physical, mental and social well-being, and not merely the absence of disease or infirmity.

—World Health Organization, 1948[1]

Health disparities exist and need to be rectified in American society. This text is intended to address this topic head-on, exploring how the problem has not been resolved and is becoming increasingly worse. This topic is particularly relevant given that the demographics in the United States are rapidly changing; in the near future, people of color will become the majority group, rather than the minority group, and healthcare needs must continue to be met without the raging disparity that leads to poor health outcomes, human suffering, and a drain on the economy. Additionally, beyond the core issues associated with health disparities and diversity, great emphasis will be placed on solutions and strategies. This text is unique in that it is not designed to speak exclusively to those individuals in the healthcare field, but to anyone who is concerned and committed to a healthy society for all people within its boundaries. This text also addresses topics, concepts, and issues intended to ensure that those in health fields understand why the rapid demographic changes currently taking place in the United States add a sense of urgency to the need for the health status gap to be closed and that diversity is essential to this process.

Furthermore, evidence-based research clearly indicates that racial/ethnic diversity in the delivery of health care improves outcomes for emerging majority populations. The discussion of diversity will be contrasted with the concept of cultural competence and will demonstrate that, although distinctly different, the two elements are intrinsically linked in efforts made toward the ultimate goal of closing the health status gap in the United States. To truly understand racial and ethnic health disparities and diversity, it is important to delve into the statistics, in terms of varying groups, and consider how these other groups fare in comparison to the White population from a health vantage point. Key indices are explored, including infant

---

1 Reprinted from Text of the Constitution of the World Health Organization, 1948. http://apps.who.int/iris/bitstream/10665/85573/1/Official_record2_eng.pdf. Copyright 1948.

and maternal mortality, morbidity, longevity, specific diseases, healthcare access, and other key concerns, over time spans, to determine whether the problem has improved or worsened. Socioeconomic factors are explored, as a primary premise of this text is that one of the main reasons for health disparities is socioeconomic status, which is also a contributing factor to lack of sufficient diversity in health care. Because this text aims to provide solutions, interviews are included with various individuals who lend their insight based on experiential knowledge.

▶ Overview of the Chapters

Chapter 2 is an exploration of the notion of health disparities. The key question is, what does the term *health disparity* really mean? This chapter also includes a historical overview of health disparities. The definition of health equity is also provided with a thorough explanation of its significance and relevance to health disparities. Chapter 3 is a candid exploration of the extent of the healthcare gap and the challenges in closing it. Initially, it was literally a Black-and-White issue; that is, the health status of Black people was compared to that of White people. This framework has changed as we have come to acknowledge the racial and ethnic diversity within the United States, but the largest gap overall is still that between Black people and White people—hence the primary focus of this text. Various groups will be categorized, with insight provided regarding the health status of each, as compared to the White population. Chapter 4 explores the link between health and education including the history of the public school system that exists today, the "achievement gap" and the link between educational achievement and health outcomes. Culture, as it relates to teaching and learning is also explored. Chapter 5 assesses health disparities by the numbers, briefly overviews the Patient Protection and Affordable Care Act (commonly referred to as Obamacare), provides healthcare reform updates, and considers health care in other nations, maternal mortality, as an example, to provide insight into suburban health issues. Men's health and the unfortunate widening of the health status gap are also discussed. Chapter 6 focuses on health disparities in urban communities. It compares the plight of the urban environment to that of the rural environment, as discussed in Chapter 7. Understanding the variables unique to each setting is useful in forming solutions toward closing the gap. Chapter 7 explores rural communities and unique issues associated with them that contribute to health disparities. The rural community warrants specific exploration because the dynamics of the healthcare gap change in this setting; these communities are composed primarily of White people living at a low socioeconomic level. Through the lens of these communities, further insight is provided as to why socioeconomic status is a key factor in understanding health disparities.

Women are generally the caretakers in families. They bear the children, participate in the workforce, and experience significant health disparities, largely due to race, ethnicity, and socioeconomic status. Chapter 8 explores key issues related to women and offers solutions to the health disparities they encounter. Chapter 9 considers the effects of health disparities on a unique population—children. Although children are discussed throughout the text, this chapter takes a serious look at their specific issues, as they are the future of the nation and perhaps will be the beneficiaries of any successes toward closing the gap. Chapter 10 covers the elderly and health equity. Key issues are explored including chronic diseases, mass incarceration of the elderly, filial piety and other relevant topics. It includes an interview with a healthcare professional who provides cogent insight regarding Nursing Homes and their relevance to the elderly population as well as how they impact their daily living. Chapter 11 looks into the future of health care, with a focus on health disparities. It offers voices, beyond this author's, in the form of interviews; reviews recommendations from a working group, with commentary by this author; and summarizes the elements of a diversity plan. Chapter 12 includes case studies pertaining to racial and ethnic health disparities. These case studies offer a look at specific scenarios, which can be explored and discussed to understand the impact of the problem on individuals and systems. Commentary is provided for most of the cases although a few are open for individual/group discussion without thoughts offered by the author.

Chapter 13 attempts to define diversity, with the key questions being, what is diversity, and who defines it? Various definitions are explored to help us understand the concept. Chapter 14 provides insight into the importance of making diversity happen and sustaining it and provides examples of "models that work." Chapter 15 includes case studies pertaining to diversity. These case studies look at specific scenarios, which can be explored and discussed in order to understand the impact of the problem on individuals and systems. Commentary is provided for each case. Chapter 16 revisits topics thoroughly explored in two books previously written by this author, *Cultural Competency for Health Administration* and *Public Health and Cultural Competency for the Health Professional*, both published by Jones and Bartlett Learning. This chapter consists of a comparative analysis of cultural competency versus diversity and offers a cogent explanation of why the two concepts are different and why both are necessary. Here, the emphasis is on the importance of cultural competency.

Health disparities present such a grave problem that when seeking a resolution, we must look beyond typical approaches. Hence, Chapter 17 offers a spiritual approach toward resolution. It is not about religion as we typically use the word, but is more a journey into self-actualization and leaves the reader, after reading the final chapter of this text, with the opportunity to reflect on all that came before it.

This final chapter, with regard to the pertinent issues of the entire text, considers the question, where do we go from here?

▶ Features of the Text

Beginning with Chapter 2, chapters generally contain the following elements: learning objectives, a list of key terms, an introduction, a chapter summary, chapter problems, and references. Chapters 4, 6, 9, and 17 are offered by contributing authors. Chapters 12 and 15 consist of case studies only.

Following the main chapters, appendices are provided to supplement the information discussed throughout the text. These resources include cultural competence assessment surveys, a sample of the elements of a diversity plan, tables and figures relevant to men's health, a table explaining criminal justice reform, additional information, and a glossary of terms. An index is also provided for the reader's convenience.

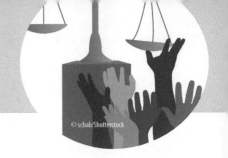
© schab/Shutterstock

CHAPTER 2

Health Disparities: The Meaning and a Historical Overview

Healthy citizens are the greatest asset any country can have.

—**Winston S. Churchill**

LEARNING OBJECTIVES

After reading this chapter, you should be able to do the following:

1. Understand the role that culture plays in health disparities.
2. List the key factors that influence the health status of various groups.
3. Explain the term emerging majority as it relates to demographic changes in the United States.
4. Discuss why the widest health status gap is between Black and White people in the United States.

▶ Introduction

Generally, **health disparity** refers to a difference or gap in **health status** between varying racial and ethnic groups. There are a number of factors to take into consideration when exploring this gap, which will be reviewed in depth throughout this text. These factors include socioeconomic and educational status, **race**, **culture**, **ethnicity**, and other population characteristics. If all of these factors are not taken into consideration when comparing the health status of different groups, then problems may arise in addressing health disparities. For example, it may be erroneously argued that one group is inherently healthier than the other, a type of bias. Or it may be assumed that one factor is the cause of a disparity, and thus solutions to the problem may be based on a myopic focus.

Moreover, it helps to consider examples in looking at this flawed approach to understanding the extent of factors that may contribute to health disparities. Specifically, it is generally understood that in the United States, which is the country of emphasis regarding health disparities in this text, the White, currently majority, population has a higher health status than do members of the African American/Black population. The latter is the largest **emerging majority** racial group if Black Hispanics are included in the group. It is appropriate to include Black Hispanics in the African American/Black group because according to the Office of Management and Budget (OMB), Hispanic is not a racial but rather an ethnic group. Therefore, Hispanic people may be Black, White, or of other racial groups. It gets a bit more complicated when discussing White Hispanic people because White Non-Hispanic people are not considered an emerging majority group; therefore, the health experiences of White Hispanic people may or may not be different than those of the White population for a number of reasons, particularly White privilege. But for Black Hispanic people, their experience, in terms of health, is very similar to that of African American/Black, Non-Hispanic people, with culture being the salient difference, which will be discussed in a later chapter. Essentially, the health status of Black people (both Hispanic and Non-Hispanic) in the United States is lower than that of the White population.

The Centers for Disease Control and Prevention (CDC) produces a document titled the "CDC Health Disparities and Inequalities Report." The 2013 report provided interesting examples of health disparities, as indicated in **BOX 2-1**.

An example of a myopic view as the rationale for the disparity between these two groups is the argument that genetics is the key factor. Some may argue that, genetically, there are illnesses that tend to exist within the Black population that contribute to their overall lower health statistics. Race continues to be one of the most politically charged subjects in American life; it involves a sociocultural component that often leads to misleading and inappropriate categorizations (Kittles & Weiss, 2003). According to an Institution of Medicine Committee Report, "genetics cannot provide a single all-purpose human classification scheme that will be adequate for addressing all of the multifaceted dimensions of health differentials" (Hernandez & Blazer, 2006). The argument of genetics, therefore, has no substantial basis as a valid and sole explanation for health disparities. There are other contributing factors to this gap, such as **socioeconomic status**, education levels, diet, and health literacy. These factors have a great impact on the gap between the health status of Black people and other emerging majority groups and that of the White population in the United States. Hence, exploring these factors in depth

---

BOX 2-1 Examples of Important Health Disparities

- In 2009, African Americans had the largest death rates from heart disease and stroke compared with other racial and ethnic populations; these disparities in deaths were also found across age groups younger than 85 years.
- From 2007 to 2010, the largest prevalence of hypertension was among adults aged 65 years and older, African American adults, U.S.-born adults, adults with less than a college education, adults who received public health insurance (18 to 64 years old), and those with diabetes, obesity, or a disability, compared with their counterparts.
- In 2008, infants of African American women had the largest death rate, which was more than twice the rate of infants of White women.
- In 2009, African Americans had the highest death rates from homicide among all racial and ethnic populations. Rates among African American males were the highest across all age groups.
- African Americans had the highest incidence and death rates from colorectal cancer in 2008 compared with all other racial and ethnic populations—despite having colorectal screening rates similar to the rates among White adults.

Factors contributing to poor health outcomes among African Americans include discrimination; cultural, linguistic, and literacy barriers; and lack of access to health care.

Data from http://www.cdc.gov/minorityhealth/populations/REMP/black.html (2015, July 31). Retrieved September 22, 2015; November 16, 2009, from http://www.omhrc.gov/templates/content.aspx?ID=3005. Data from Centers for Disease Control and Prevention. (2009). Health disparities and ethnic minority youth. Retrieved November 16, 2009, from http://www.cdc.gov /Features/HealthDisparities/

---

not only leads to a greater understanding, but also creates an opportunity to explore potential solutions. Although the solutions are complicated, they are not unachievable. The United States leads the world in healthcare spending, however, it is the only industrialized nation that does not ensure that all citizens have coverage (IOM, n.d.). As stated by the National Coalition on Health Care:

> Lack of insurance compromises the health of the uninsured because they receive less preventive care, are diagnosed at more advanced disease stages, and once diagnosed, tend to receive less therapeutic care and have higher mortality rates than insured individuals. (Institute of Medicine, 2002)

▶ Health Disparities Defined

The concept of *health disparities* has been defined in many different ways. A few formal definitions are presented in **TABLE 2-1**.

▶ A Brief Historical Overview

As previously discussed, in terms of key health indices, the health status gap between any emerging majority group and the current majority group (White people) is greatest between Black and White people. Because of the significant health disparity between Black and White people, the focus will remain on these two groups throughout this text. Some of the key indices are mortality and morbidity rates and longevity. In considering

TABLE 2-1 Varying Definitions of the Term Health Disparities in the United States

Source[a]	Definition of Health Disparities
U.S. Department of Health and Human Services, The Secretary's Advisory Committee on National Health Promotion and Disease Prevention Objectives for 2020, 2008	A particular type of health difference that is closely linked with social, economic, and/or environmental disadvantage. Health disparities adversely affect groups of people who have systematically experienced greater obstacles to health based on their racial or ethnic group; religion; socioeconomic status; gender; age; mental health; cognitive, sensory, or physical disability; sexual orientation or gender identity; geographic location; or other characteristics historically linked to discrimination or exclusion.
Dehlendorf, Bryant, Huddleston, Jacoby, & Fujimoto, 2010	In the United States, discussion of disparities has focused primarily on racial and ethnic disparities. In the international literature, and increasingly in the United States, socioeconomic status and gender disparities, disparities between disabled and non-disabled individuals, and disparities by sexual orientation have also been considered.
U.S. Department of Health and Human Services, n.d.	Differences in length and quality of life and rates and severity of disease and disability because of social position, race, ethnicity, gender, sexual orientation, education, or other factors.

[a]The full reference for each source is included in the References section at the end of this chapter.

Data from http://www.cdc.gov/minorityhealth/populations/REMP/black.html (2015, July 31). Retrieved September 22, 2015; November 16, 2009, from http://www.omhrc.gov/templates/content.aspx?ID=3005. Data from Centers for Disease Control and Prevention. (2009). Health disparities and ethnic minority youth. Retrieved November 16, 2009, from http://www.cdc.gov/Features/HealthDisparities/

longevity, going back to 1850, the average life expectancy of Black people was 21.4 years as compared to that of White people, which was 25.5 years (Talamantes, Lindeman, & Mouton, n.d.). It was a different time and lifespans were much shorter than they are today. Nevertheless, the apparent gap was due to heavier labor, inadequate medical care, poorer living standards, and greater environmental exposure for Black people. Additionally, at that time, Black people were slaves in many parts of the United States, leading to poorer health conditions. Slavery was a complex and brutal system involving many Americans, including White slavers and Black slaves. The involvement of medicine in the process is often excluded from historical discussions, but it is very important to the understanding of health disparities. According to Washington (2006), medical science was a key factor in terms of the persistence of enslavement because both physicians needed it. It was advantageous to them both economically and for medical research. Physicians were able to advance medically because of slavery.

Life on the plantation was particularly problematic in terms of health care. Slaves were fed a suboptimal diet, provided with clothing that did not provide them protection from the elements, and were forced to perform labor each day that was long and hard and without the benefit of sufficient rest. When they experienced illness, they often did not receive medication. They became ill largely because of the insufficiency of their work environments. As further stated by Washington (2006), the vulnerability of enslaved Africans was more so than that of Whites, primarily because of the slave shacks. The slaves experienced respiratory infections due to these flimsy shacks, which enabled winter cold and summer heat to enter. Their immune systems were not accustomed to the microbes relevant to pneumonias and tuberculosis.

Moving ahead chronologically, a study in 1997 revealed that White people outlived Black people by 6 years, living to 77.1 years on average, while Black people lived 71.1 years on average (Talamantes et al., n.d.). This finding leads to an obvious question: Given the ending of slavery in 1865 and a considerable difference in time, why did the gap remain? Simply put, why do White people live longer than Black people in the United States? In exploring this question further, it is important to note that there was indeed a medical civil rights movement, which allowed for integration of African Americans into healthcare environments, but still the health status gap was not closed.

▶ Medical Exploitation

Specific studies have pointed out that many Black people distrust White people, specifically in relation to health care, as many Black people feel that White institutions are powerful and experiences within them are frustrating (Levy, 1985). This belief creates a scenario of distrust when seeking health care and may impact the relationship between the healthcare provider and the patient/customer. One way that Black patients/customers may get beyond their feelings of distrust is to seek healthcare providers of the same race/ethnicity, with whom they may feel more comfortable (Kontorinakis, 2005). There is often greater understanding between people who share similar cultures, values, and positive and negative experiences (Levy, 1985). Further, a person may seek out providers of the same race/ethnicity if he or she has personally experienced, or knows of, historical instances of maltreatment from one race to another.

Unfortunately, this distrust of the medical establishment has been justified. Black people, even since the abolishment of slavery, have still fallen victim to medical exploitation and experimentation (Palmer, Wise, Horton, Adams-Campbell, & Rosenberg, 2011). Many medical atrocities have been thoroughly documented. A key example is the oft-cited Tuskegee Syphilis Study. Beginning in July 1932, the U.S. Public Health Service enrolled approximately 400 African American men with syphilis in an experiment. The men were told that they were receiving treatment. In reality, they received no treatment for their disease; they were studied to determine the effects of the disease, if left untreated, from the time of diagnosis until their death (Gamble, 1997). Treatment became available during the course of the study, but it was never given to the men (Gamble, 1997). Most of the men were poor, uneducated, and unaware that they had syphilis and were merely told that they had "bad blood." The men suffered greatly, while their loved ones (who were also unaware that the men were not being treated) watched helplessly. To add to the atrocity, their wives and children were never tested for syphilis. It was not until 1972, 40 years after the study began, that the men who survived were told that they had syphilis and had been subjects in the study. Former president Clinton would later apologize for the Tuskegee Syphilis Study, saying, Unfortunately, what has happened in the United States cannot be undone. But, it should still be discussed. Is it possible to be a unified nation when a significant portion of the people do not have trust and we continue to avoid what happened? There is shame associated with slavery in the United States and an apology is absolutely necessary.

Spencer (2010) offers a poignant response to President Clinton's words (paraphrased above): President Clinton offered an apology in 1997, which revealed the pain that individuals believe ended long ago. However, people were impacted gravely, namely African Americans. One could examine Tuskegee, as one example of many atrocities, to gain insight as to why there is a lack of trust of the medical establishment, by African Americans, which is contributing, unintentionally to the continuance of health disparities.

This study, and other forms of medical and research mistreatment, has led many Black people to distrust and fear medical care in the United States. Other forms of mistreatment, oppression, and covert and overt racism have led some members of the Black race, and members of other racial groups, to distrust the medical and public health establishments.

▶ Barriers to Seeking Care

Beyond mistrust of the medical establishment, there are other issues, such as lack of cultural competence and a shortage of Black physicians that impose a barrier for Black people in seeking medical care. The United States has a long history of lack of access to health care for non-White people. This history of unequal access and quality of care created, and continues to foster, an environment of higher morbidity and mortality rates among the various emerging majority groups. This lack of, or insufficient access to, health care in the United States has led to poorer health, **health inequality**, and a widening health status gap between the emerging majority and current majority populations. These trends have raised alarm about the impact of a skewed distribution of societal resources on social and physical well-being. Public health officials have called attention to this problem and pledged to reduce it (Adler & Stewart, 2010).

▶ Persistence of Health Disparities

A look back over the past 35 years shows acknowledgment, on behalf of the U.S. government, that the worsening health disparity gap between emerging majority and current majority populations warranted attention and resources. Various initiatives were implemented and new federal-level offices were created in an effort to address emerging majority health issues, the tremendous gap in health disparities, and the worsening emerging majority health status. In 1984 the U.S. Department of Health and Human Services released "Health, United States, 1983," a report on the health of the nation. The report documented that although the overall health of the nation showed significant progress, major disparities existed in "the burden of death and illness experienced by Black people and other minority Americans as compared with the nation's population as a whole" (Gibbons, 2005, p. 2).

Interest in health disparities has grown geometrically over the past 20 years. A primary contributor to this surge is the persistence of health disparities despite improvements in medical care and public health prevention initiatives (Adler & Stewart, 2010). The body of research on health disparities over the last 20 to 30 years increased rather significantly and especially as national attention was placed on this important issue. Within the last 20 years, one can identify several distinct eras of work on health disparities' association with socioeconomic status. Adler and Stewart (2010) describe the eras as follows, If one considers the eras, the first offers a model to consider the relationship between poverty and health, the second goes further with evidence, in terms of educational, income and occupational improvements or wealth and how these factors are related to better health outcomes. Socioeconomic status and health are linked in the third era while the fourth considers influences at various levels and the fifth considers how these factors interact.

Research in health disparities is generally considered to proceed in three generations: (1) research describing relevant disparities, (2) research that addresses the underlying causes of these disparities, and (3) investigations designed to address and resolve these disparities (Dehlendorf et al., 2010). First-generation research studies have provided an abundance of data that significant health disparities exist, including profound differences in life expectancy and cancer-related mortality both by race/ethnicity and by socioeconomic status (Adler & Rehkopf, 2008). Second-generation research studies have provided insight into pathways through which disparities occur, including individual, provider, and healthcare system factors (Kilbourne, Switzer, Human, Crowley-Matoka, & Fine, 2006). Third-generation research studies have been more limited but suggest that targeted interventions do have success at reducing health disparities (Kilbourne et al., 2006).

TABLE 2-2 highlights select and noteworthy historical U.S. government initiatives over the past 35 years to address health disparities.

TABLE 2-2 Select Noteworthy Historical U.S. Government Initiatives to Address Health Disparities	
Date	**Initiative**
April 1984	The Task Force on Black and Minority Health is established at the U.S. Department of Health and Human Services. This task force is the first coordinated and comprehensive effort facilitated by the department to investigate minority health status in comparison with the majority population.

(continues)

TABLE 2-2 Select Noteworthy Historical U.S. Government Initiatives to Address Health Disparities *(continued)*

Date	Initiative
December 1985	The U.S. Department of Health and Human Services creates the Federal Office of Minority Health. This newly formed office is charged with impacting historical health disparities by developing policy, providing important information that would inform health-related decision making, funding, and providing technical assistance to state minority entities and community-based organizations engaged in improving minority health status.
1986	With significant and increasing gaps in health status among the various racial and ethnic groups, the U.S. Department of Health and Human Services forms the Office of Minority Health. The mission of the office is to develop health policies and programs that will eliminate health disparities while protecting and improving the health of racial and ethnic minority populations.
April 1989	National Minority Health month is designated in an effort to bring greater awareness to health disparities, minority health, and racial and ethnic health status differences.
1990	Congress encourages the creation of the Office of Research on Minority Health.
February 1998	President Clinton announces an Initiative to Eliminate Racial and Ethnic Health Disparities.
September 1999	The National Institutes of Health is charged with developing a plan to reduce health disparities.
2000	The Minority Health and Health Disparities Research and Education Act is passed. The act leads to the creation of the National Center on Minority Health and Health Disparities at the National Institutes of Health.
March 2002	The Institute of Medicine's impactful, influential report "Unequal Treatment: Confronting Racial and Ethnic Disparities in Health Care" is released.
July 2002	The U.S. Department of Health and Human Services Office of Minority Health holds a National Leadership Summit on eliminating racial and ethnic disparities in health.
2009	The Secretary of the U.S. Department of Health and Human Services releases a report on health disparities and health reform.
April 2011	The U.S. Department of Health and Human Services announces a plan to reduce health disparities. The National Partnership for Action initiates a strategy to expand and strengthen community-led efforts to achieve health equity.

▶ Health Disparities and Emerging Majority Groups

Currently, health disparities have once again become a central concern in the United States and globally. Populations within the United States continue to experience marked differences in health and longevity (Adler & Stewart, 2010). This difference in health status between emerging majority groups and the White population continues to increase on the whole and has increased over time, adding to the burden of death and illness among the racial/ethnic minorities of the country.

In response to the disparities identified in the report "Health, United States, 1983," the Secretary of the U.S. Department of Health and Human Services established a task force on Black and minority health, marking the first time the U.S. government formed a group of experts to conduct a comprehensive study of minority health problems (Gibbons, 2005). In 1985 the release of the "Report of the Secretary's Task Force on Black and Minority Health" significantly raised awareness of the disparate health of the country's minority groups as compared with the White majority population (Gibbons, 2005).

The Institute of Medicine's (IOM) 2002 report "Unequal Treatment" significantly raised the level of awareness and attention given to emerging majority health and health disparities. According to the report, in 1999 Congress requested that the IOM (1) assess the extent of racial and ethnic disparities in health care, assuming that access-related factors such as insurance status and the ability to pay for care are the same; (2) identify potential sources of these disparities; and (3) suggest intervention strategies (IOM, 2002). The IOM explains the ensuing research as follows:

> To fulfill this request, an IOM committee reviewed well over 100 studies that assessed the quality of health care for various racial and ethnic minority groups while holding constant variations in insurance status, patient income, and other access-related factors. Many of these studies also controlled for other potential confounding factors, such as racial differences in the severity or stage of disease progression, the presence of comorbid illnesses, location in which care was received (e.g., public or private hospitals and health systems), and other patient demographic variables, such as age and gender. Some studies that used more rigorous research designs followed patients prospectively, using clinical data abstracted from patients' charts rather than administrative data used for insurance claims. (IOM, 2002)

The study committee reported being struck by what it found (IOM, 2002): "Even among the better-controlled studies, the vast majority [of published research] indicated that minorities are less likely than Whites to receive needed services, including clinically necessary procedures," even after correcting for access-related factors, such as insurance status. In general, the research showed the following:

- African American/Black and Black Hispanic people tend to receive a lower quality of health care across a range of disease areas (including cancer, cardiovascular disease, diabetes, mental health, and other chronic and infectious diseases) and clinical services.

- African American/Black people are more likely than are White people to receive less desirable services, such as amputation of all or part of a limb.
- Disparities are found even when clinical factors, such as stage of disease presentation, comorbidities, age, and severity of disease, are taken into account.
- Disparities are found across a range of clinical settings, including public and private hospitals, teaching and nonteaching hospitals, and so on.

Emerging majority people suffer more frequently and more severely from many diseases than do Non-Hispanic White people, and they often receive lower-quality care, which leads to poorer health outcomes. Given the diversity of the U.S. population, comparative effectiveness research should capture the health outcomes of racial and Hispanic groups and investigate whether disparities reflect variations in care or different responses to treatment (Mullins, Onukwugha, Cooke, Hussain, & Baquet, 2010). Racial and ethnic emerging majority patients are less likely to be placed in rehabilitation than are Non-Hispanic White patients, even after accounting for insurance status, suggesting existence of systemic inequalities in access. Such inequalities may have disproportionate impact on long-term functional outcomes of African American and Hispanic traumatic brain injury patients and suggest the need for an in-depth analysis of this disparity at a health policy level (Shafi et al., 2007).

Differences among racial and ethnic groups are pronounced; for example, about twice as many Black and Hispanic people report being in fair or poor health than do White people (Adler & Stewart, 2010). Differences are even greater by socioeconomic status; almost five times as many adults in poverty report fair or poor health compared with those with the highest income (Adler & Stewart, 2010). These findings are consistent with the National Healthcare Quality and Disparities Reports and suggest little progress in eliminating health disparities among emerging majority groups. The 2010 National Healthcare Quality and Disparities Report findings indicate that healthcare quality and access are suboptimal, especially for emerging majority and low-income groups (Agency for Healthcare Research and Quality, 2010). Although quality is improving, access and disparities are not improving. The reports emphasized that urgent attention is warranted to ensure improvements to quality and progress on reducing disparities with respect to certain services, geographic areas, and populations.

Thus far, the 21st century has been a period of ever-growing globalization, resulting in multiculturalism in the United States and elsewhere. The United States is considered a world leader in medical technology. Nevertheless, equity does not exist in the provision of health care because it is not distributed evenly throughout the U.S. population. Although racial and emerging majorities are fast-growing groups that will have greater numbers than the current majority, the White population, in coming years, a grim picture is provided by health statistics in terms of the health status of some emerging majority groups compared with the mainstream population.

Beyond the definitions provided in Table 2-1, health disparity is often referred to as healthcare inequality or gaps in the quality of health and health care across racial, ethnic, and socioeconomic groups. The Health Resources and Services Administration defines health disparity as "population-specific differences in the presence of disease, health outcomes or access to health care"

(Carter-Pokras & Baquet, 2002, p. 430). The focus here is disparities pertaining to the quality of care that different ethnic and racial groups receive. Reasons for disparities in access to health care, specifically, are attributed to many causes, such as low socioeconomic status, lack of insurance coverage, lack of a regular source of care, legal barriers, structural barriers, limits in the healthcare financing system, scarcity of providers, linguistic barriers, lack of health literacy among certain groups and communities, cultural barriers, and lack of diversity in the healthcare workforce. Other factors are education, segregation, and immigration status (Kosoko-Lasaki, Cook, & O'Brien, 2009). Education is significant because there is a correlation between health outcomes and years in school. There is no doubt that education impacts employment, social status, and other factors.

However, in American society, education alone may not be sufficient to explain differences in health outcomes, because African Americans with high education levels (college) also may have poorer health outcomes. Differences in health outcomes may have more to do with exposure to positive or negative healthcare practices generationally; for example, African Americans are descendants of slaves and thus may have inherited the dietary preferences of slaves that have been passed on from one generation to the next, including highly seasoned and fried foods and other preparation methods that are less healthy than the foods and methods of other groups. Research was conducted in St. Louis, Missouri, in which the eating habits of the early African Americans were explored. The following was determined:

> During slavery they subsisted on "scraps" from the master's table, second-line (imperfect) crops, and pork. Organ meats such as brains or liver, fried foods, highly salted vegetables (greens) and unusual animal parts generally discarded by the master were prepared to ingenious fashions to add flavor. Cattle and beef were usually consumed by Whites. Pig snoots, pig feet, brains, chitterlings, and tripe became the cuisine of the African American culture. (Kosoko-Lasaki et al., 2009, p. 335)

Furthermore, African Americans, who live largely in poorer socioeconomic conditions, are more apt to be first-generation college students, and may have issues associated with lack of cultural competence when seeking health care. As pointed out by LaVeist (2002):

> . . . that these disparities exist in some areas . . . suggests that the cost of care is an important consideration in clinical decisions for ethnic minority groups. Study findings that suggest the disparity is reduced for privately insured patients may also be an indication of payment-conscious clinical decisions. (p. 184)

Again, the less-than-positive health outcomes for African Americans are in part a result of eating patterns and culture; Kosoko-Lasaki et al. (2009) discuss these patterns and their cultural significance:

> A very interesting article from the 2001 *Journal of Archaeology*, entitled "Ham Hocks on Your Cornflakes" examined the role of food in the African American Identity. Excavations in Annapolis, Maryland, and 13 other sites in the Chesapeake region were explored. Findings were consistent; food remains

showed a definite pattern. Pork was much more commonly consumed than beef, and shallow water fish not typically purchased from markets where Whites typically shopped predominated. Apparently, by the late 19th century as Whites turned to beef, Blacks did not . . . . For many people, eating particular foods serves not only as a fulfilling experience, but also a liberating one—an added way of making some kind of declaration. Consumption then is at the same time a form of self-identification and communication. Blacks living under the oppression of slavery, with very few options, gathered at the end of the day for a communal meal with friends and family. They most likely found spiritual strength and regeneration through eating and camaraderie. This experience over generations became a part of the culture. (p. 335)

Hence, although education provides one with more information and insight into what it takes to be healthy, it may not be enough to override social factors and long-term exposure to cultural norms.

Segregation is also a factor in health disparity. Although the United States is extremely diverse, groups of people are largely segregated by race. According to Massey and Denton (1994), affluent Black people earning $50,000 or more per year are more segregated than are Hispanic/Latino or Asian people earning less than $15,000 per year. This finding may largely be due to the fact that many Hispanic/Latino people classify themselves as White Hispanic/Latino because Hispanic/Latino is not a race but an ethnicity; thus, they are more apt to live among White people and function as White Hispanics/Latinos. Members of various Asian groups tend to assimilate more rapidly in the United States than do other racial groups and, as a consequence, may not segregate to the same degree as African Americans. In addition, Asian and White Hispanic people have better access to credit and mortgage loans in the United States, as they face less discrimination than do Black people. Thus, Asians and White Hispanics can more easily avoid the negative outcomes of segregation and acquire homes in largely White communities where there is greater access to health care and other health-related services.

The issue of socioeconomic status and other factors are clearly documented but in terms of those individuals who are economically strong and Black, further analysis is warranted. Roeder (2019) shares some compelling examples. She shares the story of Shalone Irving, a 36-year-old African American woman who was an epidemiologist at the Centers for Disease Control and Prevention:

The deaths of mothers like Irving are devastating, private tragedies. A . . . public health crisis that's been hiding in plain sight for the last 30 years . . . For Black women far more than for White women, giving birth can amount to a death sentence. Irving's friend Raegan McDonald-Mosley, chief medical director for Planned Parenthood Federation of America, stated, There's something inherently wrong with the system that's not valuing the lives of Black women equally to white women.

Her vivid account of the stressors that impact Black people every day in the United States, no matter their economic status are compelling. There are also myths about the suburbs. There is a tendency to believe that if one lives in the suburbs, the socioeconomic status is better and therefore the health scenario is better. However, the reality as stated by Galvin (2019) is that:

Home to 1.4 million . . . The area is relatively safe, the unemployment rate is fairly low and most people have health coverage. In U.S. News' 2019 Healthiest Communities rankings—a project evaluating nearly 3,000 counties across myriad measures of health, housing, economy and more—Nassau County places 96th overall. . . . further scrutiny reveals stark disparities at the ZIP code level . . . Much of the country (has) fallen victim to this myth of wealth and wellness in the suburbs.

The bottom-line is that in urban and rural communities, there is long-established understanding that health disparities exist in these communities. But what must be understood, as further efforts toward solving the problem of lack of health equity for certain racial and ethnic emerging majority people continues, is that as pointed out in Galvin (2019) by Elizabeth Kneebone, (who was a Senior Fellow with the Brookings Institute at the time) in an analysis presented to Congress: "Among America's 100 most populous metro areas in 2015, more people lived in poverty in the suburbs than in the major cities nearby. A lack of mass transit and fragmented government resources can exacerbate the issue."

Additionally, immigration is another significant factor in health disparities primarily because many immigrant populations do not have access to health care. Although community health centers in the United States are available to serve undocumented people, the problem is that most people, including immigrant and nonimmigrant groups, are not aware of these facilities and the fact that people can be seen at these facilities regardless of their ability to pay or their immigration status. Hence, many immigrants have poorer health because they will seek care in emergency rooms or not seek care at all because they believe they will be asked for documentation that may lead to their deportation. The health disparities framework in **TABLE 2-3** provides further insight. Some of the key disparities among the various racial/ethnic groups are listed in **TABLE 2-4**.

Cultural competence is "evolving from a marginal to a mainstream healthcare policy issue and as a potential strategy to improve quality and address disparities" (Betancourt, Green, Carillo, & Park, 2005). For healthcare organizations, cultural competence strategy and training must be responsive to aims developed toward improving quality of care. Some of these aims have been developed by the Institute of Medicine, for example, and include safe, effective, patient-centered, timely, efficient, and equitable care. Furthermore, responsiveness to the national standards for culturally and linguistically appropriate services in health care, set forth by the U.S. Department of Health and Human Services Office of Minority Health, will also help in relieving health disparities (Curtis, Dreaschslin, & Sinioris, 2007). A successful example of a culturally competent system of care is described in the Child and Adolescent Service System Program, where the care and services focus on the family as the primary support and community-based approaches as part of informal support systems (e.g., churches, neighborhoods, healers). This effort also entails the introduction of choice in service, incorporation of cultural knowledge into practice and policy-making, less restrictive alternatives, and adequate cross-cultural communication to achieve goals (Cross, Bazron, Dennis, & Isaacs, 1989).

The American College of Physicians (2010) stated in their position paper that racial and ethnic disparities in health care result from the interaction of multiple complex factors, including past and current discrimination in health care, genetics, unequal educational opportunity, income and healthcare access disparities,

TABLE 2-3 Health Disparities Framework

Health—Before Care	Access to Care	Healthcare Delivery
Income levels, poverty, and other social conditions	Financial resources	Insurance coverage and type
Safety and adequacy of housing	Availability and proximity of providers	Cultural competence levels
Employment status and type of employment	Access to transportation	Patient–provider communications
Education levels	Insurance coverage	Provider discrimination or bias
Lifestyle choices—diet, exercise, tobacco, and alcohol use	Regular source of care	Differential propensities for certain diseases by racial/ethnic populations
Environmental conditions—air and water quality, pesticide exposure, green space	Language barriers	Patient preferences and adherence to treatment plans
	Legal barriers (e.g., eligibility restrictions, illegal immigrants)	Diversity of the healthcare workforce
	Prior experience with the healthcare system	Appropriateness of care
	Cultural preferences— care-seeking behaviors	Effectiveness of care
	Health literacy levels	Language barriers
	Diversity of the healthcare workforce	

Courtesy of Health Policy Institute of Chicago. (2004, September). Understanding health disparities. Retrieved from http://a5e8c023c8899218225edfa4b02e4d9734e01a28.gripelements.com/pdf/publications/healthdisparities.pdf.

cultural beliefs, and community systems. They went on to emphasize that the College believes that although improving access to quality care, reforming the healthcare delivery system, improving cultural and linguistic understanding, diversifying the healthcare workforce, and improving the inequities in the social influences of health may not fully close the disparities gap, achieving these worthy goals would dramatically improve the lives of all people and the future of the nation.

TABLE 2-4 Health Disparities at a Glance

African Americans	Hispanic Americans	American Indians/ Alaska Natives	Asian and Pacific Islanders
▪ In 2011, African American men were 1.3 times and 1.5 times, respectively, more likely to have new cases of lung and prostate cancer, as compared to Non-Hispanic White men. ▪ Have the highest cancer death rate of any racial or ethnic group. ▪ In 2010, African Americans were 30% more likely to die from heart disease than Non-Hispanic Whites. ▪ Twice as likely to have diabetes than are Whites. ▪ African Americans have 2.2 times the infant mortality rate as Non-Hispanic Whites. They are 3.5 times as likely to die as infants due to complications related to low birth weight as compared to Non-Hispanic White infants.	▪ Among Mexican American women, 77% are overweight or obese, as compared to only 64% of the Non-Hispanic White women. ▪ Hispanic women are both 40% more likely to have cervical cancer, and to die from cervical cancer as compared to Non-Hispanic White women. ▪ Among Mexican American women, 77% are overweight or obese, as compared to only 64% of the Non-Hispanic White women. ▪ Puerto Rican infants are twice as likely to die from causes related to low birth weight than are Non-Hispanic White infants.	▪ The incidence of diabetes is more than twice that of Whites. American Indians/Alaska Native women were twice as likely to die from diabetes as Non-Hispanic White women in 2013. ▪ In 2010, American Indians/ Native Americans were 2.7 times more likely to be diagnosed with end-stage renal disease than were Non-Hispanic Whites. ▪ American Indian/Alaska Native men are 1.5 times as likely to have stomach cancer as are Non-Hispanic White men, and are over twice as likely to die from the same disease.	▪ Both Asian/Pacific Islander men and women have 2.1 and 2.5 times, respectively, the incidence of liver and irritable bowel disease–related cancer as the Non-Hispanic White population. ▪ Asian/Pacific Islander men are twice as likely to die from stomach cancer compared to the Non-Hispanic White population, and Asian/Pacific Islander women are 2.6 times as likely to die from the same disease. ▪ In Hawaii, native Hawaiians have more than twice the rate of diabetes as Whites.

Wrap-Up

Chapter Summary

Racial and ethnic disparities in health care persist despite considerable progress in expanding healthcare services and improving the quality of patient care. Many factors contribute to these disparities in complex ways, but the quality of health care can be improved for all patients with a comprehensive strategy that includes ensuring that strategies are implemented to not only reduce healthcare disparities, but also to improve the efficiency and equity of care for all patients (Betancourt, Green, Carrillo, & Ananeh-Firemong, 2003). This effort includes taking into consideration the improvement of communication and comfort levels between healthcare providers and their patients/customers. Many healthcare organizations are facing dramatic demographic shifts in their customer/patient populations and, therefore, are challenged to provide quality healthcare services to an increasingly diverse patient base. This chapter has discussed complex, sensitive, and challenging issues related to health disparities, emerging majorities, and the health status gap that has historically existed in the United States between different racial groups, with special focus on the substandard health status of Black people, with insight regarding contributing factors.

Chapter Problems

1. List three factors that contribute to health disparities.
2. Explain the notion of medical exploitation in terms of Black people in the United States.
3. What are some key barriers to accessing health care? Explore potential solutions.
4. Consider the following statement: Education level is a significant determinant in health disparities because there is a correlation between years in school and health outcomes. Is this statement true or false? Why?
5. What is the difference between the terms *emerging majorities* and *minorities* as they relate to populations in the United States?
6. Are there issues in terms of health disparities/lack of health equity in suburban communities for certain racial and ethnic emerging majority groups? Explain.

References

Adler, N. E., & Rehkopf, D. H. (2008). U.S. disparities in health: Descriptions, causes, and mechanisms. *Annual Review of Public Health, 29*, 235–252.

Adler, N. E., & Stewart, J. (2010). Health disparities across the lifespan: Meaning, methods, and mechanisms. *Annals of the New York Academy of Sciences, 1186*, 5–23.

Agency for Healthcare Research and Quality. (2010). *2010 National Healthcare Disparities Report.* (AHRQ Publication No. 11-0005). Rockville, MD: U.S. Department of Health and Human Services.

American College of Physicians. (2010). *Racial and ethnic disparities in health care, Updated 2010.* Policy Paper. Philadelphia, PA: American College of Physicians.

Betancourt, J. R., Green, A. R., Carrillo, J. E., & Ananeh-Firemong, O. (2003). Defining cultural competence: A practical framework for addressing racial/ethnic disparities in health and health care. *Public Health Reports, 118*(4), 293–302.

Betancourt, J. R., Green, A. R., Carrillo, J. E., & Park, E. R. (2005). Cultural competence and health care disparities: Key perspectives and trends. *Health Affairs, 24*(2), 499–505.

Carter-Pokras, O., & Baquet, C. (2002). "What is a "health disparity"? *Public Health Reports, 117*(5), 426–434.

Cross, T., Bazron, B., Dennis, K., & Isaacs, M. (1989). *Towards a culturally competent system of care (Vol. 1)*. Washington, DC: Georgetown University Child Development Center, Child and Adolescent Service System Program Technical Assistance Center for Child and Mental Health Policy.

Curtis, E. F., Dreaschslin, J. L., & Sinioris, M. (2007). Diversity and cultural competence training in healthcare organizations. Hallmarks of success. *The Healthcare Manager, 26*(3), 255–262.

Dehlendorf, C., Bryant, A. S., Huddleston, H. G., Jacoby, V. L., & Fujimoto, V. Y. (2010). Health disparities: Definitions and measurements. *American Journal of Obstetrics and Gynecology, 202*(3), 212–213.

Galvin, G. (2019). The Suburban myth of health and wealth. *U.S. News and World Report.* Retrieved from https://www.usnews.com/news/healthiest-communities/articles/2019-03-26/long-island -and-the-suburban-myth-of-health-and-wealth

Gamble, V. (1997). Under the shadow of Tuskegee: African Americans and health care. *American Journal of Public Health, 87*(11), 1173–1778.

Gibbons, M. C. (2005). A historical overview of health disparities and the potential of eHealth solutions. *Journal of Medical Internet Research, 7*(5), e50.

Hernandez, L., & Blazer, D. (Eds.). (2006). *Genes, behavior, and the social environment: Moving beyond the nature/nurture debate.* Washington, DC: National Academies Press.

Institute of Medicine. (2002). *Unequal treatment: Confronting racial and ethnic disparities in health care.* Retrieved from https://www.nap.edu/read/12875/chapter/1

Kilbourne, A. M., Switzer, G., Human, K., Crowley-Matoka, M., & Fine, M. J. (2006). Advancing health disparities research within the health care system: A conceptual framework. *American Journal of Public Health, 96*(12), 2113–2121.

Kittles, R. A., & Weiss, K. M. (2003). Race, ancestry, and genes: Implications for defining disease risk. *Annual Review of Genomics and Human Genetics, 4*(1), 33–67.

Kontorinakis, M. (2005). The doctor-patient interaction: Addressing issues of racial and ethnic disparities in health outcomes. Retrieved from http:www.allacademic.com/meta/p23104 _index.html

Kosoko-Lasaki, S., Cook, C., & O'Brien, R. (2009). *Cultural proficiency in addressing health disparities.* Sudbury, MA: Jones and Bartlett Publishers.

LaVeist, T. (2002). *Race, ethnicity, and health: A public health reader.* San Francisco, CA: John Wiley & Sons.

Levy, D. (1985). White doctors and Black patients: Influence of race on the doctor–patient relationship. *Pediatrics, 75*(4), 639–643.

Massey, D. S., & Denton, N. A. (1994). *Handbook of prejudice, stereotyping and discrimination.* New York, NY: Psychology Press.

Mullins, C. D., Onukwugha, E., Cooke, J. L., Hussain, A., & Baquet, C. R. (2010). The potential impact of comparative effectiveness research on the health of minority populations. *Health Affairs, 29*(11), 2098–2104.

Palmer, J. R., Wise, L. A., Horton, N. J., Adams-Campbell, L. L., & Rosenberg, L. (2003, March 19). Dual effect of parity on breast cancer risk in African American women. *Journal of the National Cancer Institute.* Retrieved from http://jnci.oxfordjournals.org/content/95/6/478.full.pdf

Roeder, A. (2019, Winter). America is failing Its Black Mothers. *Magazine of the Harvard T.H. Chan School of Public Health.* Retrieved from https://www.hsph.harvard.edu/magazine/magazine _article/america-is-failing-its-black-mothers/

Institute of Medicine. Care Without Coverage—Too Little, Too Late. The National Academies Press, 2002.

Shafi, S., de la Plata, C. M., Diaz-Arrastia, R., Bransky, A., Frankel, H., Elliott, A., Parks, J., & Gentilello, L. (2007). Ethnic disparities exist in trauma care. *Journal of Trauma Injury, Infection, and Critical Care, 63*(5), 1138–1142.

Spencer, D. (2010). The legacy of Tuskegee: Investigating trust in medical research and health disparities. *Journal of the Student National Medical Association.* Retrieved from http://jsnma .org/2010/09/the-legacy-of-tuskegee-investigating-trust-in-medical-research-and-health -disparities/

Talamantes, M., Lindeman, R., & Mouton, C. (n.d.). Health and health care of Hispanic/Latino American elders. Retrieved from www.stanford.edu/group/ethnoger/hispaniclatino.html

U.S. Department of Health and Human Services. (n.d.). Public health: Five priorities. Retrieved from http://www.hrsa.gov/publichealth/

U.S. Department of Health and Human Services, The Secretary's Advisory Committee on National Health Promotion and Disease Prevention Objectives for 2020. (2008, October 28). Phase I report: Recommendations for the framework and format of Healthy People 2020 [Internet]. Section IV: Advisory Committee findings and recommendations. Retrieved from http://www .healthypeople.gov/sites/default/files/PhaseI_0.pdf

Washington, H. (2006). *Medical apartheid: The dark history of medical experimentation on Black Americans from colonial times to the present.* New York, NY: Doubleday.

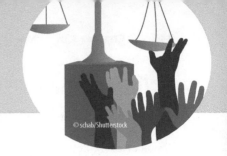

CHAPTER 3

The Extent of the Health Status Gap and Why It Has Not Been Closed

As long as poverty, injustice, and gross inequality persist in our world, none of us can truly rest.

—**Nelson Mandela**

KEY TERMS

digital divide
food desert
food injustice
food mirage

health literacy
school-to-prison pipeline
social injustice
soul food

LEARNING OBJECTIVES

After reading this chapter, you should be able to do the following:

1. Explain the connection between lack of education and health literacy.
2. Discuss social injustice and the role it plays in health disparities.
3. List socially unjust factors that impact health status in the United States.
4. Understand specific illnesses that are relevant to health disparities and specific emerging majority groups.

▶ Introduction

The healthcare industry is a business in the United States, meaning its objective is not, in and of itself, to meet the nation's health needs, but to maximize profits. Simultaneously, poverty is on the rise, leaving many people financially unable to meet their healthcare needs. At the federal, state, and local levels, efforts have been less than successful in curbing poverty trends, particularly among individuals of emerging majority groups—namely African American/Black, Black Hispanic, and Native American people. There are clear associations between health disparities and **social injustice** in a number of categories based on socioeconomic status, including food quality/availability, education, mass incarceration, and employment.

▶ Food Injustice

Race leads to significant complexities in the United States as a result of historical factors. Consequently, **food injustice** is a significant issue; particularly, individuals of low socioeconomic status may not have access to supermarkets and quality food (Bower, Thorpe, Rohde, & Gaskin, 2014). Thus, compromised health status correlates directly to low socioeconomic status. However, the matter of food injustice is not related solely to socioeconomic status; as in the Black population in the United States, there are cultural norms that play a role (Braithwaite, 1992). Although there are a number of groups that fall into the category of the emerging majority population (African American/Black, Hispanic, Native Americans/Alaska Natives, Asian American/Pacific Islander, and Latinos), for the sake of this analysis, since the health status gap is the widest between Black and White people, the emphasis will be placed on these two groups to highlight salient points.

It is a fact that African American/Black people often reside in lower-income communities (Slocum, 2010). In lower-income communities in the United States, supermarket availability is very limited, and in stores located in these communities, the quality of food is lower than that of food sold in higher-income communities (Bower et al., 2014). Also, in lower-income communities, there are often small grocery shops, known as convenience stores. These stores generally have food supplies on their shelves that are high in fat and sugar and are energy dense (Bower et al., 2014). As a result, individuals who live in communities with these types of stores as their predominant source of food acquisition will have diets of lesser quality compared with individuals who live in communities with large supermarkets that offer a great deal of food variety. This disparity/gap in the offering of quality foods has a direct impact on the health status of those who live in communities where this problem prevails (Bower et al., 2014). The old adage, "You are what you eat," therefore, becomes evident.

▶ Food Deserts and Mirages

Food deserts and **food mirages** are highly problematic and are indicative of an interface between poverty, lack of food access, and poor health outcomes (Breyer & Voss-Andreae, 2013). In the United States, healthy foods are usually acquired through large supermarkets. These types of supermarkets are typically not found in low-income neighborhoods. People living in low-income neighborhoods often have difficulty accessing the stores because of transportation issues. They are less likely to find stores such as Whole Foods and other large markets that carry healthy foods, including organic products, without traveling great distances. These types of markets are generally not in the census blocks of these neighborhoods (Galvez et al., 2008). Supermarkets are needed in low-income neighborhoods, because without them, community members lack access to healthy foods, including fruits, vegetables, and other essential items that enhance health. In short, this issue of lack of accessibility to healthy foods due to low socioeconomic status is a contributing factor to health disparities (Galvez et al., 2008).

Food Mirages

The price of food is skyrocketing in general in the United States. Consequently, even in the low-income neighborhoods where there are actual large grocery stores that include a wide selection of healthy foods, if the individuals who live in the neighborhood cannot afford to shop there, the stores are merely mirages (Breyer & Voss-Andreae, 2013). Specifically, a market may offer a choice between fresh produce and processed food. Individuals will often go into such markets and choose processed foods because they are less expensive. Based on their budgets, choosing the cheaper foods is logical. Budgets and household income are key considerations in food acquisition and quality (Breyer & Voss-Andreae, 2013). It is a complicated situation because if supermarkets build in low-income neighborhoods, the people cannot afford the food, and food mirages result. Yet, if supermarkets build outside of poor communities, individuals cannot get to them, and even if they do, they cannot afford the healthy products that are inside of them, which results in food deserts (see **TABLE 3-1**).

Foods Available in Lower-Income Communities

Unfortunately, rather than healthy foods with significant variety, in low-income communities, there are many fast-food restaurants. From a geographic exposure vantage point, in lower-income neighborhoods, which are often predominantly comprised of Black people, eating food from fast-food restaurants is expedient, convenient, and more affordable. In fact, in low-income neighborhoods, there

TABLE 3-1 Food Deserts and Mirages

Food Mirages	Food Deserts
Supermarkets build in low-income neighborhoods.	Supermarkets build outside of poor communities.
People cannot afford the food.	Individuals cannot get to them due to lack of transportation and cannot afford the food, were they to reach them, due to limited economic resources.

TABLE 3-2 Options in Low-Income Communities

Small Community Grocery Stores	Fast-Food Restaurants	Alcohol and Cigarettes
Inventory is convenient but limited.	Food is cheap and easily accessible.	These items are easily accessible in low-income communities.
Prices are higher than in supermarkets.	Individuals with limited income flock to them to feed themselves and their families.	People may turn to alcohol and cigarettes as coping mechanisms.
Access to healthy food choices is limited.	Nutritional value is questionable at best and problematic at worst.	Sellers of these items are available in excess in low-income communities.

are 2.4 fast-food restaurants per square mile compared with 1.5 in predominantly White neighborhoods (Galvez et al., 2008). It would seem that such affordability and accessibility would be positive, but the contrary is true. Obesity is a major problem in low-income communities. There is very likely a relationship between fast food and obesity, making fast food a contributing factor to the health disparities among lower-income communities and others—namely, between people of color and the White population.

The nutritional content of foods available in low-income areas is not the only consideration in this discussion. Because the produce and other food items that are accessible are not organic, much of what is available is most likely sprayed heavily with pesticides, and poultry and meat are filled with antibiotics and hormones.

TABLE 3-2 describes food options in lower-income communities.

▶ Soul Food and Diet-Related Diseases

It is important to be aware of those diseases that are food related in exploring food injustice issues and how they contribute to health disparities. Included among those diseases are the following (Purdue University, n.d.):

- Hypertension
- Cancer
- Diabetes
- Heart disease
- Obesity

When considering the health status of lower-income communities, it is clear that there is a high prevalence of such diseases. In exploring health disparities per the members of lower-income African American/Black communities, as an example, it is evident that a contributing cause of such diseases is the type of food consumed. For this population, it is necessary to consider foods still eaten today that pertain to slavery and a cultural norm that emerged from it. From a cultural vantage point, eating this type of food, affectionately known as **soul food** or "food for the soul," enables the preservation of a survivalist aspect of a group of people who experienced severe oppression and denigration in a society where they were considered less than human. Soul food was, therefore, more than just food but, a coping mechanism (Slocum, 2010). Although, for the most part, this food is fatty in content and highly salted, which increases sodium intake and can lead to hypertension and stroke, it continues to be a key aspect of food preparation for many Black/African American people (Airhihenbuwa et al., 1996).

Although most people of African descent in the United States are thought to be from West Africa, you will not find soul food eaten on the continent of Africa. As discussed previously, it was the conditions of slavery in the United States that led to this form of food preparation. Therefore, the role of food in disease processes can be appreciated by comparing the illnesses experienced by Africans to those experienced by Black/African Americans. Indeed, the marked differences found rule out the genetic factor as the cause of many illnesses in Black/African American people. It is clear that the movement of African American people from the continent of Africa, mainly West Africa, to the United States to serve as slaves, and the ensuing forms of oppression they experienced, including poor-quality food, have contributed gravely to health disparities. Unfortunately, as a consequence of the desire for Black/African American people to eat soul food, marketing efforts foster this desire, particularly in low-income communities, and fail to promote healthier choices, including organic foods and those that are more healthfully prepared (Airhihenbuwa et al., 1996).

It is unfortunate that the food preparation methods and choices of Black people in the United States, practices that continue for many, evolved from such an awful historical context involving slavery, segregation, and persecution (James, 2004). The question is, why do many Black/African American people continue this eating behavior if it is leading to negative health experiences? This is a complicated question because the problem is multifactorial. Lack of understanding, depending on one's educational level and/or nutritional insight, of the problems associated with eating food that is not prepared with health in mind is the first issue. Additionally, there are factors of socioeconomic status and food deserts and mirages, as discussed previously. For those who may want to change, accessibility and affordability of healthy foods is often the problem, depending on socioeconomic status. It is difficult to acquire whole grains, organic fruits, vegetables, and other healthy food items and, therefore, much easier to find, afford, prepare, and then consume foods that have high fat, salt, and sugar content, even if the cost is hypertension and other food-related illnesses (Jetter & Casady, 2006).

Because soul food is very tasty, it connotes a skill set in the kitchen that many Black people have passed on from generation to generation, and enjoying it is often a communal, family experience. Therefore, people who appreciate it do not want to let it go. The only way to begin to change/modify this pattern of eating would be to approach it comprehensively, from a multidimensional and multifaceted perspective, taking into consideration the interdependent nature of individual, cultural, and communal factors. Furthermore, the higher prevalence of convenience stores and other entities that mainly provide energy-dense, high-sodium-content and processed foods would need to be eliminated so as to decrease exposure, acquisition, and consumption of unhealthy foods (Smith & Morton, 2009).

In specifically looking at food-related illnesses, as mentioned previously, and continuing with the example of Black/African American people, there is a clear indication that hypertension rates are higher in this group compared with any other group, particularly White people (Centers for Disease Control and Prevention, 2015). There are other diseases, including cancer and diabetes, that relate to health disparities and food injustice. **TABLES 3-3, 3-4**, and **3-5** explore some of these illnesses and related concerns.

TABLE 3-3 Cancer-Related Health Disparities and Food Injustice	
Race	**Cancer Disparity**
Black men as compared to White men	Cancer incidence and death rates are higher among Black men (CDC, 2015).
Black women as compared to White women	Cancer death rates are higher among Black women (CDC, 2015).
Causal Relationships	
There is an inverse relationship between whole grain intake and cancer risk (Chatenoud et al., 1998).	
Since Black, low-income people often lack access to whole grain foods, their consumption of refined or processed food is most likely a contributing factor to their development of cancer (James, 2004)	
Eating fresh, organic produce protects against cancer along with antioxidants (substances believed to prevent cell damage), fiber, and other angiogenic (supportive of blood vessel development) factors. Foods high in fat, salt, and sugar contribute to cancer and other diet-related diseases. Given that many Black/African American people consume the latter, due to lack of accessibility and affordability of healthier choices, higher rates of cancer are likely the consequence (Shaw, 2006).	

Data from Centers for Disease Control and Prevention. (2015). Racial or Ethnic Variations (2015, August 20). Retrieved October 2, 2015, from http://www.cdc.gov/cancer/dcpc/data/race.htm; Chatenoud, L., Tavani, A., LaVecchia, C., Jacobs, D. Negri, E., Levi, F., and Franceschi, S. (1998). Whole grain food intake and cancer risk. *International Journal of Cancer, 77*(1), 24–28; James, D. (2004). Factors influencing food choices, dietary intake, and nutrition-related attitudes among African Americans: Application of a culturally sensitive model. *Ethnicity & Health, 9*(4), 349–367; Shaw, H. (2006). Food deserts: Towards the development of a classification. *Geografiska Annaler: Series B, Human Geography, 88*(2), 231–247.

TABLE 3-4 Diabetes-Related Health Disparities and Food Injustice	
Race	**Diabetes Disparity**
Black people as compared to White people	Black people are between 1.4 and 2.2 times more likely to have diabetes than are White people (Agency for Healthcare Research and Quality, 2001).

Causal Relationships
Diet is a key factor related to diabetes, as it plays a glycemic role (Horowitz, Colson, Hebert, & Lancaster, 2004).
Lack of access to reasonably priced, healthy food lends to difficulty for low-income Black people to adhere to specific diets necessary to stave off the problems associated with diabetes (Smith & Morton, 2009).
The local food environment provides a partial explanation for the racial and socioeconomic disparities in diabetes health outcomes (Smith & Morton, 2009).
Diabetes requires a certain degree of self-management. Lack of healthy food access inhibits the ability to do so (Horowitz et al., 2004).

TABLE 3-5 Obesity-Related Health Disparities and Food Injustice

Race	Obesity Disparity
Black people as compared to White people	Black people have a higher rate of obesity than do White people (CDC, 2014).

Causal Relationships
The high rates of obesity among the Black population is linked to socioeconomic status and the consumption of high-energy-dense, processed foods (Drewnowski & Specter, 2004).
There is a positive correlation between obesity and food stamp (Supplemental Nutrition Assistance Program) participation, which likely contributes to the high rate of obesity. (Chen, Yen, & Eastwood, 2005; Morin, 2013). Food stamps are often used to purchase foods of poor nutritional quality—the foods that are affordable and so readily available in low-income areas.

▶ Potential Solutions to Food Injustice

Ultimately, food injustice is a result of myriad factors. For example, if one considers the socioeconomic status of Black people compared with White people, the health statuses of the respective groups show some salient differences. Thus, health disparities are not the effect of differences inherent to a particular race, but of outside factors. To resolve the problem, relevant factors must be identified, including the following:

- Politics
- Education
- Culture
- Socioeconomic status (previously mentioned)

It would seem that community-based models would be most effective, as research has clearly outlined the problems, so the next step is solutions. In this chapter, K-12 education is explored, as education, or lack thereof, is one of the most critical factors in resolving the problem of health disparities.

Educational Disparities

To fully comprehend health disparities in the United States, an important topic to consider is education. In continuing to explore the two groups for which there is the widest health disparity, one notable fact is that African American/Black people are more likely to attend "high-poverty schools" than are their White counterparts (APA, n.d.). Although there are complicated reasons for the educational disparity, one of the primary issues is taxes. A significant portion of local property taxes (essentially half) is used to fund schools. Due to the lower socioeconomic status of African American/Black people at large, many do not own property, and if they do own property, it often generates less tax revenue due to its comparatively low property value. Consequently, the tax base in low-income communities where African American/Black people reside is lower, leading to less money to fund schools. Hence, the amount of money that a school receives is based on the socioeconomic status of the surrounding community. As stated by Duncan-Andrade and Morrell (2008), "We are not a nation of opportunity for all, but a nation built upon grand narratives of opportunity for all." These issues of educational disparity are relevant to many Black communities in the United States because according to the U.S. Census Bureau, Black people have the highest poverty rate and the lowest median income (DeNavas-Walt, Proctor, & Smith, 2011).

Because the schools in African American/Black neighborhoods often do not have sufficient resources compared with schools in predominantly White neighborhoods where the tax base is usually higher, African American/Black students experience an educational disadvantage, including lack of sufficient textbooks, limited (or altogether absence of) technology, and lack of equipment for labs, physical education, art, music, and other programs. Consequently, their overall curriculum is less rigorous, with lower expectations from the students and teachers as compared to their White counterparts (APA, n.d.). Unfortunately, the outcome of a lower-quality, less-resourced education is less opportunity to progress by attending college or finding decent work, which often leads to remaining in low socioeconomic status communities, perpetuating the problem from one generation to the next.

Health Literacy

As mentioned, there are serious weaknesses in the U.S. educational system that largely stem from the fact that people of lower socioeconomic status do not have access to the same educational resources as the rest of society. This disparity parallels that of the health status gap in that people of color do not fare as well in terms of education or health compared with their White counterparts, as the latter have the power and wealth in society and hence more resources available to them in both education and health.

The definition of **health literacy** is "the ability to obtain, process, and understand basic health information and services needed to make appropriate health decisions" (Institute of Medicine, 2004). Furthermore, according to an Institute of Medicine report (2001), patient-centered care is "care that is respectful of and responsive to individual patient preferences, needs, and values." This is very similar to cultural competence in that a significant number of people in the United States (1) are born in other countries (more than 34 million), (2) speak English poorly (more than 22 million), and (3) have literacy levels below what they need to understand most basic health information (more than 95 million). According to Kirsch, Jungeblut, Jenkins, and Kolstad (1993),

> Only 12 percent of adults have proficient health literacy, according to the National Assessment of Adult Literacy. In other words, nearly nine out of ten adults may lack the skills needed to manage their health and prevent disease. Fourteen percent of adults (30 million people) have below basic health literacy. These adults were more likely to report their health as poor (42 percent) and are more likely to lack health insurance (28 percent) than adults with proficient health literacy. Low literacy has been linked to poor health outcomes such as higher rates of hospitalization and less frequent use of preventive services. Both of these outcomes are associated with higher healthcare costs.

Furthermore, the problems of poverty and low educational levels lead to diminished health literacy, which impacts the health of individuals. This problem intersects deeply with culture because, often, educational attainment is intertwined with culture and language proficiency, and in the healthcare field, there is a lack of awareness of these issues. There must be accountability in the healthcare field and assurance that all involved will understand how health literacy and linguistic competence impact health, to develop creative and innovative approaches to provide patients/customers with health information. Within the context of such innovation, there must be knowledge of the fact that individuals of lower socioeconomic status, who are predominantly people of color, have less access to the Internet and other forms of technology (**digital divide**), and; therefore, innovative approaches must include different mediums for providing health information. Getting around this digital divide may include use of print sources (taking literacy levels into consideration), broadcast media such as radio and television, and one-on-one discussions with patients.

▶ The School-to-Prison Pipeline and Mass Incarceration

Although many teachers, principals, and other members of society are dedicated to improving education, there are problems, beyond financial matters, which require resolution, based on their negative impact on education. A critical issue is the **school-to-prison pipeline**, which is disruptive to the education of young people, particularly in lower-income communities. The American Civil Liberties Union (ACLU, n.d.) explains this problem as follows:

> The pipeline begins with inadequate resources in public schools. Overcrowded classrooms, a lack of qualified teachers, and insufficient funding for "extras" such as counselors, special education services, and even textbooks, lock students into second-rate educational environments.

There are some key facts to begin with in the discussion of the school-to-prison pipeline. First, Black boys are three times more likely to be suspended than White boys, and Black girls are six times more likely to be suspended than are White girls (Crenshaw, Ocen, & Nanda, 2015). This disparity in disciplinary rates represents a critical problem and the initial piece in the school-to-prison pipeline. The data show that when students are suspended from school, they are nearly three times more likely to be in contact with the juvenile justice system within the following year (Crenshaw et al., 2015).

To make matters worse, schools have implemented no-tolerance policies, which contribute to the trend of incarcerating school children. For minor infractions that would normally be handled by in-school disciplinary actions, children in the K-12 system are being arrested—another piece in the school-to-prison pipeline. A report was released by the National Association for the Advancement of Colored People (NAACP) titled "Misplaced Priorities" examining the rise in spending on prisons as compared to schools on a statewide basis (NAACP, n.d.). The report indicates that state funds are being shifted away from education and toward the criminal justice system, particularly in low-income, emerging majority populations, with the resultant outcome of destabilized communities. Young people who get second-rate educations and who are moved from school to prison may end up in a downward spiral. If branded a felon, basic rights may be taken away from them. For example, the opportunity to find a job becomes very slim, as essentially, many job applications ask whether the applicant has a felony. If the answer is yes, the individual will not be hired. Once a person is branded a felon, public housing and the receipt of food stamps are no longer options (PBS, 2014). Hence, recidivism becomes an issue, as the inability to find housing, work, or food limits options for survival and may cause individuals to resort to drastic measures.

Solution for the School-to-Prison Pipeline

Although the allocation of funds toward prisons rather than schools is outlandish, the solution to this problem is not complicated. The first step is to follow the example set by Broward County Florida School Superintendent, Robert Runcie, who decided that in his school district, there would be "appropriate responses and use of resources when responding to school-based misbehavior" (Lee, 2013). The Broward County School Board voted unanimously to sign new rules meant to drive down arrest rates of school-aged children (Reyes, 2014). This common-sense approach results in in-school disciplinary actions rather than arrests with the understanding that K-12 children must not be arrested for matters that can be handled at school. An additional solution would be to focus on state budgets to ensure that funds are not disproportionately allocated to prisons rather than to public schools. Public schools, particularly in low-income communities, need more funding, which would lead to the improvement of educational facilities.

Reasons for the School-to-Prison Pipeline

The question that comes to mind is, why would there be a school-to-prison pipeline in the first place? What kind of society would imprison its children rather than try to redirect them with positive reinforcement? What kind of society would allocate more resources toward prisons than toward their educational system? The answers are complicated. Private prisons need high incarceration rates for contracted private companies. They are businesses traded on the New York Stock Exchange. To achieve the often 90 to 100 percent occupancy rates required per contracts, they rely on the following:

- Mandatory minimum sentences
- Felony plea bargains
- The three-strikes law
- Immigration detainment
- Arrests of young people in schools

Given the focus of this discussion, namely the school-to-prison pipeline, the final point—arrests of young people in schools—should stand out. Prisoners are available labor, lending to significant profits. In fact, private prisons are now advertising their facilities as an alternative to the hiring of low-wage workers outside of the country. Chris Hedges, in a report titled "The Prison State of America" (2014), describes the prison work force as follows:

> The prison work force is guaranteed not to have car problems, there is no need for babysitters, and the workers will be on time for work and available whenever needed. Furthermore, they are not paid overtime, do not have sick time or any paid leave, do not receive benefits, social security or pensions, nor are they permitted to form unions or strike. If they complain, their punishment might be isolation. This is quite a readily available work force of about one million prisoners.

Hedges proceeds to identify some of the subcontractors, namely major corporations who sell electronics, food, cosmetics, clothing, and beyond. Prisoners also produce military helmets, uniforms, pants, shirts, ammunition belts, ID tags, and tents. For this labor, federal prisoners are paid as much as $1.25 per hour, which is far below the federal minimum wage (see **TABLE 3-6**). In terms of state prison labor, prisoners may earn as little as 17 cents an hour.

TABLE 3-6 Federal Prison Wages		
Hourly Rate	**Items Produced**	**Prisoners Work Through Subcontractors (Major Corporations)**
As much as $1.25 per hour	Examples: Military helmets, uniforms, pants, shirts, ammunition belts, ID tags, and tents	Microsoft, AT&T, Chevron, Nintendo, Starbucks, Bank of America, IBM, Victoria's Secret, Eddie Bauer, Wendy's, Proctor & Gamble, Johnson & Johnson, Fruit of the Loom, Motorola, Macy's, Sara Lee, Texas Instruments, Caterpillar, Hewlett-Packard, Nortel, Nordstrom's, Revlon, Pierre Cardin, Target, JCPenney, Quaker Oats

Data from Hedges, C. (2014, December 28). The prison state of America. Truthdig. Retrieved from http://www.truthdig.com /report/item/the_prison_state_of_america_20141228

The unfortunate reality is that prisoners need to earn money. As documented in Hedges's report, they need money to pay for essential, basic commissary items such as toilet paper, shoes, extra blankets, soap, deodorant, and sometimes electricity, room, and board. Given the paltry pay they receive, they often have to take out prison loans for medication, legal and medical fees, prison sentencing fees, and other expenses. Imagine that while in prison, the prisoners are accruing debt, which leads to owing fees when they are released. Most likely, if they are felons, they will have a tremendously difficult time finding a job and if they find work, payments are taken from their minimal paychecks to pay their prison debts. Hence, they must live in poverty, which leads to all of the concerns associated with such conditions, including poor food quality and accessibility, neighborhoods where the quality of education is low, and health illiteracy and the resultant health problems. The inevitable outcome is the continued health disparity, as the bulk of individuals who are experiencing the school-to-prison pipeline and mass incarceration are emerging majorities.

The Solution for Prison Profiteering

The solution to this prison profiteering situation is to remove the vested interest in incarcerating emerging majorities by stopping corporations from using prisoners as cheap labor with little to no pay. This corporate practice is a sinister form of greed, leading to an increase in corporate profit that can be likened to slavery in form and practice. Ending this practice is one of many solutions that can help reduce the health disparities gap.

▶ Interview With a K-12 Administrator

In exploring potential solutions to the problem of educational disparities in the United States contributing to health disparities, input from educators and administrators who have firsthand knowledge regarding education is imperative. The following interview with Dr. Adrienne Chew, who served as a public high school principal in Philadelphia for 8 years, provides an interesting perspective into the provision of education in a low-income community. This interview has been condensed and edited.

DR. ROSE: The first question is, what is your background, educationally, and your primary field of study?

DR. CHEW: My background originally was fine arts and art education. I studied at Boston University. I have a bachelor of fine arts degree in art education and painting. I also have a master's degree in special education and a doctor of education (EdD) in educational leadership.

DR. ROSE: Where did you acquire your master's in special education?

DR. CHEW: At Antioch University in Ohio, and the EdD in educational leadership is from Nova Southeastern University in Florida.

DR. ROSE: How and why did you become a principal? Did you serve at a middle or high school and for how long?

DR. CHEW: I was an art teacher and there was someone in my life who was a principal. I was, at that time, academic coaching and an art teacher. This person expressed to me that I had the qualities to go into leadership. In my early years, I kept experiencing getting laid off because of budget cuts, and they were always attacking art programs. Every time this happened, I used it as an opportunity for growth and would go back and get another degree or certification—that sort of thing. I got my principal certification. Ultimately, I became a high school assistant principal. Some new, small-model schools were opened in South Philadelphia and I became the founding principal at one of the new schools.

DR. ROSE: So you were a high school principal? What was the name of the school? Where was this school located, and how long were you there?

DR. CHEW: The Academy at Colombo in South Philadelphia. I was there for 8 years.

DR. ROSE: Tell me a little bit about the community. Was this a lower socioeconomic community?

DR. CHEW: Yes. South Philadelphia is populated with higher-income populations right now. But since the school was a magnet, it draws students from all over the city. It's a Title I school, so income-wise it was a mix.

DR. ROSE: Can you explain Title I?

DR. CHEW: Title I means that you receive federal funds for students to use for educational purposes, instructional materials, and those types of services.

DR. ROSE: What were the demographics, roughly? I don't need the specifics.

DR. CHEW: We were a "grow a grade school" first of all, so when I opened the school, we opened with approximately 125 students. Even with the number equaling 125, I noticed that we always had a higher percentage of African Americans—I would say around 50 percent. We also had a high population of Asian students, then White students, and then other. 50 percent, 30 percent, and the rest—

DR. ROSE: In terms of the Asian students, as an example, would you know what nations they were from? China, Japan, etc.?

DR. CHEW: Yes. Chinese, Vietnamese, Cambodian, and Indian. We did not have too many Japanese students.

DR. ROSE: And what about Hispanic students, in terms of nationality?

DR. CHEW: Puerto Rican and Mexicans—a lot of immigrant families without green cards. A lot of times when those students would do very well and graduate, their big thing was going to college and getting financial aid. It was very hard for them and they were not able to qualify.

DR. ROSE: As I explore the social justice issues in our society, my goal is to avoid reiterating all of the problems, but we have to start there. What would you say were some of the most significant problems at your school?

DR. CHEW: In terms of cultural issues?

DR. ROSE: Well, no. More so as a school, within the context of the community. Were there any problems that you think were relevant? For example, if we look at the Baltimore situation right now [referring to police killing of teenager Freddie Gray and the ensuing riots], we're looking at a very significantly low-income community. We are looking at an extremely high unemployment rate in that community. Many of the people have lost their housing due to the subprime mortgage situation. There are a lot of vacant homes and the community has a very high crime rate, and so when we see what's happening, we can kind of connect that to the situation that exists in that community from a socioeconomic vantage point. So the schools have a problem as a result of that. The children literally walked out of school recently, high school students, and participated in a riot. So the question is, in the school that you were working at, did you have any kind of problems communitywide, and so forth?

DR. CHEW: The schools that I worked at were high-performing schools. The students were admitted. You had to apply to both of the schools where I was the principal. You had to have scores in the 88th percentile or higher in both reading and math to get in. Our students came to us with academic ability and also a view of where they wanted to go. They challenged us in terms of what we could offer them in terms of a good education but were also aware of their neighborhoods and their particular situation. I had students whose mothers or fathers or siblings had been incarcerated or they were from foster families or they were living in a way where it was hard, but the motivation that you see in certain high-performing students I think puts them at an advantage in terms of dealing with certain strife because they are able to look at it, analyze it in a certain way, and see it through.

I had students walk out of my school in protest, but they were always part of a peaceful movement. I had students where they would send text messages about their going to have a flash mob. They would provide me with a heads-up to say this is what is going to happen, Dr. Chew, so I was able to be proactive. They were more concerned for themselves and the welfare of the other students. We had graduation rates of almost 100 percent in the first 2 years. The problem was how to maintain that or exceed it. Yes. We had students who were suicidal or who sometimes would get caught up in the violence of the streets—gang fights, threats, etc.—the same problems that happen in nonmagnet schools. But we were able to get a pulse on it, work through them and resolve them through talking and bringing parents in and working through issues. Those problems that were out there, I think we were able to work through a lot earlier and easier than some other high schools.

DR. ROSE: As one who has been a principal who has experienced success with your school and students, if you had the opportunity to advise the administrators at the school in Baltimore where the students walked out in protest, what would be your advice to resolve some of the issues specific to education?

DR. CHEW: Well, our counselor-to-student ratios went down over time. The principal has to be a communicator. Advise students of certain behaviors through assemblies; guide them. You have to teach students how to be an audience. Share with them. Allow them the opportunity to voice their opinion. I don't like the word train, but you do have to guide them and get their opinions about what they think is going on. I let them know that if they are wearing a Colombo shirt that they are representing the school. You have to have class buy-in and governance at the school. You have to have a number of different types of assemblies and recognition. You have to distribute leadership among staff and students as well.

DR. ROSE: I think that is a very good point. That happened, assemblies, when I was a student and it was important. It seems that essentially what you are saying is that the schools have to be very student focused. My next question is, what is your perspective regarding standardized testing? Is it helpful in terms of improving/helping or making the scenario better in public education in the United States, particularly in lower socioeconomic communities?

DR. CHEW: I think there has to be a measure. There is always going to be a measure. It is just the nature of the game. However, if colleges change, like some of them are, and they are not really going to be looking at standardized testing or SAT scores, then that should take the pressure off of a high school or even a middle school to put this whole perspective in place that our school has to perform well. There is always going to be an indicator. For example, in Philadelphia, there was a benchmark exam, and then with the benchmark exam there was the Pennsylvania System of School Assessment (PSSA) exam, and now they have the Keystone Exam. The problem that they're running into right now is that they said by a certain date, for certain years, everyone had to be proficient in order to graduate. My opinion is that we have to look at this and be realistic. If you have a standardized test, that's wonderful. You want to know where your students are, maybe to readjust instruction, align differently advanced placement. We always did well in certain areas rather than others. We always did well in government politics, American history, AP English, and Spanish was great. We had students that scored well. But the question becomes, is it going to benefit our students in low-income areas? Is it going to leave more behind than those who advance?

Dr. Rose: Private schools are not required to participate in standardized testing. For example, in Florida, there was the Florida Comprehensive Assessment Test (FCAT). The students at the private schools did not take those tests or participate in common core, which is in effect now. The students go on and attend college and etc. Why then are standardized tests or common core needed in public and not private schools?

Dr. Chew: I think for funding. Because they are playing the game of government and in order to get funding, you are going to have to show what your school is doing and not doing. That's one reason why I think it's driven there. But for me, I think what is happening in schools that are not testing and still doing well—it's what they are teaching. It's how they are teaching it and it's authentic literacy. They are reading and they are writing. You know, that's what's going on.

Dr. Rose: So you are saying that they are not teaching to the tests?

Dr. Chew: Yes. If you go back to the "little red school house"—well they weren't actually red—but the emphasis was basically on reading literacy, across all subjects.

Dr. Rose: Right. And it's critical. Now you said something that is really important. It's a question that I've been grappling with and I've been asking so many people. You're the first one that I think has hit the nail on the head in regard to why the standardized testing is happening. So I need a little bit of elaboration on that. So you are saying that the basis for standardized testing, one of the key factors, is because of funding? Are you saying that this is so that the schools can get federal funding? Do they need those test scores in order to get that?

Dr. Chew: Right. It is so that schools can get funding, I believe, and get ranked. Some schools don't believe in ranking. There was a time here in Philadelphia where the independent schools refused ranking. And you know that the schools were great. It's to rank. It's to fund. It's also a way to look at what teachers are doing. And I don't know if this is always the right thing to do because sometimes I think you lose good teachers this way. But, it's a way to also monitor what teachers are doing in classrooms.

Dr. Rose: All right. So the curriculum is based on the test.

Dr. Chew: And the teachers are getting points or losing points in terms of their evaluation, if their classroom is not performing well. The reason that they have benchmark scores is because they want to monitor whether you are teaching to the common core or whatever curriculum that the school district is using.

DR. ROSE: So the scores are essentially a way of evaluating them?

DR. CHEW: It's a way of evaluating your schools, your teachers, your district. It's a way for the state to say Philadelphia is doing well or not doing well. It's all about funding. You talk about this gap. It's the opportunity gap that we have here. You know, resources. They know that you are not performing well and you need money. Are we going to get the funding that we need because now they see that the resources are so different in inner city schools in Philadelphia than they are somewhere else, like in the suburbs, that don't have this problem?

DR. ROSE: Right. So the resources don't necessarily follow suit when it is determined that the scores are low.

DR. CHEW: Exactly. Not always but sometimes they do because there used to be this thing where, in Philadelphia, if your school is doing well, then you didn't get as much money as another school got. But still, all in all, whatever money one school was getting versus another, was the money enough to do what was necessary? I believe you are still looking at your bigger, broader, socioeconomic issues, which is the community; these are your opportunity gaps. What resources are they getting in the community? What happens to our families that are falling apart? Michelle Alexander's whole big thing on mass incarceration brings this to the forefront.

DR. ROSE: That's my next question for you.

DR. CHEW: It's like a whole big thing here going on. Where are our kids coming from? What are they seeing? Why are they angry? Do they have a right to be angry? Of course they do. We saw anger all over Baltimore. And the anger is in a certain segment of that population down there. There's this whole thing with the haves and the have-nots—grabbing stuff. That stuff that they were grabbing, is that going to make their life better? No, it's not, but for that moment it's some sort of satisfaction—now I can get something that I can't have.

DR. ROSE: Right, which would not be attainable normally for them. So in some ways, it's an opportunity. It's not clearly understood, but it's an opportunity for that moment in time to be a have—to have things that you can't normally have.

DR. CHEW: That's how I see it. How many jobs were lost? A senior center burned to the ground. They didn't think about the long term. It was just that moment to release. There were a lot of people who would say no to this. There were community leaders there, long-term residents for which this is where they live and who saw this happen before and know that the outcome is not going to be what they think it's going to be, but the opposite. But nobody was able to listen because they were so caught up in that moment of excitement or riot or demonstration.

DR. ROSE: So in regard to the school-to-prison pipeline, because you did mention Michelle Alexander [author of the book entitled *The New Jim Crow: Mass Incarceration in the Age of Colorblindness*] and mass incarceration. What are your thoughts about the school-to-prison pipeline? Why is this happening? How would you explain it? How are these children ending up in prison? What's happening inside of a school that allows a K-12 child to be arrested—so that we have a significant number of children going to prison from school? How is that happening? How are these children ending up in prison? You are in the school, inside the physical building. I need a visual on this. What happens inside of the school that allows a child to be arrested? How does it happen? As a principal, what is your understanding of how a K-12 child is arrested so that we have significant numbers of children going to prison from school? How does this manifest?

DR. CHEW: It's because, well we know about the whole thing; we know about the communities and the parents. I think the principals in their daily work have to establish and sustain a harmonious culture that celebrates diversity and promotes multicultural communal activities. When we talk about diversity, and even within our Black community, there are many Black people that come from different cultures and speak different languages. Okay. Your school culture has to reflect that they are welcome.

DR. ROSE: Right. Cultural competency.

DR. CHEW: What are the messages that are put in that school from day one, so the kindergarten child to the 12th grader gets the same message? Also, parents have to make sure that the children come to school. As a principal, in addition to scores, I also looked at attendance. Are we creating a sense of belonging for our students at early ages? Are our teachers aware or unaware? What level do we want to get them to? We want inspired teachers. There are certain behaviors that teachers have to have. Teachers have to be culturally responsive. Do we have the best teachers in our underperforming schools? Does the kid like their teacher? If teachers are unaware of their behaviors, then they are not being culturally responsive. If they are not aware of their behaviors, then they are not communicating the content of their subject matter. Are you knowledgeable and strong in your content? This is all about having good teacher training programs. Do we have the best teachers in underperforming schools? Do the kids like their teacher?

DR. ROSE: But it is my understanding that when these school-to-prison pipeline scenarios take place that for minor infractions—let's just say that the teacher has some of these qualities and is inspired but the child does something in school, maybe hits another child and the school has a zero-tolerance policy. Rather than sending the child to the principal's office, they will call the police and actually have the child arrested.

DR. CHEW: That's unacceptable.

DR. ROSE: How does that transpire? Do principals have policies regarding this?

DR. CHEW: There are policies that are in place at all schools. The kid comes into the building with a weapon. There is a policy for that. It used to be that if a child brought a weapon or drugs to school, whether it was a first or second offense, you'd be sent to another school. Now, they are doing it differently. They are reviewing the data. They will put you on a plan. You are getting support from a counselor or other mentoring-type program so that I think it is wonderful that kids aren't getting kicked out or suspended for long periods of time.

DR. ROSE: So I am still trying to understand what policies get the child to jail? I hear what you are saying that you would have counseling and steps and so forth, but yet we are seeing substantial numbers of children that are going to jail, so what I'm trying to get at is at what point does it go from in-school handling to the child going out of the building in handcuffs?

DR. CHEW: It's leadership. It's the leadership approach.

DR. ROSE: But I guess it also has to do with policy because the school may have a policy that says if a child is found with a weapon, he or she has to be arrested or if a child hits another child he or she has to be arrested. Is it a fact that there can be policies to that effect?

DR. CHEW: Depending on your school, policy may be your best leverage when you have a very large school. It's your approach. Cell phone policy—3,000 students. There's a student with a cell phone. The parent comes to school and wants the child to have the cell phone back. There are all kinds of nasty name-calling. That's my child. That's the principal's policy, in writing. You don't know what that student is going to do with the cell phone. Depending on your school, in which you know that climate and culture, you have to put out that fire. Instructional climate and safety. Those things have to be there. When you're dealing with 3,000 students, if I side on policy, I don't have error. For smaller schools, things may be different. I'm not favoring one student or one situation over another, which we can do, but it's hard to do when you have a lot of students. When you have a small number of students, it's easier, to have a nurturing culture. You do things differently and you don't have so many students that you are sending off. I've had to reassign students to a disciplinary school because of drugs or what have you. There are some situations where you can implement a so-called lesson. The point is that you are not going to sell drugs in my building.

DR. ROSE: All right. So I have three more questions for you. The first is STEM. Many educators are arguing the point that rather than a focus on the humanities, that STEM should be the focal point right now, particularly in terms of lower socioeconomic students. How do you feel about that?

DR. CHEW: I think it's great. Opportunities for students to become engaged in science, technology, engineering, and math—beautiful. I'm all for it. The opportunity is there. STEM is critical. It's essential. What is technology going to look like 10 years from now? Why would we not want our students to know everything that they can possibly know regarding STEM? We want our students to have opportunities to be part of the highest paying fields, in terms of careers, that they can have. Because that is where the money is in terms of careers.

DR. ROSE: Right. That's true. In the lower socioeconomic neighborhoods, one of the biggest problems is resources. Do you think the schools are resourced sufficiently for students to experience STEM at the levels that they should?

DR. CHEW: I can't speak for every school. I know that in budgets, most schools are putting an emphasis on getting technology. I know in Philadelphia, they have schools that are specifically focused on science, engineering, and math.

DR. ROSE: Are those magnet schools?

DR. CHEW: Yes. It also depends on, if you want to discuss high schools, the kind of teachers that are hired. Are teachers skilled in delivering STEM? Physics teachers, robotics—

DR. ROSE: Okay, excellent. What are your thoughts about some schools eliminating physical education?

DR. CHEW: It is essential to the curriculum. It provides a sense of belonging. Some students are athletic and need that type of program. I think it is very important along with health education. A half-year of PE and a half-year of health education. There are things that kids must be able to do—collaboration, learning—

DR. ROSE: Yes. The team aspect is very critical. There is an intellectual component to it as well.

DR. CHEW: Good leadership and good schools have it.

DR. ROSE: Lastly, critical pedagogy, particularly hip-hop pedagogy. It is becoming a key component these days in schools where low socioeconomic status students attend, or at least the desire to see this in schools. What are your thoughts about this?

DR. CHEW: I think it's wonderful. The students must be able to tell you what they know. If they want to sing about it, write about it, deliver it, then you know they know it. I'm all for it. Teaching science through hip-hop. Slam poetry. Once again, it's expression. These kids, their ears have been trained. It's poetry. It's wonderful. They are expressing and moving—they are engaged, they respond. It engages the learner. They are able to express what is on their minds, their hearts. You learn if they are hungry, if they are a foster child. Once they are able to express themselves and get that stuff out of the way, you allow other info to enter.

DR. ROSE: So students who experience hip-hop pedagogy in high school and then they get to college and it is not embraced, then what? Would hip-hop pedagogy then be a part of the curriculum around all subjects? Is it to be the curriculum for the children or extra-curricular? Do you agree that for "some" children, this is the way they learn?

DR. CHEW: It can't be all hip-hop. You still have to play the game of preparation for school. I see a combination of hip-hop pedagogy. Students should have their major and the remaining classes would be in their core subject. Maybe a hip-hop school would be an approach. I think it would be wonderful. In Philadelphia, they have a String Theory school. They have a Rock School of Dance also here in Philadelphia. They have SLA, which is the Science and Leadership Academy, which is inquiry based. Most students in these institutes are still doing a lot of reading and writing. At the core of it all there has to be literacy. Our kids have to be literate. Hip-hop is argumentative. When I express myself, I'm giving you my viewpoint. The question is can they write it? Can they read it, in a traditional manner?

DR. ROSE: Excellent! Thank you!

Interview Summary

In the preceding interview, Dr. Chew offers valuable insight into some key factors to ensure that schools work for K-12 children in lower socioeconomic communities. From the vantage point of teachers, she discusses quality. She highlights policy in terms of management of big schools as well as the need for STEM (science, technology, engineering, and math). These are the kinds of solutions that need to be focused on to enhance the educational experience for children, particularly in the K-12 environment. Educational achievement, at this level, will lead students to move forward to achieve higher education and consequently become educated, preparing them to lead quality lives, earn money, and take care of their health. These accomplishments will surely contribute to closing the health status gap.

However, there is the problem of when it doesn't go well. When students are not in high-performing schools, are in lower socioeconomic communities, and policies reek of social injustice, children are positioned to enter the school-to-prison pipeline rather than the school-to-college pipeline. This inevitably leads to negative experiences in overall life outcomes, including health disparities. Hence, it is important to explore this issue with an eye toward solutions.

Wrap-Up

Chapter Summary

Social injustice plays a critical role in the perpetuation of health disparities in the United States. Issues such as food injustice, in its various forms, and health literacy must be addressed. There is a lack of quality education and health literacy in low socioeconomic status communities, primarily among people of color. In terms of educational disparities, the school-to-prison pipeline and prison profiteering must end as necessary steps toward reducing health disparities. **FIGURE 3-1** provides insight into what must happen to solve the problem of health inequity from an ideal standpoint.

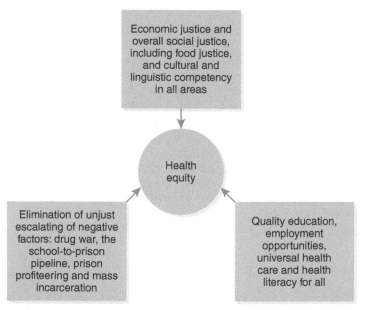

FIGURE 3-1 An ideal solution toward health equity.

Chapter Problems

1. Explain why low health literacy is a result of poor education in the United States.
2. Health disparities, health literacy, and social injustice are all-important issues that people in the healthcare field should understand. Why?
3. There are specific differences between food mirages and food deserts. Explain.
4. List three diet-related diseases that are specifically contributing to health disparities among people of color.
5. Per the Dr. Chew interview, name one solution that she points out toward improving the K-12 educational system in lower socioeconomic communities.

References

Agency for Healthcare Research and Quality. (2001). Diabetes disparities among racial and ethnic minorities. Retrieved from http://archive.ahrq.gov/research/findings/factsheets/diabetes/diabdisp/diabdisp.html

Airhihenbuwa, C., Kumanyika, S., Agurs, T., Lowe, A., Saunders, D., & Morssink, C. (1996). Cultural aspects of African American eating patterns. *Ethnicity & Health, 1*(3), 245–260.

American Civil Liberties Union. (n.d.). School-to-prison pipeline. Retrieved from https://www.aclu.org/racial-justice/what-school-to-prison-pipeline

American Psychological Association. (n.d.). Ethnic and racial minorities and socioeconomic status. Retrieved from http:www.apa.org/pi/ses/resources/publications/factsheet-erm.aspx

Bower, K., Thorpe, R., Rohde, C., & Gaskin, D. (2014). The intersection of neighborhood racial segregation, poverty, and urban communities and their impact on food store availability in the United States. *Preventive Medicine, 58*, 33–39.

Braithwaite, R. (1992). *Health issues in the Black community.* San Francisco, CA: Jossey-Bass.

Breyer, B., & Voss-Andreae, A. (2013). Food mirages: Geographic and economic barriers to healthful food access in Portland, Oregon. *Health & Place*, 131–139.

Centers for Disease Control and Prevention. (2015). Racial or ethnic variations. Retrieved from http://www.cdc.gov/cancer/dcpc/data/race.htm

Chatenoud, L., Tavani, A., LaVecchia, C., Jacobs, D., Negri, E., Levi, F., & Franceschi, S. (1998). Whole grain food intake and cancer risk. *International Journal of Cancer, 77*(1), 24–28.

Chen, Z., Yen, S. T., & Eastwod, D. B. (2005). Effects of food participation on body weight and obesity. *American Journal of Agricultural Economics, 87*(5), 1167–1173.

Crenshaw, W., Ocen, P., & Nanda, J. (2015). Black girls matter: Pushed out, overpoliced and underprotected. Retrieved from http://www.law.columbia.edu/null/download?&exclusive=filemgr.download&file_id=613546

Denavas-Walt, C., Proctor, B., & Smith, J. (2011). Income, poverty and health insurance coverage in the United States: 2010. United States Census Bureau. Retrieved from www.census.gov/prod/2011pubs/p60-239.pdf

Drewnowski, A., & Specter, S. E. (2004). Poverty and obesity: The role of energy density and energy costs. *The American Journal of Clinical Nutrition, 79*(1), 6–16.

Duncan-Andrade, J., & Morrell, E. (2008). *The art of critical pedagogy: Possibilities for moving from theory to practice in urban schools.* New York: Peter Lang.

Galvez, M., Morland, K., Raines, C., Kobil, J., Siskind, J., Godbold, J., & Brenner, B. (2008). Race and food store availability in an inner city neighborhood. *Public Health Nutrition, 11*(6), 624–631.

Hedges, C. (2014, December 28). The prison state of America. Truthdig Retrieved from http://www.truthdig.com/report/item/the_prison_state_of_america_20141228

Horowitz, C., Colson, C., Hebert, P., & Lancaster, K. (2004). Barriers to buying healthy foods for people with diabetes: Evidence of environmental disparities. *American Journal of Public Health, 94*(9), 1549–1554.

Institute of Medicine. (2001). *Crossing the quality chasm: A new health system for the 21st century: Formulating new rules to redesign and improve care.* Washington, DC: National Academies Press.

Institute of Medicine. (2004). *In the nation's compelling interest: Ensuring diversity in the healthcare workforce.* Washington, DC: The National Academies Press.

James, D. (2004). Factors influencing food choices, dietary intake, and nutrition-related attitudes among African Americans: Application of a culturally sensitive model. *Ethnicity & Health, 9*(4), 349–367.

Jetter, K., & Cassady, D. (2006). The availability and cost of healthier food alternatives. *American Journal of Preventive Medicine, 30*(1), 38–44.

Kirsch, I. S., Jungeblut, A., Jenkins, L., & Kolstad, A. (1993). *Adult literacy in America: A first look at the results of the national adult literacy survey (NALS).* Washington, DC: National Center for Education Statistics, U.S. Department of Education.

Lee, M. (2013, November 5). South Florida squeezes school-to-prison pipeline. Juvenile Justice Information Exchange. Retrieved from http://jjie.org/south-florida-squeezes-school-to-prison-pipeline/105628/

Mandela, N. (n.d.) Retrieved from https://www.brainyquote.com/quotes/nelson_mandela_737776

Morin, R. (2013, July 12). The politics and demographics of food stamp recipients. Pew Research Center. Retrieved from http://www.pewresearch.org/fact-tank/2013/07/12/the-politics-and-demo-graphics-of-food-stamp-recipients

National Association for the Advancement of Colored People. (n.d.). Misplaced priorities: A new report from NAACP. Retrieved from http://www.naacp.org/pages/misplaced-priorities

PBS (2014). Michelle Alexander: "A System of Racial and Social Control." Retrieved from http://www.pbs.org/wgbh/frontline/article/michelle-alexander-a-system-of-racial-and-social-control/4

Purdue University. (n.d.). Diet-related diseases. Retrieved from http://www.four-h.purdue.edu/foods/Diet-Related%20Diseases.htm

Reyes, R. (2014). Bold lesson: Florida district swaps cops for counseling. Retrieved from http://www.nbcnews.com/news/latino/bold-lesson-florida-school-district-swaps-cops-counseling-n13936

Shaw, H. (2006). Food deserts: Towards the development of a classification. *Geografiska Annaler B Geografiska Annaler, Series B: Human Geography, 88*(2), 231–247.

Slocum, R. (2010). Race in the study of food. *Progress in Human Geography, 35*(3), 303–327.

Smith, C., & Morton, L. (2009). Rural food deserts: Low-income perspectives on food access in Minnesota and Iowa. *Journal of Nutrition Education and Behavior, 41*(3), 176–187.

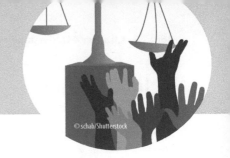
© schab/Shutterstock

CHAPTER 4

Understanding the Impact of Urban Education on Urban Health

Dr. Courtney Rose and
Dr. Edmund Adjapong

KEY TERMS

achievement gap
Brown v. Board of Education
colorblindness
common school system
cultural capital
cultural incongruence
culturally relevant pedagogy

demographic imperative
hip-hop pedagogy
pedagogy
reality pedagogy
tracking
virtual professional learning network
  (VPLN)

LEARNING OBJECTIVES

After reading this chapter, you should be able to do the following:

1. Describe the link between health and education.
2. Understand the history of the development of the public school system that exists in America today.
3. Define the "achievement gap" and how it has been used to perpetuate beliefs about particular groups' educational abilities and outcomes.
4. Identify and explain the link between educational achievement and health outcomes.
5. Explain the role of culture in as it relates to teaching and learning.

▶ Introduction

The link between education and health is well-known and highly researched. Access to both health care and education are closely tied to, and mitigated by, one's geographic location and socio-economic status. Those holding higher paying jobs, which is closely linked to educational attainment, have the ability to live and move to locations in closer proximity to better schools, more nutritional food sources, transportation, and health services (Virginia Commonwealth University Center on Society and Health, 2014). Additionally, one's ability to engage in educational processes is closely linked to their health status. Chronic illness and poor nutrition impact attendance rates, concentration and cognitive skills, all of which deeply impact the degree to which students are able to absorb and process information (Zimmerman & Woolf, 2014).

Looking at the relationship between health and education from the other end, decades of studies show that higher levels of academic achievement have positive impacts on individual's health behaviors and health usage. Specifically, education fosters the development of cognitive skills, problem-solving abilities, and personality traits, among others, that mediate the relationship between health and education (Ross & Wu, 1995; Zimmerman & Woolf, 2014). Most notably, the hard skills acquired in school (i.e., reading comprehension and argumentation) increases individual's health literacy making it easier for them to understand their health needs, read and interpret instructions, and advocate for their own health needs and those in their families and communities. Unfortunately, another similarity between health and education is the gap between the quality of services and outcomes that exists between various groups of the population, often drawn along racial and socio-economic lines rooted in historical and systemic practices and policies intended to limit access and opportunity. In this chapter, the authors explore the academic **achievement gap** and the history of the American schooling system, providing insight into the root causes of the education gap as well as potential avenues for long-term change toward educational, and by association, health equity.

Mind the Gap

In the increasingly test-based approach to education, the "achievement gap" has become one of the biggest buzzwords within the field of education. This gap disproportionately affects students in predominantly African American and Latino populations, and in low-income urban areas. Since the inception of the compulsory American schooling system, various laws, mandated policies, curricular designs, and education reform agendas became enmeshed in deficit-based constructions of difference and diversity. These have been used to limit access to educational opportunities and resources for those in historically marginalized and underserved populations (Anderson, 1988; Kliebard, 2004; Nasaw, 1979). Historically, constructions of race, gender, (dis)ability, and social class have been used to establish a cultural norm rooted in the ideals of a White, middle-/upper-class, male-dominated society (Delpit, 1988; Gay, 2000; Irizarry, 2009). Within this framing, perceived social and cultural differences resulted in the continuous labeling of those who deviate from, or are not able to fit within, the "norm" as "socially and/or culturally deprived," in need of fixing, or in some extreme cases, removal from the system altogether.

How Did We Get Here?

Historians in the fields of Education and Sociology explore the development of the **common school system**, which was the precursor to the compulsory public education system currently functioning within American society today. Fearing the consequences of granting the right to vote to the "common man," those in power quickly moved to develop a system of education that would work to socialize and civilize the children of the poor whose education was previously the responsibility of the family (primarily the mother) to provide. Using compulsory taxation of the people, the government publicly funded their schools, claiming that it was the only way to guarantee "protection from the rapacity of the unschooled" (Nasaw, 1979, Ch.3, Campaigning for School Taxes, para.8). Through various reform movements, proponents of the common schooling system constantly worked to ensure that resources (monetary, material, and human) were used efficiently. This resulted in multiple "reform efforts," which limited access to various components of the curriculum to those it was deemed unnecessary for, particularly as the use of various tests and sorting tools became popular methods to determine one's intellectual capacity and projected future place in society. Thus, social mobility, or the ability for one to "pull themselves up by their bootstraps," was limited for many, thereby reproducing existing social stratification and protecting the elite positions of those in power (Nasaw, 1979).

Within this movement, the education of recently freed Black slaves, and poor Whites, particularly in the South, became a major area of contention among proponents of the common schooling movement. Fearing both the overeducated *and* uneducated freed Black man, the majority of schools initially designed for this population provided training in service-oriented, and largely manual, labor that continued to limit them to work in the homes, fields, and later, factories of White America (Nasaw, 1979). Therefore, some argue that from its inception, compulsory public education as it exists today was never intended for the inclusion of African Americans, or other racial/ethnic groups, and the basic infrastructure of American society works to perpetuate the subjugation and exclusion of the majority of members in these groups (Adjapong, 2019).

The Sorting Game

One can trace current practices in the use of testing to the introduction of intelligence testing. Initially used in France, the IQ test was brought to the United States as a means of determining the "innate intelligence" of individuals and detecting the "genetically inferior" (Kamin, 1974). Through the use of these tests, intelligence became closely attributed to those of Western European descent with a disproportionate number of poor people and those of Eastern European, Native American, and African descent determined unintelligent. Linking intelligence and genetics in this manner, IQ testing becomes a means of justifying social inequity and the persistent gap between rich and poor. Even more disturbing, IQ testing is historically linked to the Eugenics movement within the United States with some states passing laws to sterilize those determined to be "feeble-minded" and ultimately the passing of the Immigration Act of 1924, which restricted immigration from Southern and Eastern Europe (Kamin, 1974).

The "science" behind Intelligence Quotient (IQ) testing became the basis for segregating students into two tracks: (1) those educated to work in service and manual labor and (2) those educated for higher education and prestigious careers (Kamin, 1974). Traces of this same system are clearly visible in the **tracking** practices, often labeled "ability grouping," that exist within the American public school system today and acts as a covert way of pushing disproportionate numbers of students of color, particularly Black and Latinx students, out of high-level and college-preparatory courses (Gamoran et al., 1995). In response to arguments of intentionally discriminatory actions, many look to the law to define the circumstances in which test use may be discriminatory or otherwise inappropriate. Under the equal protection clause of the 14th Amendment landmark cases have been filed intending to show testing practices and policies were intentionally discriminatory and/or act to preserve the effects of prior discrimination.

Presently, these tests are no longer used to justify historical claims of *inferiority* along socially constructed lines of difference such as race, class, or gender. However, they are still widely used to measure student learning, assess learning disabilities and/or giftedness, and explain/predict educational outcomes. Given that the culture of schools is grounded in the social norms of dominant White culture of society, the standard of teaching and learning remains tipped in favor of similar cultural norms. Not surprisingly there remains an ever-widening gap between the performance of students from low-income and diverse racial/ethnic groups and a simultaneous over-representation of these students in special education and remedial courses. It is through the increased use of test performance as a predictor of future success, and the subsequent tracking and labeling practices, that are associated with it that lead many students to internalize their scores to a degree in which they essentially embody them in their day-to-day lives.

In many schools the language of the testing culture becomes entrenched in daily functioning. Students are no longer "learning," they are trying to "achieve mastery" or at the very least "reach proficiency." Classrooms are covered in posters and charts outlining "what smart and/or good students do" complete with various mnemonic devices to help students memorize and remember them when it all has to come down for state testing. Additionally, in preparation for each subject-area assessment, teachers are often asked to devote a portion of their class time to "differentiated instruction," which involves breaking their classes down to performance-based groups, determined by their scores on tests and quizzes given throughout the school year, to target specific skills and concepts for specific students.

In the case of testing culture, a stigma arises in the form of rewards and consequences based on students' ability to perform on a standardized task on which great value is placed collectively by the group and broader educational systems. Regardless of student, teacher, and family buy-ins, the students' performance on these tests are used to place them in future classes, determine their access to resources and opportunities and serve as a predictor for future success on the same task the following year. Thus, even the well-intentioned teacher finds her/himself facing a moral dilemma of rebelling against, and resisting the notion of, standardization while also preparing their students to compete within a system that lives and breathes by it. Similarly, any parent/guardian wishing to guide their children to academic success must either concede to these testing practices, hiring tutors and test prep coaches beginning as early as third grade or removing their students from the public school system altogether into private schools where testing does not function as a rigid gatekeeper marketed as a tool for accountability but in actuality functioning to keep many opportunities out of reach for specific populations.

From Achievement Gap to Opportunity Gap

Although the achievement gap itself is discussed very clearly as a matter of inequality between racial groups, dominant narratives in the public conversation attempt to shift the problem out of the sphere of race matters to one of social class and family values. Shifting the dialogue in this manner reframes the issue as inequality of *engagement with and performance in* education. This places the root cause of the problem in the families themselves as factors such as family structure, parenting styles, and neighborhood characteristics are used to explain the persistence of unequal levels of academic achievement across racial lines (Burchinal et al, 2008; Dotterer, Iruka, & Pungello, 2012). Beginning in the first few years of a child's life, the burden is placed on single, low-income, working parents (largely mothers and predominantly people of color) to educate themselves on the various types of educational/childcare programs that would better prepare their children for the K-12 experience. Additionally, research comparing experiences across racial groups within similar social class backgrounds, researchers and scholars find that cultural differences in parenting styles also contribute to the inequalities in school readiness as children from some racially and culturally diverse home environments are deemed unready to engage with the learning environments as compared to their White counterparts (Dotterer, Iruka, & Pungello, 2012).

However, contrary to these views are those presented by scholars and researchers who maintain that it is not inequality of *engagement and performance*, but rather inequality, and more accurately inequity, of *opportunity to access* quality education (Walters, 2001; Ladson-Billings, 2006; Milner, 2012). Running parallel to the aforementioned research, scholars holding this position, place the root of the problem in the various *systems* of society. They present the argument that through legal and political moves the state intentionally shifted the onus of achieving equity within education from the schools to the people while simultaneously justifying the discriminatory actions of those in powerful positions (Walters, 2001; De Vito, 2007). These researchers and scholars agree that there is a difference in the approaches and values given to the educational experiences of parents living in low-income, urban environments, and their children as compared to their middle and upper class, suburban counterparts. However, they find that it is impossible to discuss these disparities without explicitly exploring matters of race relations (Ladson-Billings, 2006; Milner, 2012).

Similar to the work of those researchers focusing solely on social class, these scholars begin their exploration of the problem in the late fifties and early sixties. However, they explore more closely what was going on within the legal and political spheres of society, highlighting major Supreme Court cases that allowed particular regions to continue to essentially deny the right to education to various racial and ethnic groups (De Vito, 2007). In their initial work of applying Critical Race Theory to education, educational researchers Gloria Ladson-Billings and William Tate (1995) examine the emphasis on property rights within American society. Noting the priority of protecting *property* in the years leading up to the development of the constitution and the construction of enslaved Black people as such property to White owners, Ladson-Billings and Tate (1995), note the lack of incentive to protect the *human* rights of Black people, even after the abolishment of slavery. Although many counter this argument by pointing to the various "victories" within civil rights litigation, particularly the widely debated **Brown v. Board of Education** decision, educational and legal scholars point to the ambiguity that exists within much of this legislation that often leads to slow progress, and in many cases none at all (Crenshaw, 1988; Ladson-Billings, 2004).

(Mis)Interpreting *Brown v. Board of Education*

As previously mentioned, increased emphasis and importance on student test scores highlights the variations in performance across both racial and socioeconomic lines, which has come to be known as the "achievement gap." Sociologists and educational researchers hold varying views on the central causes of this gap in student outcomes, however many link it back to the foundations on which the very system was built (Ladson-Billings, 2012). In a country with a long history of racism and racial inequity, the integration of African-American students into the educational system may have had adverse effects in terms of psychological well being and overall acquisition of resources (physical, financial, and human) (Ladson-Billings, 2012; Payne, 2008). Therefore, the central question is whether or not Black students have become more disadvantaged in the decades following the famous *Brown v. Board of Education* decision that found it unconstitutional to segregate schools based on race. Specifically, while the integration of schools was presented as an opportunity to "level the playing field for all students", research points to evidence that it actually resulted in more costs than benefits for students of color within this country, particularly Black students.

Schools and educational curriculum are some of the primary tools used by the governing body of society, particularly in America, in terms of socializing citizens (all members of society must attend and all members spend the majority of their formative years within the walls of schools). Additionally, in societies in which academic success is the predominant path to economic success (Kingston, 2001, p.88) it is logical to presume that those with high stakes in the economy want to ensure that their positions are secure. Therefore, in discussing the integration of two groups historically grounded in two very different social and cultural backgrounds, such as African American and White students, it is necessary to explore the manner in which one group's social and **cultural capital** becomes a barrier in a world dominated by the other.

Questions concerning the overall intent and consequences of desegregation of schools per the *Brown* decision have generally focused on comparing the culture of the schools that Black students attended pre-*Brown* with that of racially integrated schools post-*Brown*. While few would suggest that the American education system go back to the overtly segregated circumstances of the pre-*Brown* era, there is a need to address the negative effects that African American/Black students experience due to the common (mis)interpretation of the language used in the decision itself. Gloria Ladson-Billings (2004) summarizes the argument in her comparison of the *Brown* decision to that of a musician landing on a wrong note in the middle of a performance. She uses this image to "convey the problem of good intentions gone awry" as "one wrong note does not destroy or invalidate an entire performance, but it does create a kind of dissonance that is more less evident depending on one's vantage point" (Ladson-Billings, 2004, p. 3).

Those advocating for desegregation within the public schools had good intentions of creating an equal playing field, particularly the families of African American students who wanted to ensure that their children received the same level of access to high-quality educational facilities, materials, and experiences. However, in fighting for *equal* access they unintentionally fueled the belief held by those in dominant circles of society that African-American students/students of color are inferior to White students and, some argue, ultimately did more damage than good (Ladson-Billings, 2004; Blanchett, Mumford & Beachum, 2005; Horsford, 2010). In this regard, existing research asserts that the issues stemming from school segregation were due to systemic and institutionalized racism, which extended beyond the school system itself and permeated throughout society as a whole. Therefore, since these underlying issues were not directly addressed and blame was instead placed on African Americans (and other racial/ethnic groups) themselves, long-term change that would benefit these historically marginalized groups would be difficult to achieve (Massey & Denton, 1993; Ladson-Billings, 2004; Blanchett, Mumford & Beachum, 2005).

Predominantly African American schools in the pre-*Brown* era provided supportive environments in which educators provided students with the skills and knowledge they needed in order to be successful in navigating the racially stratified system in which they lived (Horsford, 2010). Educational historians acknowledge the lower quality of the materials and facilities provided to African-American educators, however, the strong levels of care, trust, and understanding between educators, students, and families allowed for African American students to flourish within these racially segregated neighborhood schools. Additionally, the strong presence of African-American teachers and administrators during this time provided African-American students with role models that could relate to the racism and inequity that the students experienced outside of the school walls (Ladson-Billings, 2004; Horsford, 2010). Thus, at this time schools and educators held a strong value within the African-American community, going to great lengths in order to enrich the curriculum with experiences that would help their students build the same skills that their White counterparts were receiving (afterschool programs and clubs focused on drama, speech, and scholastic accomplishment as examples) (Walker, 2000).

Subsequently, with the passing of the *Brown* decision came a steep decline in the number of African American teachers present in schools, as African American students were bused out to White working-class schools and their neighborhood schools shut down. Environments within these mixed-race schools provided students with an opportunity to learn how to communicate and work with members of other races; however, since the underlying institutionalized racism within society was never addressed, within-school segregation was common practice (Ladson-Billings, 2004; Wells et al, 2005). The post-*Brown* era brought with it the tendency to track more White students into high-level or gifted courses, in some cases as early as Kindergarten (Wells et al, 2005).

Additionally, faced with educating students from diverse racial and cultural backgrounds, it became common to push for a culture built on **'colorblindness'** in which racial and cultural differences were ignored to emphasize similarities between and among students. This practice often left students to navigate the harsh realities of a racially stratified society on their own (Wells et al, 2005). Finally, desegregation found more funds and resources moving out of the African American community and into the White schools in which the students would be integrated. However, due to the policies and systemic practices within housing, banking, and other federal agencies, as well as the various methods in which White schools were able to work around the policies that would force full integration, many African Americans could not afford to follow these resources in order to place their students within these schools (Massey & Denton, 1993; Blanchett, Mumford & Beachum, 2005). In this regard, the newly-integrated schools within the new system *appeared* colorblind on the surface, but little attention was given to addressing the underlying, lasting consequences of segregation (i.e., Black underachievement and internalized messages of racial inferiority/superiority) (Omi & Winant, 1994), and worked under the assumption that simply placing White and Black students together would be enough to achieve educational equality. In addition to the practices in this section, the testing culture and practices mentioned earlier in this chapter provide a key example of a practice that continues to impact students and educators today, and is one that has long-lasting impacts reaching far back into America's segregated past.

Lasting Impact of Segregation

Placing heavier emphasis on the intangible psychological factors for Black people, in the *Brown* decision the Supreme Court argued that the racially segregated learning environment "generates a feeling of inferiority as to their status in the community that may affect their hearts and minds in a way unlikely to ever be undone" (*Brown I*, p. 7). The 1954 *Brown* decision presented the foundation for the debate between the colorblind/performance-based approach and the race-/culture-conscious approach. However vague language in the *Brown* decision, which placed the onus on local authorities and courts to determine the best methods of achieving these principles based on contextual factors largely associated with geographical location, exposed the tension around the explicit use of race, and later culture, as a factor in the process.

Desegregation, as it was outlined in *Brown,* is no longer an effective process through which educational equality can be accomplished within American society. As Bell (2004) argues race-based power hierarchies, built around White over Black conceptions of superiority, are too highly entrenched within the systemic functioning of American society. The myth of *Brown* assumes that simply creating "diverse" learning environments will automatically promote a more welcoming and accepting society, rectifying past discrimination. However, without addressing the underlying assumptions about race, true equality cannot be achieved. The colorblind mentality fails to recognize that although the Constitution aims to protect *individuals*, its creators did not have *all* individuals in mind, a fact that becomes much more noticeable in the shifting demographic landscape of today's public education system.

Current Demographic Landscape of America's Public Education System

Recent data from the National Center for Education Statistics (NCES) and U.S. Department of Education (USDOE) project that students of color will constitute the majority of the student population, accounting for 56% of the student population as soon as 2024 (USDOE, 2016). The national poverty rate for school-age children (ages 5–17) remains around 20%, with recent data showing increases in 41 states between 2000 and 2014 (Kena et al, 2016). The image of the "traditional family" is also shifting with a greater number of students coming from homes headed by single parents, those with different sexual orientations and a wide variety of other family structures. Additionally, across the nation, there is an increase in homes in which English is not the primary or dominant language spoken, with some schools reporting up to 100 different languages spoken in the early 2000s (Ukpokodu, 2002). By the 2013–14 school year, 9.3% of public school students were English Language Learners (ELLs) (Kena et al, 2016).

Amidst this changing demographic landscape, the K-12 teacher workforce remains largely racially, culturally, linguistically, and socioeconomically homogeneous (Villegas & Irvine, 2010). Statistical data shows the teacher workforce is over 80% White, English-speaking, middle-class und from suburban or rural communities (Gay, 2000; Lowenstein; 2005). Although research shows evidence that teacher education programs are attempting to diversify their applicant and student pools, projected data suggest the teaching force will remain primarily homogeneous for a long time (Cochran-Smith, 2003). Explicit attention to the challenges of this **demographic imperative** is critical in order to improve the educational opportunities and outcomes for students who do not fit within the White, patriarchal, middle-class norms.

The demographic implications for education go beyond gaps in numerical representation between students and teachers. Looking beyond the numbers there are also marked differences in the biographies and lived experiences of many teachers and the diverse students in their classrooms. Teachers coming from middle-class, suburban environments who speak only English and teaching in urban environments serving students who are racially, linguistically, and socioeconomically diverse will likely have different cultural frames of reference and perspectives through which to interpret and make sense of the world (Banks et al, 2005). This **cultural incongruence**, or difference in the cultural frames of reference and daily lived realities, can limit these teachers' capacity to function as role models for many of their students or act as cultural brokers/agents for students capable of assisting students in bridging home and school experiences (Villegas & Irvine, 2010).

Perhaps most alarmingly, dominant discourses that frame "diversity" as "deficit" often cause White middle-class teachers to view cultural diversity as obstacles to be overcome resulting in lowered expectations or fears about working with different cultural and life experiences, particularly in traditionally underserved areas (Banks et al, 2005; Ladson-Billings, 1999; Nieto, 2005). This construction of difference is a discursive practice that remains central to debates within teacher education concerning how to prepare teachers for diverse populations. Data pointing to the "demographic imperative," or persistent, and widening, gap between a student body that is increasingly racially/ethnically, linguistically, and socio-economically diverse and a teaching force that remains predominantly White, female, middle-class, and English-speaking produces an increased sense of urgency in how to approach teacher education, presenting varied perspectives on the best practices in preparing effective educators for *all* students (Banks et al, 2005; Ladson-Billings, 1999; Lowenstein, 2009; Zeichner, 2003).

Bridging In-School and Out-of-School Selves

In response to the demographic imperative, professional organizations and institutions whose primary missions are concerned with the preparation of teachers have taken official action toward the redesigning of teacher education programs, curriculum and practice. In 1972 the American Association of Colleges for Teacher Education (AACTE) formed one of the first commissions on multicultural teacher education, making three assertions: (1) cultural diversity is a valuable resource, (2) multicultural education is education that preserves and extends the resource of cultural diversity rather than merely tolerating it or making it "melt away," and (3) a commitment to cultural pluralism ought to permeate all aspects of teacher preparation programs in this country (Banks et al, 2002; Cochran-Smith, 2003). In 1976, the National Council for the Accreditation of Teacher Education (NCATE) added multicultural education and teaching for diversity to its standards.

Subsequently, all institutions seeking accreditation were required to show evidence that they were planning for the incorporation of multicultural content by 1979 and then provided within all teacher education programs by 1981 (Cochran-Smith, 2003a). A prominent thread throughout multicultural teacher education research focuses on this urgent need to (re)structure university-based programs for the development and implementation of more effective multicultural teacher education courses and programs. Looking to existing research documenting the work of successful educators of diverse populations (i.e., Ladson-Billings' Dreamkeepers) as well as the damaging discourses and practices impacting the educational experiences of culturally diverse students, scholars contributing to this work identify key components in the transformation of formal teacher education for diversity.

Culturally Relevant/Responsive Education

Literature looking at the larger structural issues in formal university-based teacher education programs highlight the common practice of segregating explicit discussions of culture, race, and diversity to single courses within programs. These courses may be optional and not required for completion of degree programs and send the message that attention to diversity is optional, or only important once other content-specific skills are mastered (Cochran-Smith, 1991; Ladson-Billings, 2000; Villegas & Lucas, 2002). Additionally, detaching these courses from the rest of the curriculum makes it difficult for concepts covered within them to be reinforced enough to make a lasting impact on future practice once teachers enter the classroom (Villegas & Lucas, 2002).

Instead, proponents of critical multicultural and culturally relevant pedagogical practices call for a shift in the design of teacher education programs that integrate issues of cultural relevance and diversity throughout the entire program. Aligning directly to the core tenets of culturally relevant **pedagogy**, Villegas & Lucas (2002) identify six strands necessary in the development of the culturally relevant educator:

1. socio-cultural consciousness
2. affirming attitudes toward students from culturally diverse backgrounds
3. commitment and skills to act as agents of change
4. constructivist views of learning
5. learning about students and
6. culturally relevant teaching practices

Using these six strands can serve "as an organizing framework" through which to build a vision for a program that infuses attention to diversity throughout the curriculum and gives "conceptual coherence to the preparation of teachers for diversity" (Villegas & Lucas, 2002, p. 30).

Transforming teacher education programs through some of the strategies suggested by Cochran-Smith (1991) and Villegas and Lucas (2002) helps to address some issues that teachers experience as they attempt to take what they have learned back into their K-12 classrooms. Transforming teacher education in this way may encourage pre-service teachers to adopt situated pedagogies that more explicitly address issues of race, class, and gender and create more culturally congruent teaching and learning environments for culturally diverse students (Ladson-Billings, 2000). Teachers need opportunities to develop the necessary cross-cultural competency or sociopolitical awareness required in the construction of culturally affirming and meaningful curriculum, instruction and interactional patterns that are connected to students' prior experiences and culturally-specific ways of learning and knowing (Banks et al, 2005; Gay, 2000; Ladson-Billings, 1999).

Hip-Hop Pedagogy

Hip-hop pedagogy is an approach to teaching and learning that focuses on utilizing the creative elements of hip-hop, the culture of students, within educational spaces (Adjapong & Emdin, 2015; Adjapong, 2017). To encourage educators to be culturally relevant as it relates to students who identify as part of the hip-hop generation, educators must utilize pedagogical approaches that are rooted in hip hop culture. First, it is imperative to recognize that hip-hop is more than a genre of music. Since its conception in the South Bronx during the 1970s, hip-hop has been identified as culture has impacted and empowered youth populations across the globe, especially youth who identify as part of groups who have been historically marginalized by systems (Adjapong & Emdin, 2015; Dunley, 2000). Hip-hop is a culture that has been in existence for over 40 years. Hip-hop was birthed the midst of a social and economic crisis in the Bronx and was an effort to build strong communal ties in times of economic and social hardship. Urban youth attended block parties to escape their unfortunate realities. Hip-hop pedagogy draws from the frameworks of **culturally relevant pedagogy** (Ladson-Billings, 1994) and **reality pedagogy** (Emdin, 2016). From culturally relevant pedagogy, hip-hop pedagogy draws a focus on understanding the youth culture that is exhibited in students' communities and the use of an understanding students' youth culture and their communities in improving teacher effectiveness. Culturally relevant pedagogy encourages teachers to immerse themselves so deeply in the culture of students through actual engagement with the students, that it becomes second nature to find ways to develop students' interest in, and natural affinity for learning content. From reality pedagogy, hip-hop pedagogy draws a focus on the teacher learning about the authentic realities of students and teaching, utilizing students' authentic realities and culture to better engage them. Reality pedagogy provides teachers with practical tools to become proximal with students to engage in dialogue where teachers can learn from the experiences of students who have traditionally been marginalized by school systems as it relates to science education.

Ultimately, if teachers are invested in using Hip-hop pedagogical practices that are directly anchored in the realities of students it allows for the formation of "weak ties" and "strong ties" between teachers and students. Coleman (1988) suggests that there are links between individuals and groups within every social network that are categorized as "strong ties" or "weak ties." "Strong ties" correspond to the connections individuals or groups who are "friends" have in common.

While, weak ties correspond to "acquaintances" who do not have much in com-mon that would normally connect them (Easley & Kleinberg, 2010). Students of the hip-hop generation who participate in the same culture (hip-hop) would be known to have "strong ties" because they share the same cultural practices. Teach-ers who do not identify as part of the hip-hop generation, while teaching students who do identify as part of the hip-hop generation would be known as having "weak ties" with their students because the teacher does not share the same cultural prac-tices with students, but the teacher engages with students on a daily basis, which encourages a "weak tie." When teachers use teaching approaches that are anchored in the culture and realities of their students it provides an opportunity for the teacher to gain insight on the students' cultural practices and develop the "weak ties" that already exist into "strong ties" over time. Coleman (1998) refers to these connections ("weak ties" and "strong ties") as dense networks and describes them as close-knit networks that facilitate trust and cooperative exchanges. The creation of these dense networks between students and the educator can allow for a positive exchange of content to students and provide a space for educators to authentically learn about the realities of their students. Ultimately, if educators position them-selves to understand the complexities of youth culture (i.e., hip-hop culture), they will have a better understanding of students and have a deeper understanding of how their students participate and navigate in the world, through their cultural lens.

Social Media and Education

Technology has transformed human life through improved communication, social networking, the ease to access information, and improved entertainment to name a few. In education, technology is used as a tool to improve student learn-ing and to make content more accessible. While there are many applications of technology in education and within classrooms, limited consideration is given to how technology, specifically social media, can impact teachers' learning and pro-fessional development. Many educators in the 21st century use various forms of technology as part of their daily teaching practices and as part of their personal lives. Many teachers turn to **Virtual Professional Learning Networks (VPLN)** found on social media platforms to learn and to grow professionally. A VPLN as a uniquely personalized space where participants can engage in dialogue with a network of individuals from around the world via social media platforms such as Twitter (and other social media platforms) to support one another's continuous professional learning. Garrison (2007) describes an online PLN as a synchronous or asynchronous online platform for individuals to collaboratively engage in criti-cal thinking and discussions around specific issues (Trinkle, 2009). VPLNs consist of global virtual learning networks that enable participants to share diverse, global perspectives on teaching strategies and educational issues. VPLNs are mainly found on Twitter with educators and other stakeholders using hashtags to engage in conversation and share materials. While there are shortcomings of traditional professional development for educators, through their participation in VPLNs they are provided opportunities to meet their specific professional learning needs (Krutka, Carpenter & Trust, 2017). Some argue that VPLNs provide educators with the opportunity to use social media platforms as a tool to interact with colleagues and experts who share similar interests and concerns while transcending spatial boundaries using an electronic device as simple as a cell phone (Gee, 2004). Further, Twitter chats (of VPLNs) occur often during the same scheduled time each week allowing educators to plan in advance to participate, given their busy schedules or even plan to participate in multiple VPLN's that cater to their multiple of specific needs (Conner, Pope & Galloway, 2009). Through virtual interactions with colleagues and experts, educators can access and share a variety of tools, including skills, habits, resources, ideas, and information that will support their daily practice (Krutka, Carpenter & Trust, 2016).

Wrap-Up

Chapter Summary

Education is widely-documented as one of the primary social determinants of health. Education has an effect on income level, healthy eating habits, access to healthier neighborhoods, and can create opportunities for overall better health. While access to education is a constitutional right, as discussed in this chapter, access to adequate and effective education that caters towards students' needs is limited for groups who have historically been marginalized. Similarly, access to affordable and adequate health care is also limited for groups who have historically been marginalized. To provide equitable access to both adequate opportunities to attain an education and for health care for all, there must be a restructuring of both systems.

In education, as with health care, this restructuring requires an explicit acknowledgement and discussion of the historical missteps in law, policy, and practice that have given way to existing discriminatory practices. Recent shifts in teacher education and pedagogy/curricular designs center these discussions as issues of race and culture and are integral components in the development of culturally relevant educators and their practice. Additionally, finding new ways to incorporate technology and communication styles, instructional materials, and other practices of engagement rooted in youth culture, help to bridge students' personal and academic identities, creating stronger ties to the educational environment. In doing so, it is possible to see a shift from viewing culturally, racially, and ethnically diverse students as being culturally deprived to being culture rich, providing valuable insights, perspectives, and experiences through which to enhance the learning community and to create more welcoming and equitable experiences for all.

Chapter Problems

1. Describe the link between education and health.
2. The 1954 *Brown v. Board of Education* decision declared segregated schools as unconstitutional, however the authors discussed the ways in which *Brown* actually resulted in numerous and long-lasting negative results. List and briefly describe at least two negative consequences of *Brown* mentioned in this chapter and their impact on one's educational experience.
3. Describe what culturally relevant pedagogy looks like in practice.

References

Adjapong, E. S., & Emdin, C. (2015). Rethinking pedagogy in urban spaces: Implementing hip-hop pedagogy in the urban science classroom. *Journal of Urban Learning Teaching and Research, 66*(11), 66–76.

Adjapong, E. S. (2017). Bridging Theory and Practice in the Urban Science Classroom A Framework for Hip-Hop Pedagogy. *Critical Education, 8*(15), 5–22.

Anderson, J. D. (1988). *The education of blacks in the south, 1860-1935*. United States: The University of North Carolina Press.

Banks, J. A., Cochran-Smith, M., Moll, L., Richert, A., Zeichner, K., LePage, P., … McDonald, M. (2005). Teaching diverse learners. In L. Darling-Hammond & J. Bransford (Eds.), *Preparing teachers for a changing world: What teachers should learn and be able to do* (pp. 232–274). San Fransisco, CA: Jossey-Bass.

Blanchett, W. J., Mumford, V., & Beachum, F. (2005). Urban school failure and disproportionality in a post-brown era: Benign neglect of the constitutional rights of students of color. *Remedial and Special Education, 26*(2), 70–81. doi: 10.1177/07419325050260020201

Burchinal, M., Nelson, L., Carlson, M., & Brooks-Gunn, J. (2008). Neighborhood characteristics, and child care type and quality. *Early Education and Development, 19*(5), 702–725.

Cochran-Smith, M. (1991). Learning to teach against the grain. *Harvard Educational Review, 61*(3), 279–311. doi:10.17763/haer.61.3.q671413614502746

Coleman, J. S. (1988). Social capital in the creation of human capital. *American journal of sociology*, S95–S120.

Conner, J., Pope, D., & Galloway, M. (2009). Success with less stress. *Educational Leadership, 67*(4), 54–58.

Crenshaw, K. W. (1988). Race, reform, and retrenchment: Transformation and legitimation in antidiscrimination law. *Harvard Law Review,* 1331–1387.

Delpit, L. (1988). The silenced dialogue: Power and pedagogy in educating other people's children. *Harvard Educational Review, 58*(3), 280–299. doi:10.17763/haer.58.3.c43481778r528qw4

De Vito, D. (2007). The gap between the real and the ideal: The right to education amid fiscal equity legislation in a democratic culture. *Ethics and Education, 2*(2), 173–180.

Dotterer, A. M., Iruka, I. U., & Pungello, E. (2012). Parenting, race, and socioeconomic status: Links to school readiness. *Family Relations, 61*(4), 657–670.

Dunley, T. (2000, May 12). The colour barrier is no more. So whose music is it anyway? Montreal Gazette, p. A1.

Easley, D., & Kleinberg, J. (2010). Networks, crowds, and markets (Vol. 8). Cambridge: Cambridge University press.

Emdin, C. (2016). *For White Folks Who Teach in the Hood… and the Rest of Y'all Too:Reality Pedagogy and Urban Education*. Beacon Press.

Fordham, S., & Ogbu, J. U. (1986). Black students' school success: Coping with the "burden of 'acting white'". *The Urban Review, 18*(3), 176–206. doi: 10.1007/BF01112192

Gamoran, A., Nystrand, M., Berends, M., & LePore, P. C. (1995). An organizational analysis of the effects of ability grouping. *American Educational Research Journal, 32*(687–715).

Garrison, D. R. (2007). Online community of inquiry review: Social, cognitive, and teaching presence issues. *Journal of Asynchronous Learning Networks,* 11(1), 61–72.

Gay, G. (2000). *Culturally responsive teaching: Theory, research, and practice*. New York: Teachers' College Press.

Gee, J. P. (2004). *An introduction to discourse analysis: Theory and method*. Routledge.

Horsford, S. D. (2010). Black superintendents on education black students in separate and unequal contexts. *Urban Review, 42*, 58–79. doi: 10.1007/s11256-009-0119-0

Irizarry, J. G. (2009). Representin': Drawing from hip-hop and urban youth culture to inform teacher education. *Education and Urban Society, 41*(4), 489–515. doi:10.1177/0013124508331154

Kamin, L. J. (1974). *The science and politics of I.Q.* Oxford, England: Lawrence Erlbaum.

Kena, G., Hussar, W., McFarland, J., de Brey, C., Musu-Gillette, L., Wang, X., … Dunlop Velez, E. (2016). *The condition of education 2016 (NCES 2016-144)*. Retrieved from https://nces.ed.gov /pubs2016/2016144.pdf

Kingston, P. W. (2001). The unfulfilled promise of cultural capital theory. *Sociology of Education, 74*, 88–99. Retrieved from www.jstor.org/stable/2673255

Kliebard, H. M. (2004). *The struggle for the American curriculum, 1893-1958* (2nd ed.). New York: Routledge.

Krutka, D. G., & Carpenter, J. P. (2017). Enriching professional learning networks: A framework for identification, reflection, and intention. *TechTrends, 61*(3), 246–252.

Ladson-Billings, G. (1994). *The Dreamkeepers: Successful teaching for African-American students.* John Wiley & Sons.

Ladson-Billings, G. (2000). Fighting for our lives preparing teachers to teach African American students. *Journal of Teacher Education, 51*(3), 206–214.

Ladson-Billings, G. (2004). Landing on the wrong note: The price we paid for Brown. *Educational Researcher, 33*(7), 3–13. Retrieved from www.jstor.org/stable/3700092

Ladson-Billings, G. (2006). From the achievement gap to the education debt: Understanding achievement in US schools. *Educational Researcher, 35*(7), 3–12.

Ladson-Billings, G. (2012). Through a glass darkly: The persistence of race in education research and scholarship. *Educational Researcher, 41*(4), 115–120.

Ladson-Billings, G. J. (1999). Preparing teachers for diverse student populations: A critical race theory perspective. *Review of Research in Education, 24*, 211–247.

Ladson-Billings, G., & Tate, W. (1995). Toward a critical race theory of education. *Teachers College Record, 97*(1), 47–68.

Lowenstein, K. L. (2009). The work of Multicultural teacher education: Reconceptualizing white teacher candidates as learners. *Review of Educational Research, 79*(1), 163–196. doi:10.3102/0034654308326161

Massey, D. S. & Denton, N. A. (1993). *American apartheid: Segregation and the making of the underclass* (Chps 2 & 3). Cambridge, MA: Harvard University Press.

Milner, H. R. (2012). Beyond a test score: Explaining opportunity gaps in educational practice. *Journal of Black Studies, 20*(10), 1–26. doi: 10.1177/0021934712442539

Nasaw, D. (1979). *Schooled to order: A social history of public schooling in the united states.* New York: Oxford University Press.

Nieto, S. (2005). Schools for a new majority: The role of teacher education in hard times. *The New Educator, 1*(1), 27–43. doi:10.1080/15476880490447797

Omi, M., & Winant, H. (1993). On the theoretical status of the concept of race. *Race, Identity and Representation in Education*, 3–10.

Payne, C. M. (2008). *So much reform, so little change: The persistence of failure in urban schools.* Cambridge, MA: Harvard Educational Publishing Group.

Ravitch, D. (2010). *The death and life of the great American school system: How testing and choice are undermining education.* New York: Basic Books

Ross, C. E., & Wu, C. (1995). The links between education and health. *American Sociological Review, 60*(5), 719–745. doi:10.2307/2096319

Trinkle, C. (2009). Twitter as a professional learning community. *School Library Monthly, 26*(4), 22–23.

U.S. Department of Education, Office of Planning, Evaluation and Policy Development, Policy and Program Studies Service. (2016). *The state of racial diversity in the educator workforce.* Retrieved from http://www2.ed.gov/rschstat/eval/highered/racial-diversity/state-racial-diversity -workforce.pdf.

Villegas, A. M., & Lucas, T. (2002). Preparing culturally responsive teachers: Rethinking the curriculum. *Journal of Teacher Education, 53*(1), 20–32. doi:10.1177/0022487102053001003

Walker, V. S. (2000). Valued segregated schools for African American children in the south, 1935-1969: A review of common themes and characteristics. *Review of Educational Research, 70*(3), 253–285. doi: 10.3102/00346543070003253

Walters, P. B. (2001). Educational access and the state: Historical continuities and discontinuities in racial inequality in American education. *Sociology of Education*, 35–49.

Wells, A. S., Holme, J. J., Revilla, A. T., & Atanda, A. K. (2005). How desegregation changed us: The effects of racially mixed schools on students and society. *Columbia University.* http://cms.tc .columbia.edu/i/a/782_ASWells, 41504.

Zeichner, K. (2003). The adequacies and inadequacies of three current strategies to recruit, prepare and retain the best teachers for all students. *Teachers College Record, 105*(3), 490–519.

Zimmerman, E., & Woolf, S. H. (2014, June 5). *Understanding the Relationship between Education and Health* [Discussion Paper, Institute of Medicine]. Washington, D.C.

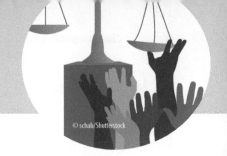
© schab/Shutterstock

CHAPTER 5

Health Disparities by the Numbers and Obamacare

Health is more than absence of disease; it is about economics, education, environment, empowerment, and community. The health and well-being of the people is critically dependent upon the health system that serves them. It must provide the best possible health with the least disparities and respond equally well to everyone.

—Joycelyn Elders

KEY TERMS

digital divide
healthcare exchanges
individual mandate
leading causes of death
life expectancy

medicaid
medicare
obamacare
patient protection and affordable
   care act

LEARNING OBJECTIVES

After reading this chapter, you should be able to do the following:

1. Discuss the basic details of the Patient Protection and Affordable Care Act.
2. Understand the difference between the Patient Protection and Affordable Care Act and Obamacare.
3. Explain the difference between Medicaid and Medicare.
4. Describe healthcare exchanges.

▸ Introduction

A number of key indicators validate the fact that there is a significant health disparity between various racial groups and the ethnic group, Hispanic, and the White population. Statistics relating to the Hispanic/Latino group are usually convoluted by virtue of Hispanic not being a racial group. Within this group, there are racial groups. For example, a person may be Black Hispanic or White Hispanic. Often, data are presented as Non-Hispanic Whites, which merely indicates that White people in said data do not speak Spanish, and if they do, perhaps they are from Spain (European). Yet, there are, for example, White people who speak Spanish with origins from Latin America and Black people who speak Spanish with origins from Latin America. This imprecise manner of classifying the groups confounds the Hispanic/Latino data because it gives the impression that individuals from these two particular groups have equivalent health experiences /outcomes. The reality is that Black Hispanics have a similar healthcare experience to the African American/Black group and White Hispanics have a similar experience to the White Non-Hispanic group. Consequently, all Hispanic/Latino data in this chapter are presented with the term *ethnic group* as a reminder that a comparison is being drawn between racial groups and an ethnic group that contains myriad racial groups.

▸ Health Status Gap

TABLES 5-1 and **5-2** provide a glimpse of the health status gap based upon selected health indicators. The widest gap is between Asian Americans/Pacific Islanders and African Americans, in terms of **life expectancy** at birth (see Table 5-1).

Health insurance is a critical factor in terms of health status. People of color comprise a significant percentage of the U.S. population, as indicated in Table 5-2. The majority of the uninsured are people of color, also referred to in this text as emerging majorities. The new healthcare law, titled the **Patient Protection and Affordable Care Act**, often abbreviated as the Affordable Care Act (ACA) and also known as **Obamacare**, has helped to assuage the problem of lack of access to health insurance but has not resolved the problem, as discussed in more detail later in this chapter.

TABLE 5-1 Health Insurance Coverage of Non-elderly Population by Race				
African American	**White**	**Native American**	**Asian American/Pacific Islander**	**Hispanic/ Latino (Ethnic Group)**
74.8* (2016)	78.5*	76.9 (2010)	86.5 (2010)	81.8* (2016)

Peterson Kaiser Health System Tracker. (n.d.). Life Expectancy at birth (in years), by race/ethnicity. Retrieved from https://www .healthsystemtracker.org/indicator/health-well-being/life-expectancy/; The Henry J. Kaiser Family Foundation. (n.d.). Life expectancy at birth (in years), by race/ethnicity. Retrieved from http://kff.org/other/state-indicator/life-expectancy-by-re/

TABLE 5-2 Healthcare Insurance Coverage of Total Non-Elderly Population by Racial/Ethnic Group, 2014

Category	Percentage
Asian	10%
White Americans	9%
African Americans/Blacks	13%
Latinos/Hispanics (ethnic group)	21%
Native Americans/Alaska Natives	21%

Data from Center for American Progress. (2014). Health Insurance Coverage of Nonelderly Population by Race/Ethnicity, 2014. Retrieved from: https://www.kff.org/report-section/key-facts-on-health-and-health-care-by-race-and-ethnicity-section-4-health-coverage/

▶ Leading Causes of Death

There are some commonalities regarding the 10 **leading causes of death** among the racial and ethnic groups. **TABLE 5-3** provides insight, although there is variation by year. Data are scarce regarding recent information for each group. However, it is clear that the various emerging majority groups are suffering from similar issues. What is different is the impact of these diseases and the lifespan of individuals who suffer from and, subsequently, die from them. African American/Black people have the shortest lifespan, in comparison to all other groups, which is largely associated with socioeconomic status, access to care, and other factors such as diet, opportunities available for exercise, access to necessary treatment or preventive measures, and community/environmental concerns largely stemming from economic, environmental, and social injustice.

TABLE 5-3 Ten Leading Causes of Death by Race, Emerging Majority Groups, and Ethnic Group

African Americans (2013)	Native Americans/ Alaska Natives (2013)	Asian Americans or Pacific Islanders (2010)	Hispanics/ Latinos (2010) (Ethnic Group)	Whites (2007)
Heart disease	Heart disease	Cancer	Cancer	Heart disease
Cancer	Cancer	Heart disease	Heart disease	Cancer

(continues)

TABLE 5-3 Ten Leading Causes of Death by Race, Emerging Majority Groups, and Ethnic Group *(continued)*				
African Americans (2013)	**Native Americans/ Alaska Natives (2013)**	**Asian Americans or Pacific Islanders (2010)**	**Hispanics/ Latinos (2010) (Ethnic Group)**	**Whites (2007)**
Stroke	Unintentional injuries	Stroke	Unintentional injuries	Chronic lower respiratory disease
Unintentional injuries	Diabetes	Unintentional injuries	Stroke	Stroke
Diabetes	Chronic liver disease and cirrhosis	Diabetes	Diabetes	Unintentional injuries
Chronic lower respiratory disease	Chronic lower respiratory disease	Influenza and pneumonia	Chronic liver disease	Alzheimer disease
Nephritis, nephrotic syndrome, and nephrosis	Stroke	Chronic lower respiratory disease	Chronic lower respiratory disease	Diabetes
Homicide	Suicide	Nephritis, nephrotic syndrome, and nephrosis	Alzheimer disease	Influenza and pneumonia
Sepsis	Influenza and pneumonia	Alzheimer disease	Nephritis, nephrotic syndrome, and nephrosis	Nephritis, nephrotic syndrome, and nephrosis
Alzheimer disease	Nephritis, nephrotic syndrome, nephrosis	Suicide	Influenza and pneumonia	Suicide

Mathews, T. J., MacDorman, M. F., Thoma, M. E., & Division of Vital Statistics. (2015, August 6). Infant mortality statistics from the 2013 period linked birth/infant death data set. *National Vital Statistics Reports, 64*(9). Retrieved from http://www.cdc.gov/nchs /data/nvsr/nvsr65/nvsr65_02.pdf

Year	Black/ African American	White	Native Hawaiian or Other Pacific Islander	Asian	Hispanic/ Latino (Ethnic Group)
2016	11.4	4.9	7.4	3.6	5.0

TABLE 5-4 Infant Mortality (Deaths Occurring to Infants Younger Than 1 Year of Age per 1,000 Live Births) by Race and Ethnicity (2016)

Centers for Disease Control and Prevention. Infant Mortality Rates by Race and Ethnicity, 2016. Retrieved from: https://www.cdc.gov/reproductivehealth/maternalinfanthealth/infantmortality.htm#chart

▶ Infant Mortality

The infant mortality rate provides an indication of the health status of mothers and children. **TABLE 5-4** highlights the fact that African American people experience the highest infant mortality rate, followed by Native Americans/Alaska Natives. According to the Central Intelligence Agency of the United States (2009), there are other nations across the world that have lower infant mortality rates than that of African American people in the United States. The overall infant mortality rate for the United States, by the CIA's estimates, is 5.87, which is higher than the rate for the White population in the United States. But, the infant mortality rate is nearly double, at 11.2, for the African American population in the United States. This is a gap that must be closed.

Black Men's Health

Black men have particular concerns that are relevant in terms of the issues related to health disparities. Hence, the detail presented here is mainly related to Black men. For further insight into the health status of Black men (and other racial groups of men), including the leading causes of death, see data provided in Appendix XV. Although the detail is rather disconcerting, the optimistic news, per researchers for the Men's Health Network (2013), is that when men are actively engaged in learning about their health, they are willing and active participants in the healthcare system (Lamas, R. Giorgianni, S. and Nwaiwu, C., 2019).

▶ Solutions

Per the Men's Health research Networks Executive Summary entitled *Providing for and Influencing the Care of Boys and Men in America*, based on the Dialogue at a conference on men's health in May, 2013 (Men's Health Braintrust, 2013) there are key areas for activity and advocacy to enhance the intersection of male patients and providers which are as follows:

■ Education of boys about health and wellness needs to have a greater emphasis in primary and secondary education.

- Institutes of higher education should offer educational and career tracks in male gender-focused areas related to psychosocial, environmental, and life-style skills.
- Healthcare provider education and training need to incorporate core curriculum elements in the area of comprehensive men's health.
- These should include content in pathophysiologic, psychosocial, communication and treatment considerations relevant to the needs of male patients across the lifespan.
- As the Medical Home continues to evolve and become implemented, practitioners should consider ways to address the "Doctor for Guys" gap. Serious and thoughtful consideration should be given to transforming the discipline of men's health to focus on meeting men's life-long comprehensive needs in a gender-appropriate manner.
- Provider professional organizations, voluntary health associations, public sector policy makers and private sector commercial and service organizations should encourage, implement and evaluate additional approaches to engaging boys and men in wellness and health care.
- Producers, advertisers, mass media advisors, and policy makers should increase the male-centric media outreach intended for boys and men that encourage men to view active engagement in health and wellness as part of modern masculinity.
- Foundations, public sector, and commercial private sector stakeholders should give consideration to programs that do outreach, education and screening for boys and men.
- Organizations and groups that sponsor life-style programs that attract boys and men should begin to incorporate health and wellness related participation in the programs with the goal of showing how health is part of masculinity.

Additionally, health providers and product managers should embrace men as target audiences and offer male-centric services. For the most part, all health indices serve as documentation of this tremendous health status gap, which needs to be closed in the United States, particularly the gaping hole between Black and White people. Federal efforts toward improving health care, especially access and quality of care, are sorely needed; hence the Affordable Care Act, mentioned above, also known as Obamacare, is now law. Below is an overview of this law with insight regarding its potential impact on closing the health status gap in the United States.

▶ Obamacare

The Affordable Care Act is a federal statute that was signed into U.S. law by President Barack Obama on March 23, 2010. The question is whether this new law has had a positive impact in contributing to the reduction of health disparities. Leonard (2015), in her article "Study: Obamacare Hasn't Solved Health Care Disparities," describes the law's results, stating, among other findings, the following:

> The Affordable Care Act increased insurance availability for the poor by expanding Medicaid eligibility to more people based on their income level. The law originally intended for all states to expand Medicaid, but

the Supreme Court ruled in 2012 that states could choose not to do so. Twenty-two states currently have not expanded the program.

During an interview with Dr. Donna Shalala, former Secretary of Department of Health and Human Services, who held that role longer than any other person in U.S. history, Shalala stated the following:

> I don't think there is a lot of reform in healthcare reform. What I do think is that it is a substantial increase in coverage. We're going to get close to most Americans having health insurance. So this bill is largely about coverage. (Rose, 2013, p. 68)

Donna Shalala served her term at the pleasure of President Clinton. The implication of her statement appears accurate. Although there were some changes indicated in the healthcare reform bill that are viewed by some as helpful (e.g., young people may stay on their parents' insurance until age 26 years, and one can no longer be denied insurance coverage based on preexisting conditions), the fact of the matter is that the system is still profit driven. Health corporations continue to provide the insurance; hence premiums are paid to private corporations, creating profit for them and other profit-making entities (e.g., providers of healthcare equipment and supplies) for every dime spent on health care. Consequently, the logical conclusion is that perhaps there is a vested interest in people being sick, rather than well, with a constant need to seek health care. If one sells widgets, then the seller wants individuals to constantly need widgets. If one sells health care, then the seller wants individuals to constantly need health care.

Although the goal here is not to provide a comparative analysis of the healthcare "system" in the United States to systems in other nations, a brief summary of other industrialized nation's healthcare systems (to be discussed later in this chapter) will suggest that the U.S. system is a for-profit healthcare system with the bottom line acting as a key factor, perhaps conjoined with the goal of improving the well-being and optimal health status of the people. All other industrialized nations have universal health care, in various forms, with profit making deemphasized and a greater focus on preventive care. Those who are against universal health care will point out all of the negatives they can find regarding these other nations' approaches (e.g., long waiting lines, higher taxes). Lower-income individuals often seek care in an emergency department in the United States, because they do not have health insurance or a private doctor in their community to serve them. The wait time in most emergency departments is unbelievably long and the cost to the patient and the facility is high. Consequently, the United States must have a vested interest in the health of all people, regardless of race, income, ethnicity, and all other diverse factors, without profit as a motive.

As stated by Adriann Barboa of Strong Families New Mexico, a group that supports policies related to diversity, "although people have insurance they still have hard choices" (Leonard, 2015). Leonard (2015) elaborates, drawing from the results of a survey conducted by the Alliance for a Just Society, on the challenges faced by many people who do have insurance:

> [People] struggle with monthly premiums, copays and deductibles. Many who don't obtain coverage under Medicaid expansion still have limited incomes. For this group, the healthcare law offers insurance through

healthcare marketplaces, called exchanges, where Americans can buy coverage that can be offset by tax subsidies. The survey also showed that Americans are struggling with technical access and language barriers when it comes to obtaining insurance coverage.

Barboa reports that New Mexican families tell her they must decide between medication and food, despite the state's expansion of Medicaid, as the state of New Mexico has one of the highest poverty levels in the nation (Leonard, 2015).

Healthcare Reform Update

Although there was a great deal of discussion about healthcare reform and the repeal of Obamacare, since Barack Obama left office, this has not happened. There were several new bills that were introduced, in both the House and the Senate, however, none were passed. Nevertheless, there was one significant change and that was the **individual mandate** removal, per a tax bill that was passed in 2017. Consequently, the penalty repeal will take effect in 2019. Hence, if a person did not have insurance in 2019, he/she will not have to pay a penalty. The individual mandate required that all individual (citizens and legal residents) in the United Sates have health insurance. If one did not secure health insurance, he/she would be penalized, financially, as assessed by the IRS. Exemptions from said penalty were possible, if individuals met specific requirements.

Some states actually retained the penalty, but at the federal level, this is no longer the case. Otherwise, the ACA remains intact. It is important to continue to observe all activities surrounding healthcare reform, as candidates for the upcoming election in 2020 are all focusing in various ways on potential changes.

▶ The Digital Divide

When the healthcare reform law, which is commonly known as Obamacare, was first introduced, one of the biggest problems was that the primary mechanism for signing up for health care was through an online platform. This process was very problematic initially due to issues with online access based on poor design. Additionally, the notion of the **digital divide** surfaced as a key problem, as many of the individuals in greatest need of health care do not have access to computers. Measures were put in place to have individuals sign up in person or by telephone, but nevertheless, there remained an issue. The digital divide refers to the notion that in lower socioeconomic status communities, individuals may not have computers. They are likely to have cell phones that allow basic access to the Internet, but more complicated endeavors such as signing up for health care may be problematic. The problem is not just about having a computer but also understanding the process of going to a website. It seems that these factors should have been taken into consideration, and failure to do so indicated a lack of understanding of the implications of being poor in the United States, from a technological vantage point.

Leonard's article also mentions language and immigration barriers and access to care due to health disparities. As mentioned previously, some individuals choose to continue to use the emergency department for care since they do not have personal doctors. Health-seeking behaviors are different among racial groups, and consequently, having healthcare insurance alone may not be useful without cultural understanding of individuals' and communities' perceived notions about health care along with the provision of culturally and linguistically competent health education materials. As pointed out by Donna Shalala in the interview mentioned earlier regarding the varied demographics associated with people in American society and healthcare reform, "So that means that health care has to change along with it. Both who provides the health care and how they provide it" (Rose, 2015).

▶ Insight From an Academic— Dr. Robert Fullilove

In an interview conducted with Dr. Robert Fullilove, he offered insight regarding Obamacare. Dr. Fullilove is the Associate Dean for Community and Minority Affairs, Professor of Clinical Sociomedical Sciences, and Co-director of the Cities Research Group at the Mailman School of Public Health, Columbia University. He has authored numerous articles in the area of minority health.

DR. ROSE: What is your perspective regarding healthcare reform, given the rapidly changing demographics in the United States?

DR. FULLILOVE: I think that so much of what we worry about with respect to access to health care really reflects the high cost of health care. As long as it requires money to take care of any one of a variety of medical conditions and as long as the kind of preventive medicine we would like to propose as a cornerstone for how we would want to practice public health depends on someone being able to pay the cost for seeing a physician, we are not going to realize our goals and perspective on providing quality health care for everyone. The cost of dealing with diseases like hypertension, cardiovascular disease, or conditions like obesity is so high that the only way we're going to bring the costs under control would be to sort of aggressively push the kinds of programs and priorities that are at the core of public health. To achieve this, a legislative shift in the government's philosophy as being an absolute essential cornerstone for the creation of a system of public health in the United States, in general, and the promotion of the kind of program that will reduce health disparities is.

DR. ROSE: So in terms of Obamacare, should it have gone further?

DR. FULLILOVE: I've worked in government, in the federal government, for 5 years, and worked in state government, in the state of New Jersey, for 3, and what I know is, no law is ever perfect. No law at the moment of its writing and its passage and signing by either the president or governor is ever perfect. It always requires toning, shifting, cutting, editing.... I think this law is the creation of an important precedent. I think the law is imperfect for a wide variety of reasons, but I think that now that the precedent has been established, our capacity to alter, shape, and edit the laws so that it actually does meet a variety of different needs... rather dramatically improved... so I see it as a start, not as a finish. I don't think the law will cover all of the needs that the American people have, but I do believe it is a start.

Dr. Fullilove's comments regarding Obamacare highlight some of the concerns and benefits regarding this relatively new law. The key, however, is to ensure that people understand it. To a certain degree, some people are not aware, as an example, that the Patient Protection and Affordable Care Act, the Affordable Care Act, and Obamacare are all terms used to describe the same law.

▶ What Is the Difference Between the Patient Protection and Affordable Care Act, the Affordable Care Act, and Obamacare?

Recently, a reporter asked individuals on various streets in a city in the United States whether they thought the Affordable Care Act or Obamacare was better. Many tried to give explanations as to why they preferred one over the other, but what became clear is that most did not know the two are one and the same. The name of the law that emerged as a result of healthcare reform is the Patient Protection and Affordable Care Act. The short version of that name is the Affordable Care Act, which is further abbreviated to ACA. Originally, those who were adamantly against healthcare reform, before it became law and because the notion of creating a new law emerged from President Obama, nicknamed it Obamacare. There was resistance to this name at first, but ultimately President Obama embraced it, so many refer to the law as Obamacare. In this text, the term Affordable Care Act or ACA will be used from this point on.

President Obama signed the ACA into law on March 23, 2010. This law has a significant impact on health care in the United States in that it mandates that all Americans have some type of health insurance, whether it is through their employer, **Medicaid**, **Medicare**, or other means. There are many people in the United States who do not have healthcare insurance, so the discussion surrounding healthcare reform has been about trying to rectify that problem. Some people in the United States believe that everyone should have health insurance, while others do not hold this belief. This disagreement has led to a very serious debate in the United States, which continues even though the ACA has been passed and is now the law of the land.

Before the ACA, in the United States, individuals' health insurance was generally based on their employment, with the most common exceptions being Medicaid and Medicare. If an individual is employed and if his or her employer offers health insurance, then the individual will pay a premium, deducted from his or her paycheck, for health insurance through a company selected by his or her employer. This system seems simple but can be quite complicated and costly because the employee may have a spouse and other dependent family members who need coverage, making the employee's premium unaffordable. Prior to the ACA, there may have been issues that prevented coverage, such as preexisting medical conditions. Also, for all employees to receive coverage in this way, employers have to offer it, which is not always the case. Consequently, before the ACA, there were individuals in the United States who just did not have health insurance coverage. The following is a partial list of some of the categories of the uninsured:

- Individuals who are unemployed and not eligible for Medicaid or Medicare and who cannot afford private insurance
- Individuals who are employed but whose employers do not offer health insurance

- Individuals who are employed but opt out of health insurance because they can't afford the premium
- Individuals who were denied insurance coverage because they had a preexisting condition
- Individuals who do not want health insurance and opt out of purchasing it

The intention of the ACA is to, on a mandatory basis, provide more individuals with access to affordable health insurance, no matter their employment status. Although the full details of the law will not be covered here, some details are important to review, beginning with the fact that it enables individuals who are not receiving health insurance coverage through their employers to have access to insurance at potentially affordable prices. Of course, for this to happen, a significant number of people must buy insurance, as the idea is that a higher number of participants will lead to reduced premiums. Health insurance offered must meet the minimum standards set by the law. If individuals do not have health insurance, they will have to pay a penalty. If an individual cannot afford to pay for health insurance coverage and is not eligible for Medicaid, he or she may be eligible for a government subsidy to assist with the premium in the form of a tax credit or Medicaid expansion (if states choose to do so). Key decisions related to aspects of the law are state based, such as whether a state decides to participate in Medicaid expansion or whether the state chooses to establish health insurance exchanges (discussed in the next section). The Medicaid expansion aspect of the law was challenged on a constitutional basis, at which time it was deemed by the Supreme Court that states could opt out of this segment of the law, and many did.

One aspect of the law that appeals to young people is that they can continue to receive health insurance coverage through their parents' plan until they are 26 years old. As an example, college students graduate and often, currently, are unable to find employment. As a result, they are unable to secure health insurance on their own. Remaining on their parents' health insurance until they are 26 years old bides time for either gaining employment, positioning themselves to pay for their own health insurance, or, if they meet the Medicaid requirements, ultimately taking that route offered through the ACA.

▶ The Health Insurance Exchange Marketplace

The health insurance exchange marketplace (**healthcare exchanges**) is an online market that was launched on October 1, 2013. The launch was not smooth, but to avoid the political trap associated with discussion of the who, how, when, and why of that problem, this discussion will focus only on what the marketplace is. Basically, the online marketplace is where individuals can go to review coverage options and ultimately choose a health insurance plan from competitive providers. The online tool includes a calculator for determining prices and subsidy eligibility and a review of the various plan options. Individuals who are not insured are required to buy one of these plans if they have no other means to participate in a qualifying plan. Those individuals who have insurance through their employers may also enroll if they find a plan in the marketplace that is better suited to them, although they will not be eligible for subsidies.

Subsidies are assistance that the government will provide to individuals to help with the purchase of insurance, if it is determined that one is eligible. Failure to enroll in a plan will lead to a penalty unless an individual is granted a waiver/exemption. The initial deadline to enroll was January 2014, although some necessary extensions were made at that time. Private insurance companies offer the insurance plans. The plans have different premiums, deductibles, and co-pays. This online approach enables the consumer to explore options and choose his or her health insurance plan based on affordability and other factors such as coverage needs.

▶ Medicaid and Medicare

President Lyndon Johnson signed Medicaid and Medicare into law on July 30, 1965. Medicaid is a program for low-income individuals, including children, and is means tested (income based). The federal government provides oversight for Medicaid, but states determine eligibility and administer their own program. Medicare is a program that originated for Americans over 65 years of age and for individuals with long-term disability or end-stage renal disease. Many seniors rely on Medicare to take care of chronic, long-term illnesses such as arthritis, diabetes, Parkinson disease, and Alzheimer disease. This program covers services of doctors and the use of pharmaceutical drugs. A significant percentage of individuals over 65 years of age rely on Medicare Advantage. Advantage is the private care option of Medicare.

Eligibility guidelines for Medicaid are set by states and are income based, primarily for the poor. Age, pregnancy status, disability, citizenship, and other factors may be considered. States are provided with matching funds from the federal government and cannot receive those funds unless they are providing services to those who meet the established categories. Therefore, if a person is receiving AFDC, which is Aid to Families With Dependent Children, he or she is eligible for Medicaid. To receive matching funds, the state must provide Medicaid services to individuals in that category. Also, in terms of children, if a child's family is living at or below 133 percent of the poverty level, the family is eligible for Medicaid. These qualification standards are mere examples, although there are many more in terms of necessary categories for which Medicaid services must be provided in order for states to receive federal matching funds. Individuals who are covered by Medicaid are not required to secure insurance coverage through the healthcare exchange, under the ACA. The federal government provides oversight, although it is administered by state. The federal government also ensures that certain services are covered, including inpatient and outpatient hospital care, prenatal care, vaccines, and services by doctors and beyond.

▶ Examples of Healthcare Systems in Other Nations

Many countries have some form of universal health care. In some systems, the provision of health care is compulsory and is subsidized by the government and usually involves public insurance plans. An example of such a system is the United Kingdom's National Health Plan. Other nations in Europe, and beyond, also have some form of universal health care. Examples include Australia, New Zealand,

France, Canada, Saudi Arabia, Oman, Costa Rica, Kyrgyzstan, and Cuba. For illustrative purposes, brief overviews of a few healthcare systems in specific nations are presented in the following discussion, with a focus on the healthcare provisions afforded to the nations' citizens, per information from the World Bank (n.d.). The ACA is not universal health care.

Brazil

Brazil provides free health coverage for all, as it is considered a right to have it. There is a private and a public healthcare system called the Sistema Único de Saúde (*Unified Health System* in English). It is a nationalized program that includes primary health care. Also included are public and contracted hospitals. These facilities deliver specialty care. The poor and the middle class receive public health care, and the wealthy receive private health care, hence it is based on socioeconomic status. One may argue that this is a system in which the wealthy have more options than do the poor. Although that may be the case, the reality is that all individuals have access to care, no matter their economic status. The question, which goes beyond the scope of this overview, is the quality of said care, particularly in terms of the poor as compared to the wealthy, who can afford private care.

Chile

In Chile, per their constitution, health protection is considered a right. Public and private health care are available. Wealthy people can purchase insurance. The options are the Instituciones de Salud Previsional (ISAPRE; *Health Insurance Institutions* in English) or receiving health coverage through their employer. Public health care is funded by taxes at a rate of 7 percent, and the system is titled Fondo Nacional de Salud (FONASA; *National Health Trust* in English). So in this case, similar to Brazil, there are options available to the wealthy that are not available to the poor. However, again, the key is access. All persons have access to care, no matter their economic status. Toward that end, if people encounter a health situation, they may seek out assistance without the worry or concern of how to pay for it, as coverage is built into their healthcare system for all.

Canada

Canada has universal health care, which is paid for by income taxes and sales tax. All citizens of Canada have health care. The doctors are all private in Canada, as compared to the United Kingdom's universal health system, in which the doctors are public employees. In this system, interestingly, the doctors bill the government. Doctors do not bill the patients. There are no co-pays, so patients do not have concerns about payments to their doctors or related bills.

In the preceding examples, each nation is different and has to come up with a healthcare system or plan that works for its people. It seems that the most important aspect of any healthcare plan is accessibility. If an individual is ill and must see a doctor, there needs to be a comfort level that no barriers exist to seeking care. Furthermore, affordability is a necessity. If one needs to access care, is there a means to pay for it? Universal health coverage removes that concern, as taxes are collected from each individual to cover the care of both those who are able to contribute and those who cannot. This notion has an altruistic ring to it. There is an indication inherent in societies that have chosen this route that health care is a right, and therefore the provision of it to all, no matter their socioeconomic status, must and will happen.

▶ A Potential Solution Toward Closing the Health Status Gap

A creative idea to help ease the problems associated with health care in the United States, particularly for emerging majority groups, would be an "Emerging Majority Health Corps." This initiative would entail a targeted effort of recruiting individuals from emerging majority groups who, in the early stages of their K-12 education, show a significant interest in the sciences and medicine. Students would be trained and prepared to study necessary subjects for college premedical (and other health professions) entry, with scholarships available to them upon acceptance for admission. A portion of healthcare premiums provided to health corporations could be used to subsidize those scholarships along with government funding. Low-interest loans would also be useful to assist with the process for those students who fall short of necessary funding (for undergraduate and graduate professional schools), above what is provided through scholarships and government funding. Loan forgiveness options, based on length of dedicated service, would be an important component of the process. Non-taxed, loan forgiveness options, based on length of dedicated service, would be an important component of the process.

Undergraduate Emerging Majority Health Corps students would attend graduate and professional schools with health careers and medicine as the intended outcome. Upon completion of medical or other health professional schools, students would be required to serve in low-income, emerging majority communities, where there is significant health disparity, for a designated number of years, with the goal being to assist in closing the health status gap. There is currently a similar program in place, but it does not require that the participants be a member of emerging majority groups. This qualification is critical, as research has shown repeatedly that individuals prefer to receive healthcare treatment from people who look like them. Since graduates would have been committed to this process by becoming an Emerging Majority Health Corps member, they would be assured of hire in emerging majority communities at various healthcare facilities, both private and public (e.g., Federally Qualified Community Health Centers).

It does not seem that the solution to closing the gap and improving diversity in health care requires rocket scientists coming up with solutions through complex thinking beyond the capability of U.S. minds. It appears that there merely needs to be a commitment to improving the health of all individuals in society, no matter their race, ethnicity, or socioeconomic status—but with due recognition of the fact that some groups are suffering more than others in regard to health care, at rates that are much higher than those of the current majority group based on key health indicators and diseases. If solutions are not found, then soon, since emerging majority groups will be the majority, the majority of Americans will be suffering from inadequate health care at higher rates than their White counterparts. Everyone deserves optimal care, and efforts must be tailored to make sure this happens.

Given that there is a campaign in progress, at the time of this writing, toward electing a new president of the United States, perhaps the matter of closing the health status gap will be tackled again, particularly for low-income communities where the gap is the widest as compared to the White population. Many have felt disappointed that this issue was not addressed more fervently under the Obama administration, particularly for Black, poor people who have the lowest health status in the United States. Bedard (2015) reports the feelings of the first Black governor of Virginia, Douglas Wilder, as Wilder describes in his book *Son of Virginia*, as follows (Bedard, 2015):

> Wilder charged that Black America is worse off under Obama. Describing what voters told him during Obama's reelection campaign, Wilder wrote, "I was distressed by the deep well of unhappiness I felt as voters repeatedly described the ways in which they were worse off than they'd been at the beginning of President Obama's term."

Clearly, there are varying opinions about this perspective from one politician to another, particularly in terms of health. Solutions perhaps are in the minds and actions of forthcoming leaders, but in the meantime, the people who are suffering will continue to do so and remain seriously behind in terms of optimal health. This inability to ensure the health of all is a disgrace to the United States, which is unfortunate given that it is touted to be the wealthiest nation in the world.

Wrap-Up

Chapter Summary

The health status gap is wide, particularly for Black people as compared to the White population. Key indicators such as life expectancy, infant mortality rate, and leading causes of death tell the story. In fact, the unfortunate reality is that the health status gap is widening. Per Zimmerman and Anderson (2019) per a recent study:

> Improving health equity often figures as an important goal for communities, thought leaders, and policy makers in public health. Yet, this analysis suggests that across the past 25 years, the promise of improving health equity has not been met. Greater or different efforts than those tried in the past will have to be mustered if health equity is to improve. Performance tracking of health equity may help to keep policy makers accountable to making the necessary changes.

The problem must be solved. According to Nielson (2019):

Annual health survey (Centers for Disease Control and Prevention, 1993–2017), approx. 5.5 million Americans ages 18–64. CDC recommended questions (reliable indicators):

Over the last 30 days, how many healthy days have you had? On a scale of 1 to 5, how would you rate your overall health? Findings: Americans' self-reported health declined since 1993. Race, gender and income play a bigger role in predicting health outcomes now vs. 1993. White men-highest income bracket: healthiest group.

The results are disheartening as Nielson (2019) further points out per the researchers that "Results of this analysis suggest that there has been a clear lack of progress on health equity during the past 25 years in the United States."

The question is whether or not healthcare reform, specifically the ACA, is contributing to the solution and whether recent changes (e.g., elimination of the individual mandate) will have an impact, as well as other reform efforts under consideration. A brief overview of the ACA provides the opportunity to ponder this. Brief insight is provided as to how other nations have tackled the problem, including health care for all, through universal coverage. An idea, the Emerging Majority Health Corps, is provided to perhaps stimulate more ideas toward other potential solutions.

Chapter Problems

1.   What are the key aspects of the Affordable Care Act (ACA)?
2.   What is the difference between the Affordable Care Act, the Patient Protection and Affordable Care Act, and Obamacare?
3.   Would an Emerging Majority Health Corps, as described in this chapter, be a useful effort toward reducing health disparities? Why or why not?
4.   What is the difference between Medicaid and Medicare?
5.   Explain the digital divide and its relevance to ACA?
6.   What do you suggest to raise awareness of good health care for Black men and men in general?

References

Bedard, P. (2015, October 5). Virginia's first Black governor says Obama ignored Blacks. *Washington Examiner*. Retrieved from http://www.washingtonexaminer.com/virginias-first-black-governor -says-obama-ignored-blacks/article/2573231

Central Intelligence Agency. (2009). *The world factbook*. Retrieved from https://www.cia.gov /library/publications/the-world-factbook/docs/profileguide.html

Elders, J. (n.d.). Retrieved from https://www.inspiringquotes.us/author/6286-joycelyn-elders

Fadich, A., Llamas, R. P., Giorgianni, S., Stephenson, C. & Nwaiwu, C. (2018). 2016 Survey of State-Level Health Resources for Men and Boys: Identification of Inadvertent and Remediable Service and Health Disparity. *American Journal of Men's Health, 12*(4), 1131–1137.

Leonard, K. (2015). Study: Obamacare hasn't solved health care disparities. U.S. News and World Report. Retrieved from http://www.usnews.com/news/blogs/data-mine/2015/04/09/study -obamacare-hasnt-solved-health-care-disparities

Men's Health Brain Trust. (2013). Executive Summary-providing for and influencing the care of boys and [4] men in America: A report by the Men's Health Braintrust based on the dialogue on Men's Health, Patients and Providers Workgroup Conference, May 2013. Retrieved from: http://www.menshealthnetwork.org/library/Dialogue2summary.pdf?embedded=true

Nielson, S. (2019). The gap between rich and poor Americans' Health is widening.

NPR. Retrieved from: https://www.npr.org/sections/health-shots/2019/06/28/736938334/the-gap -between-rich-and-poor-americans-health-is-widening

Rose, P. (2013). *Cultural competency for the Health Professional.* Burlington, MA: Jones & Bartlett Learning.

The World Bank. (n.d.). Universal Health Coverage Study Series (UNICO). Retrieved from http://www.worldbank.org/en/topic/health/publication/universal-health-coverage-study-series

Zimmerman, F., and Anderson, N. (2019). Trends in Health Equity in the United States by Race/Ethnicity, Sex, and Income, 1993-2017. *JAMA Netw Open, 2*(6):e196386. doi:10.1001/jamanetworkopen.2019.6386 Retrieved from: https://jamanetwork.com/journals/jamanetworkopen/fullarticle/2736934?utm_source=For_The_Media&utm_medium=referral&utm_campaign=ftm_links&utm_term=062819

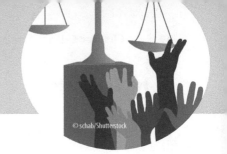

CHAPTER 6

Health Disparities in Urban Communities: The Issues, Concerns, and Solutions

Anthony E. Munroe

KEY TERMS

population health   urban communities
poverty

LEARNING OBJECTIVES

After reading this chapter you should be able to:

1. Define health disparity.
2. Explain how social determinants of health are mostly responsible for health inequities.

▶ Introduction

Fifty three years ago, in March 1966, during the Medical Committee for Human Rights meeting at the University of Chicago, Dr. Martin Luther King, Jr., who at that time was the head of the Southern Christian Leadership Conference, spoke about the disparities in health care among Blacks. These many years later, we continue to experience significant health disparities in communities of color, especially **urban communities** of African Americans and Hispanics.

As we examine health disparities, particularly in urban communities, it is important to recognize the social, political, and economic implications. Such disparities, particularly among urban communities of color, give us some insight into the "social justice platform into health care and access to quality healthcare services" (Braveman, 2006). In this chapter we will discuss health disparities, socioeconomic status, determinants of health, **poverty**, access to quality healthcare services, and the types of providers who typically serve minority urban communities. These are all major factors and issues worth reviewing to better understand the complex nature of health disparities in urban communities. We will take a case study look at Chicago, Illinois, as we review health disparities in urban neighborhoods and communities.

▶ The Issues, Concerns, and Solutions Relating to Health Disparities

In the United States, health disparities are well documented among various groups, as defined by race/ethnicity, type of community (e.g., rural, urban), gender, economic status, and other group dynamics. Groups not identified as the White majority tend to have poorer health, higher mortality and morbidity rates, and less access to quality healthcare services. Health disparities can fundamentally refer to the differences in health status across various populations as influenced by numerous factors. Some of the factors are behavioral—for instance, whether one uses tobacco products such as cigarettes, overconsumes alcohol, does not or cannot exercise, or has limited access to healthy food options.

The term *health disparities* appears to represent a concept that can be intuitively understood, yet there is much controversy about its exact meaning (Dehlendorf, Bryant, Huddleston, Jacoby, & Fujimoto, 2010). A central aspect of the most accepted definitions is that not all differences in health status between groups are considered to be disparities; rather, only differences that systematically and negatively impact less advantaged groups are classified as disparities (Braveman, 2006). The Kaiser Family Foundation (2012) offers the following definitions:

> "Health disparity," generally refers to a higher burden of illness, injury, disability, or mortality experienced by one population group relative to another group. A "healthcare disparity" typically refers to differences between groups in health coverage, access to care, and quality of care. While disparities are commonly viewed through the lens of race and ethnicity, they occur across many dimensions, including socioeconomic status, age, location, gender, disability status, and sexual orientation.

The most concise and accessible definition of health disparities/inequalities/equity was articulated by Margaret Whitehead in the early 1990s as differences in health that "are not only unnecessary and avoidable but, in addition, are considered unfair and unjust" (Braveman, 2006, p. 168).

In the 2012 report titled "Disparities in Health and Health Care," the Kaiser Family Foundation offers historical insight into the issue of health disparities in the United States:

> Health and healthcare disparities first gained significant federal rec-
> ognition with the release of two Surgeon General's reports in 2000 that
> showed disparities in tobacco use and access to mental health services
> by race and ethnicity. These reports were followed with the first major
> legislation focused on reduction of disparities, the Minority Health and
> Health Disparities Research and Education Act of 2000, which created the
> National Center for Minority Health and Health Disparities and autho-
> rized AHRQ [Agency for Healthcare Research and Quality] to regularly
> measure progress on reduction of disparities. Soon after, the Institute of
> Medicine released two seminal reports documenting racial and ethnic dis-
> parities in access to and quality of care. Over the last decade, awareness of
> disparities has increased at all levels of government and among the general
> public, although substantial gaps in awareness remain, particularly among
> the public.

The National Institutes of Health (NIH, 2010) cites the following disparities in its "Health Disparities" fact sheet:

> By 1980, average life expectancy in America had reached 74 years—
> 25 years longer than at the beginning of the 20th century. However, African
> Americans, Hispanic Americans, American Indians, Asian Americans,
> and Native Hawaiians/Other Pacific Islanders, who represented 25% of
> the U.S. population, continued to experience significant health disparities,
> including shorter life expectancy and higher rates of diabetes, cancer, heart
> disease, stroke, substance abuse, infant mortality, and low birth weight
>
> There was a growing awareness that racial and ethnic minority groups
> experienced poorer health compared to the overall population of the
> country. Scientists believed that the disparities were a result of a complex
> interaction between factors such as biology and the environment, as well
> as specific behaviors that could not be meaningfully addressed due to a
> shortage of racial and ethnic minority health professionals, discrimina-
> tion, and inequities in income, education, and access to health care.
>
> In 1985, a Task Force on Black and Minority Health convened by the
> Secretary, DHHS, asked the NIH to determine why minorities were expe-
> riencing higher rates of diseases, disability, and death than the overall U.S.
> population and to work to eliminate such health disparities. (NIH, 2016)

According to Thomson (2011), "Urbanites are also at above-average risk of violence, accidents, polluted air and water and shortages of green space and nutritious food— all with potentially unhealthy consequences, especially for the poor." Many urban communities are plagued with insufficient resources, crumbling schools, housing that is substandard, and other environmental and social factors that create enormous stress and unhealthy living conditions. There are a number of such communities in the city of Chicago, which we will examine later in this chapter.

▶ Health and Health Disparities

The Institute of Medicine's (IOM) report, *Unequal Treatment: Confronting Racial and Ethnic Disparities in Health Care*, significantly raised the level of awareness and attention given to minority health and health disparities. According to the report, in 1999, Congress requested that the IOM (1) assess the extent of racial and ethnic disparities in health care, assuming that access-related factors such as insurance status and the ability to pay for care are the same, (2) identify potential sources of these disparities, and (3) suggest intervention strategies (IOM, 2002a). The IOM (2002b) explains the effects of its report:

> To fulfill this request, an IOM study committee reviewed well over 100 studies that assessed the quality of health care for various racial and ethnic minority groups, while holding constant variations in insurance status, patient income, and other access-related factors. Many of these studies also controlled for other potential confounding factors, such as racial differences in the severity or stage of disease progression, the presence of comorbid illnesses, where care is received (e.g., public or private hospitals and health systems), and other patient demographic variables, such as age and gender. Some studies that employed more rigorous research designs followed patients prospectively, using clinical data abstracted from patients' charts, rather than administrative data used for insurance claims. (p. 2)

Health disparities have a variety of contributing factors or determinants. Socioeconomic status, insurance coverage, poverty, race, ethnicity, language barriers, disability, educational level, and gender are some of the determinants that can impact health disparities. The gaps in health status and mortality between Whites and ethnic minorities (particularly African Americans and Hispanics) have been well documented, and much hard data about these discrepancies have been collected (Dresher-Burke, 2010). When compared with Whites, African Americans have higher rates of diabetes, infant mortality, and many other conditions; they are sicker and also have a higher mortality rate (Dresher-Burke, 2010).

Health disparities frequently refer to disparities in health care, including differential access to screening and/or treatment options, or unequal availability of culturally or linguistically knowledgeable and sensitive health personnel (Adler & Stewart, 2010). It is conceivable that health policy and public health funding decisions can be made depending upon the perspective and definition approach used by the legislators and decision makers. How one defines *health disparities* or *health equity* can have important policy implications with practical consequences (Braveman, 2006).

Much of the discrepancy in health care can be accounted for by social factors; namely, lower income and lower rates of health insurance are associated with worse health. However, even after controlling for socioeconomic conditions, Whites enjoy better health and have lower mortality rates (Dresher-Burke, 2010). The causes of health disparities are varied and not always clear, but most researchers agree that disparities are a reflection of social and economic inequities and political injustice (Whitman, Shah, & Benjamins, 2011). While there probably is very little overt racism, many physicians (who are usually White) and other healthcare providers harbor unconscious biases toward racial groups different from their own (Dresher-Burke, 2010). Researchers have suggested that as a result of systematic and historical differential treatment, African Americans have a low level of trust in the medical establishment, causing them to seek medical care and undergo recommended medical procedures less often (Dresher-Burke, 2010). To make meaningful strides in closing the health gap, the issue must be honestly addressed and physicians should receive extensive cultural competence training (Dresher-Burke, 2010).

According to the Kaiser Family Foundation's 2012 report on "Disparities in Health and Health Care," "The Affordable Care Act (ACA) advances efforts to reduce health and healthcare disparities and to improve health and health care for vulnerable populations." The report goes on to state the following:

> These provisions affect multiple dimensions of health and health care, including health coverage, access to care, delivery system reforms, provider supply and capacity, and public health and prevention efforts. Some of the provisions explicitly focus on disparities, whereas others have broader goals with important benefits for vulnerable populations. In addition, the ACA increases federal priorities to address disparities by elevating the National Center for Minority Health and Healthcare Disparities to an institute within the NIH and creating Offices of Minority Health within key HHS agencies to coordinate disparity reduction efforts.
>
> Health coverage expansions that will significantly increase coverage options for low- and moderate-income populations and reduce the number of uninsured are a major component of the ACA. The ACA establishes a new continuum of coverage options that includes an expansion of Medicaid to a national eligibility floor of 138% FPL [federal poverty level] ($26,344 for a family of three in 2012) and the creation of new Health Benefit Exchanges with tax credits for individuals up to 400% FPL ($76,300 for a family of three in 2012). These expansions will help reduce wide variations in access to health coverage across states and significantly increase availability of coverage for low- and moderate-income populations. These expansions are particularly significant for people of color, who make up a disproportionate share of the uninsured and of low-income populations. Roughly 60% of non-elderly uninsured Blacks, Hispanics, and American Indians/Alaska Natives have income below the Medicaid expansion limit of 138% FPL and over 90% have incomes below 400% FPL (**FIGURE 6-1**). However, non-citizens will continue to face specific eligibility restrictions for Medicaid coverage and targeted outreach and enrollment efforts will be key for translating eligibility into coverage, particularly for vulnerable populations.

The ACA includes provisions to increase access to providers, promote workforce diversity and cultural competence, strengthen data collection and research efforts, and expand prevention and public health efforts. For example, the ACA expands funding for community health centers, which are an important source of coverage

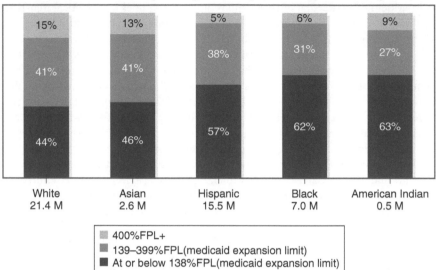

Distribution of coverage among non-elderly uninsured by race/ethnicity:

White 21.4 M	Asian 2.6 M	Hispanic 15.5 M	Black 7.0 M	American Indian 0.5 M
15%	13%	5%	6%	9%
41%	41%	38%	31%	27%
44%	46%	57%	62%	63%

- 400%FPL+
- 139–399%FPL(medicaid expansion limit)
- At or below 138%FPL(medicaid expansion limit)

The federal poverty level was $18,530 for a family of three in 2011. Asian group includes Pacific Islanders. American Indian group includes Aleutian Eslimos. Two or more races excluded. Data may not total 100% due to rounding.

FIGURE 6-1 Income of Uninsured by Race/Ethnicity, 2011.

Reproduced from Kaiser Family Foundation. 2012. Focus on Health Care Disparities, Dec. 2012. Publication # 8396.

for low-income individuals and people of color, and temporarily increases Medicaid payments for primary care services. The ACA also provides increased funding to support training of healthcare professionals and support for cultural competence training and education materials. The ACA strengthens data collection and research efforts by requiring all federally funded health programs and population surveys to collect and report data on race, ethnicity, primary language, and supporting a number of disparities research efforts. Lastly, the ACA includes a wide array of prevention and public health initiatives, including a national oral health education campaign with an emphasis on racial and ethnic disparities, and permanently reauthorizes the Indian Health Care Improvement Reauthorization Extension Act of 2009, which includes provisions designed to address the health and healthcare needs of American Indians and Alaska Natives, including preventive programs (Kaiser Family Foundation, 2012).

▶ Life Expectancy: Chicago

The Office of Disease Prevention and Health Promotion's Healthy People 2020 program (2016) states the following:

> Health starts in our homes, schools, workplaces, neighborhoods, and communities. We know that taking care of ourselves by eating well and staying active, not smoking, getting the recommended immunizations and screening tests, and seeing a doctor when we are sick all influence

our health. Our health is also determined in part by access to social and economic opportunities; the resources and supports available in our homes, neighborhoods, and communities; the quality of our schooling; the safety of our workplaces; the cleanliness of our water, food, and air; and the nature of our social interactions and relationships. The conditions in which we live explain in part why some Americans are healthier than others and why Americans more generally are not as healthy as they could be.

Hunt, Tran, and Whitman (2015) highlight the health disparity issue in Chicago:

In Chicago, the highest life expectancy was observed among Hispanics at 84.6 and the lowest life expectancy was observed among Blacks at 71.7—a difference of about 13 years. Life expectancy varied substantially across the 77 community areas of Chicago, from a low of 68.2 to a high of 83.3—a difference of 15 years. There were strong correlations between life expectancy and the racial, ethnic, and socioeconomic distributions among the community areas.

There is a strong, negative correlation between the proportion of Black residents in a community area and the life expectancy (-0.75; $p < .0001$). Conversely, there is a strong, positive relationship between the proportion of White residents and life expectancy (0.75; $p < .0001$). The correlation is positive and smaller but statistically significant for Hispanic people (0.49; $p < .001$).

Whitman et al. (2011) review the research done on health disparities in Chicago:

Recent analyses of health conditions in Chicago reveal that Blacks fare worse than Whites or Hispanics on a variety of indicators, including stroke, diabetes, breast cancer mortality, and maternal smoking. These analyses also show a strong, negative, and statistically significant correlation between these conditions and median household income at the community level (at the city level for breast cancer). There is extensive support in the literature for the relationship between socioeconomic status and poor health.

▶ Determinants of Health

The World Health Organization (n.d.) describes determinants of health as follows:

The social determinants of health are the conditions in which people are born, grow, live, work and age. These circumstances are shaped by the distribution of money, power and resources at global, national and local levels. The social determinants of health are mostly responsible for health inequities—the unfair and avoidable differences in health status seen within and between countries.

Access to affordable healthy foods is one determinant of health. As Thomson (2011) states, "The concept of food deserts has been around for about 20 years and has been gaining currency in tandem with rising public consciousness of the effect—for good or ill—of eating habits on health."

As Ritter and Graham (2017) assert, "Socioeconomic status is one of the most important predictors of health. Socioeconomic status is typically measured by educational attainment, income, wealth, occupation, or a combination of these factors" (p. 14). These factors have a large impact on the social conditions in which individuals live. The Centers for Disease Control and Prevention (2016) provides a useful overview of the social determinants of health:

> Conditions in the places where people live, learn, work, and play affect a wide range of health risks and outcomes. These conditions are known as social determinants of health (SDOH). We know that poverty limits access to healthy foods and safe neighborhoods and that more education is a predictor of better health. We also know that differences in health are striking in communities with poor SDOH such as unstable housing, low income, unsafe neighborhoods, or substandard education. By applying what we know about SDOH, we can not only improve individual and **population health** but also advance health equity.

Rose (2013), drawing from the article "Health Disparities Across the Lifespan: Meaning, Methods, and Mechanisms" by Adler and Stewart, describes the health status gap that exists between socioeconomic groups in the United States:

> Racially, ethnically and socioeconomically, there are significant differences, essentially stemming from the reality that those who had education less than the others had the worst health. Considering levels of education, even if one had average levels of education, they were not as healthy as those individuals who had high levels of wealth and education. Along racial and ethnic lines, Black and Hispanic people indicated fair or poor health, as compared to White people. Poverty is indicated as a clear factor in terms of health as five time as many adults who are poor, as compared to the wealthiest individuals, report that their health is either fair or poor.

▶ Poverty

Ritter and Graham (2017) describe the additional health challenges faced by those living in poor urban environments:

> Members of minority cultures are more likely to live in poor neighborhoods. These neighborhoods often have poor performing schools, high crime rates, substandard housing, few healthcare providers and pharmacies, more alcohol and tobacco advertising, and limited access to grocery stores with healthy food choices. These social determinants of health can accumulate over the course of a life and can be detrimental to physical and emotional health. (p. 297)

According to Ritter and Graham (2017), "Poverty is higher among certain racial and ethnic groups and is a contributing factor to health disparities because poverty affects many factors, including where people live and their access to health care" (p. 18). Higher socioeconomic status is generally associated with better health. The effects of higher socioeconomic status can include improved access to health-enhancing resources, improved access to health care, and a greater likelihood of living in a healthier neighborhood (Ritter & Graham, 2017). According to the Agency for Healthcare Research and Quality (AHRQ, 2011), "Despite improvements, differences persist in healthcare quality among racial and ethnic minority groups. People in low-income families also experience poorer quality care."

Ritter and Graham (2017) explain the effect that one's neighborhood has on health:

> There is little doubt that neighborhood characteristics are important elements associated with health. Residents of socially and economically deprived communities experience worse health outcomes on average than those living in more prosperous neighborhoods. Neighborhoods may influence health through relatively short-term influences on behaviors, attitudes, and healthcare utilization, thereby affecting health conditions that are more immediate. Neighborhoods also can influence health on a long-term basis through "weathering," whereby the accumulated stress, lower environmental quality, and limited resources of poorer communities experienced over many years negatively affects the health of residents. (p. 297)

▶ Access to Care and Community-Based Providers

According to the Kaiser Family Foundation (2012), some populations are at a distinct disadvantage in accessing health care in the United States:

> Hispanics, Blacks, and American Indians/Alaska Natives as well as low-income individuals all are much more likely to be uninsured relative to Whites and those with higher incomes. Low-income individuals and people of color also face increased barriers to accessing care, receive poorer quality care, and ultimately experience worse health outcomes

Nash (2016) defines population health as the (a) distribution of health outcomes within a population, (b) health determinants that influence this distribution, and (c) policies and inventions that affect those determinants. Population health outcomes can be improved by focusing on these determinants. Determinants of health include individual behavior, social influences, physical environment, medical care, public health policy, and intervention.

The limited availability of healthcare providers in some communities can serve as an impediment to health care, as the Kaiser Family Foundation (2008) explains:

> Despite efforts since the 1970s to increase the number of health professionals in medically underserved areas, members of racial/ethnic minority groups are still underrepresented in the healthcare workforce and are more likely than Whites to live in neighborhoods that lack adequate health resources. For example, 28% of Latinos and 22% of African Americans

report having little or no choice in where to seek care, while only 15% of Whites report this difficulty. African Americans and Latinos are also twice as likely as Whites to rely upon a hospital outpatient department as their regular source of care, rather than a doctor's office where opportunities for continuity of care and patient-centered care are greater. This is a result of many factors, including the higher rates of uninsured and the limited availability of primary care physicians in some communities of color

These disparities in healthcare availability, accessibility, and affordability lead to distinct problems in underserved populations. The AHRQ (2011) cites the following findings from a review of U.S. healthcare reports for the year of 2010:

- Blacks and American Indians and Alaska Natives received worse care than Whites for about 40% of measures.
- Asians received worse care than Whites for about 20% of measures.
- Hispanics received worse care than Non-Hispanic Whites for about 60% of core measures.
- Poor people received worse care than higher-income people for about 80% of core measures.

Addressing disparities in health and health care is important not only from a social justice standpoint, but also for improving the health of all Americans by achieving improvements in overall quality of care and population health. Moreover, health disparities are costly, resulting in added healthcare costs, lost work productivity, and premature death. Kaiser Family Foundation (2012) notes the following:

Recent analysis estimates that 30% of direct medical costs for Blacks, Hispanics, and Asian Americans are excess costs due to health inequities (**FIGURE 6-2**) and that, overall, the economy loses an estimated $309 billion per year due to the direct and indirect costs of disparities.

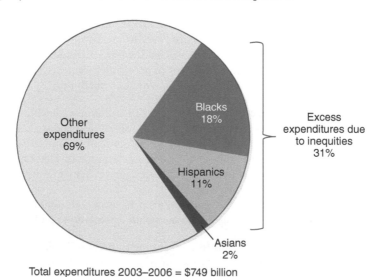

Total expenditures 2003–2006 = $749 billion

FIGURE 6-2 Excess Medical Expenditures Due to Health Inequities.

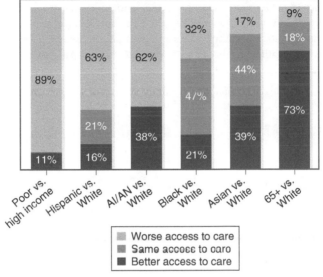

NOTES: AI/AN = American Indian or Alaska Native.

FIGURE 6-3 Disparities in Access to Care.

Reproduced from Kaiser Family Foundation. (2012). *Disparities in health and health care: Five key questions and answers.* Retrieved from https://kaiserfamilyfoundation.files.wordpress.com/2013/01/8396.pdf

In sum, the Kaiser Family Foundation (2012) offers the following insights:

> In its 2011 reports on healthcare quality and disparities, the Agency for Healthcare Research and Quality (AHRQ) finds that low-income individuals and people of color experience more barriers to care (**FIGURE 6-3**) and receive poorer quality care. Moreover, other research shows that individuals with limited English proficiency are less likely than those who are English proficient to seek care even when insured. Research also finds differing patient experiences and levels of satisfaction by race, gender, education levels, and language.

▶ Solutions

As stated by the Centers for Disease Control and Prevention (2011), "The future health of the nation will be determined to a large extent by how effectively we work with communities to reduce and eliminate health disparities between non-minority and minority populations experiencing disproportionate burdens of disease, disability, and premature death." Further, comprehensive efforts must be made to address and resolve the fundamental and historic social and economic issues that continue to plague urban, poor communities—especially communities of color. Access to good and strong schools, housing, jobs, transportation, social services, caring and high-quality healthcare providers and institutions, healthy food options, and clean and safe environments with parks, as well as living environments free of toxic waste, are all key. Violence of any and all forms in the urban community is a major concern that must be resolved with strong leadership and cooperation of all, including the community, community leaders, elected officials, public safety, law enforcement, and policy makers.

Finally, health disparities must remain a national to local priority that gets the support and resources necessary to make a marked difference. As the U.S. population grows and continues to become represented by more people of color, it is in the nation's best interest to elevate health disparities to prominent and significant priority.

Wrap-Up

Chapter Summary

This chapter focused on health disparities and healthcare disparities by explaining the difference between these terms in relationship to racial and ethnic groups in urban communities. Key areas of exploration include socioeconomic status, determinants of health, poverty, access to quality healthcare services, providers that serve urban communities, and other key issues. In terms of life expectancy, per race and ethnicity, Chicago is used as a case study to provide insight based on comparative analyses. Solutions are provided that will be helpful in reducing/eliminating health inequities with an emphasis on why this must be a national priority in the United States as the nation continues to become more diverse based on rapidly increasing numbers of people of color.

Chapter Problems

1. Explain the difference between the terms *health disparity* and *healthcare disparity*.
2. List the above-average risks that urbanites experience.
3. What provisions are included in the Affordable Care Act that aim to reduce health disparities?
4. In the city of Chicago, Black people fare worse than White or Hispanic people fare on a variety of indicators. List at least three of the indicators and provide a brief explanation as to why these disparities exist.
5. Why is it important for health disparities to remain a national to local priority?

References

Adler, N. E., & Stewart, J. (2010). Health disparities across the lifespan: Meaning, methods, and mechanisms. *Annals of the New York Academy of Sciences, 1186*, 5–23.

Agency for Healthcare Research and Quality. (2011, March). *Disparities in healthcare quality among racial and ethnic minority groups: Selected findings from the 2010 national healthcare quality and disparities reports*. Retrieved from http://archive.ahrq.gov/research/findings/nhqrdr/nhqrdr10/minority.html

Braveman, P. (2006). Health disparities and health equity: Concepts and measurement. *Annual Review of Public Health, 27*, 167–194.

Centers for Disease Control and Prevention, Office of Minority Health and Health Equity. (2011). Our guiding principle. Retrieved from http://www.cdc.gov/stltpublichealth/hop/pdfs/OMHHE_Factsheet.pdf

Centers for Disease Control and Prevention. (2016). Social determinants of health: Know what affects health. Retrieved from http://www.cdc.gov/socialdeterminants/

Dehlendorf, C., Bryant, A. S., Huddleston, H. G., Jacoby, V. L., & Fujimoto, V. Y. (2010). Health disparities: Definitions and measurements. *American Journal of Obstetrics and Gynecology, 202*(3), 212–213.

Dresher-Burke, K. (2010). *Health disparities in the United States: Social class, race, ethnicity, and health*. Donald A. Barr Reviewed by Krista Dresher-Burke. *The Journal of Sociology & Social Welfare, 37*(1), Article 13.

Hunt, B. R., Tran, G., & Whitman, S. (2015). Life expectancy varies in local communities in Chicago: Racial and spatial disparities and correlates. *Journal of Racial and Ethnic Health Disparities, 2*(4), 425–433.

Institute of Medicine. (2002a). *Unequal treatment: Confronting racial and ethnic disparities in health care*. Washington, DC: Author.

Institute of Medicine. (2002b). *Unequal treatment: What healthcare providers need to know about racial and ethnic disparities in healthcare*. Washington, DC: National Academies Press.

Institute of Medicine. (2006). *Examining the health disparities research plan of the National Institutes of Health: Unfinished business*. Washington, DC: National Academies Press.

Kaiser Family Foundation. (2008). Eliminating racial/ethnic disparities in health care: What are the options? Retrieved from http://kff.org/disparities-policy/issue-brief/eliminating-racialethnic-disparities-in-health-care-what/

Kaiser Family Foundation. (2012). *Disparities in health and health care: Five key questions and answers*. Retrieved from https://kaiserfamilyfoundation.files.wordpress.com/2013/01/8396.pdf

McDonough, J. E., Gibbs, B. K., Scott-Harris, J. L., Kronebur002ch, K., Navarro, A. M., & Taylor, T. (2004). *A state policy agenda to eliminate racial and ethnic health disparities*. New York, NY: The Commonwealth Fund.

Nash, D. B., (2016). *Population health* (2nd ed.). Burlington, MA: Jones & Bartlett Learning.

National Institutes of Health. (2010). Health disparities. Retrieved from https://report.nih.gov/nihfactsheets/viewfactsheet.aspx?csid=124

Office of Disease Prevention and Health Promotion. (2016). Social determinants of health. Healthy People 2020. Retrieved from https://www.healthypeople.gov/2020/topics-objectives/topic/social-determinants-of-health

Ritter, L. A., & Graham, D. H. (2017). *Multicultural health* (2nd ed.). Burlington, MA: Jones & Bartlett Learning.

Rose, P. (2013). *Cultural competency for the health professional*. Burlington, MA: Jones & Bartlett Learning.

Thomson, S. C. (2011). Urban health care: Disparities abound. *Health Progress, 92*(6), 4–7.

Whitman, S., Shah, A. M., & Benjamins, M. (2011). *Urban health: Combating disparities with local data*. New York, NY: Oxford University Press.

World Health Organization. (n.d.). What are social determinants of health? Retrieved from http://www.who.int/social_determinants/sdh_definition/en/

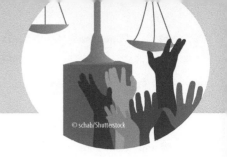

CHAPTER 7

Health Disparities in Rural Communities

While the existing array of strategies is better than doing nothing, it has not prevented the sharpening of rural/remote access as a policy issue. Something different and additional will have to be done in [the] future if rural/remote access is to be improved.

—**Barer and Stoddart**[1]

KEY TERMS

access to care
geographic isolation
migrant and seasonal agricultural
  worker (MSAW)
obesity

overweight
risky behaviors
rural health
seasonal farmworker

LEARNING OBJECTIVES

After reading this chapter, you should be able to do the following:

1. Explain some of the key issues regarding health disparities and rural communities.
2. Delineate health issues that impact migrant and seasonal agricultural workers.
3. List risky behaviors that members of rural communities may participate in.
4. Discuss how socioeconomic status impacts the health status of individuals in rural communities.
5. Identify some of the controversies associated with undocumented workers and immigration reform perspectives.

1   The Society of Rural Physicians of Canada. Comment on "Improving Access to Needed Medical Services in Rural and Remote Canadian Communities: Recruitment and Retention Revisited" by Morris L. Barer and Greg L Stoddart The Society 1999 http://www.srpc.ca/librarydocs/Comonbs.PDF

▶ Introduction

Although health disparities in urban communities are usually the focal point of this issue, there are serious problems unique to rural communities that contribute to the overall health status gap. According to the U.S. Department of Health and Human Services (2002), health disparities are the "differences in [the] incidence, prevalence, morbidity, mortality and burden of diseases and other adverse health conditions that exist among specific population groups in the United States." There are very specific risk factors that contribute to poor health conditions for people living in rural environments. Some of them are as follows per the Rural Health Information Hub (RHIhub, 2014):

- Geographic isolation
- Lower socioeconomic status
- Higher rates of risky health behaviors
- Limited job opportunities

Urban areas suffer greatly in terms of illnesses/disease, but the situation relating to **rural health**—that is, the health of individuals living in rural communities—is still graver. A key factor is lack of **access to care**. Due to **geographic isolation**, there are often limited health resources and providers in rural environments—hence, lack of access to care. Furthermore, many people in rural communities are unable to find work. The U.S. Department of Agriculture (2016) offers the following rural employment statistics:

> Employment grew more than 1 percent in rural areas during the year that ended in the second quarter of 2015. This is a marked improvement from previous years of very slow growth or decline. Nonetheless, rural employment in mid-2015 was still 3.2 percent below its pre-recession peak in 2007 (p. 1).

Lack of, or slow, employment growth translates to lack of health insurance in many instances, unless individuals have reached the poverty level and are eligible for Medicaid or are eligible for Medicare based on their age (i.e., are 65 years or older). The other option is seeking healthcare insurance through options created by the Patient Protection and Affordable Care Act.

▶ Risky Behaviors

Some of the **risky behaviors** that individuals in rural communities participate in that may impact their health are smoking, heavy alcohol consumption, and abstention from regular exercise, according to the Georgetown University Health Policy Institute (2003). The experience of **overweight** and **obesity** is also a significant issue. Additionally, the population makeup of people in rural communities is quite different from that in urban communities. The RHIhub (2014) describes the challenges facing this population as follows:

> Several studies have shown that rural residents are older, poorer, and have fewer physicians to care for them. This inequality is intensified as rural residents are less likely to have employer-provided healthcare coverage,

TABLE 7-1 Rural Versus Urban Life Expectancy (per 100,000 People)

Life Expectancy	Rural Communities	Urban Counties
All	76.8	78.8
Male	74.1	76.2
Female	79.7	81.3
White	77.2	79.2
Black	72.8	74.2
Native American and Alaska Native	74.8	85.8
Asian and Pacific Islander	84.9	86.9
Hispanic (Ethnicity)	82.2	83.1

Data from Singh, G. K., & Siahpush, M. (2014). Widening rural-urban disparities in life expectancy, U.S., 1969–2009. *American Journal of Preventive Medicine, 46*(2), 19–29.

and if they are poor, often are not covered by Medicaid. Federal and state agencies and membership organizations are working to diminish these disparities and keep rural America healthy and strong. Some provide funding, information, and technical assistance to be used at the state, regional, and local level, while others inform state and federal legislators to help them understand the issues affecting health care in rural America.

In general, as illustrated in **TABLE 7-1**, the life expectancy for members of rural communities are generally lower than for members of urban communities across all racial, ethnic, and gender categories.

▶ Migrant Farmworkers

Another group to consider when assessing health disparities in rural communities is **migrant and seasonal agricultural workers (MSAWs)**. Their health status is adversely affected by myriad issues, including hazardous work environments, poverty, low wages, inadequate housing, limited availability of clean water and septic systems, limited access and continuity of care, lack of insurance, and cultural and language barriers (RHIhub, 2015). According to RHIhub (2015), MSAWs face unique health issues:

> MSAW populations experience serious health problems including diabetes, malnutrition, infectious diseases, pesticide poisoning, and injuries from work related machinery. These critical health issues are exacerbated

by the migratory culture of this population group, which makes it difficult to develop a relationship with a healthcare provider, maintain treatment regimens, and track health records.

Migrant farmworkers may face an additional challenge in that a significant number are undocumented immigrants and lack authorization to work in the United States (Kandel, 2008). The estimated number of agricultural workers in the United States is approximately 2.5 million, with most residing and working in the state of California (Hansen & Donohoe, 2003), although this number varies. Mehta et al. (2000) point out that, "According to the U.S. Department of Labor's National Agricultural Workers Survey (NAWS), approximately 1.4 million of these farm laborers are MSFWs [migrant seasonal farmworkers]." Other estimates have reported that between 3 and 5 million MSAWs and their dependents (including husbands, wives, children, and other family members) live in the United States (Colt, Stallones, & Cameron, 2001). Larson (2013), citing the definitions provided by the Migrant Health Program of the Bureau of Primary Health Care, U.S. Department of Health and Human Services, clarifies the qualifications of these categories:

> A **seasonal farmworker**... [is] "an individual whose principal employment is in agriculture on a seasonal basis, who has been so employed within the last twenty-four months." A migrant farmworker meets the same definition but "establishes for the purposes of such employment a temporary abode." p. 2

Essentially, MSAWs provide labor that fortifies the U.S. fruit and labor industry (Mobed, Gold, & Schenker, 1992).

▶ Health Issues

Mobed et al. (1992) explain some of the health issues that impact MSAWs:

> Potential farm work-related health problems include accidents, pesticide-related illnesses, musculoskeletal and soft-tissue disorders, dermatitis, noninfectious respiratory conditions, reproductive health problems, health problems of children of farm workers, climate-caused illnesses, communicable diseases, bladder and kidney disorders, and eye and ear problems (p. 1 abstract).

Because the population of MSAWs is constantly moving, longitudinal studies have been limited. Hansen and Donohoe (2003) point out some of the same issues as those previously stated and also include infectious diseases (including bacterial, fungal, and parasitic infections), heat stress, respiratory conditions, reproductive issues, oral health concerns, cancer, and social and mental health problems. Federal dollars are provided to assist with some of this population's many health issues, with services provided by Federally Qualified Health Centers (FQHCs). FQHCs receive funding from the Health Resources Services Administration, per the Public Health Service Act, Section 330. These grants enable the provision of health care to individuals regardless of either their ability to pay or their immigration status. The community health centers accept Medicare, Medicaid, and other forms of insurance.

▶ The Tragic Health Status of MSAWs

What is taking place in America regarding MSAWs is a tragedy. Although there is concern expressed regarding undocumented immigrants, including the belief among some people that undocumented immigrants should be removed from the United States or made legal citizens, immigration reform has yet to occur. This situation causes political consternation between various factions and is extremely controversial. Many of the people purporting that immigrants must enter the country on a documented status and maintain such clearance fail to acknowledge that there is complicity in employing undocumented migrants. Employers of MSAWs enjoy the fruits of the MSAWs' labor—literally, in some cases—but pay them minimally and do not ensure that they have access to health care. There must be admission and understanding that MSAWs are a benefit to the U.S. economy, particularly in terms of the fruit and vegetable market, which is a tremendous industry. MSAWs are grossly underpaid despite the intensity of their labor. For example, one key health issue, birth and neonatal problems, exemplifies the intensity of their labor, as explained by Hansen and Donohoe (2003):

> Prolonged standing and bending, overexertion, dehydration, poor nutrition, and pesticide or chemical exposure contribute to an increased risk of spontaneous abortion, premature delivery, fetal malformation and growth retardation, and abnormal postnatal development. Moreover, low socioeconomic status; frequently young maternal age; and late, little, or no prenatal care increase risks to mother and child. (p. 158)

These conditions have led to an infant mortality rate that is approximately twice the national average (Slesinger, Christenson, & Cautley, 1986). Furthermore, in a study regarding California migrant women, stillbirth was the outcome for 24 percent of the women (De la Torre & Rush, 1989).

▶ Solutions to Improve the Health Status of Migrant Farmworkers

In terms of solutions, Hansen and Donohoe (2003) recommend the following to improve the health status of MSAWs:

- Create a stronger public health infrastructure.
- Enroll more healthcare providers to work with underserved populations.
- Employ more community outreach workers.
- Train bilingual and bicultural healthcare providers.
- Encourage alternative healthcare delivery methods (e.g., "healthcare vans").
- Implement more advanced information-tracking systems that can be networked among clinicians.
- Increase preventive health services such as dental care, family planning, accident prevention, and detection and control of chronic diseases.
- Broaden legislation and protection through improved U.S. Department of Labor, Occupational Safety and Health Administration, and Environmental

Protection Agency standards to eliminate overcrowded and unsanitary living conditions and workplace hazards and exposures.

- Create a system of universal access to care.
- Improve education among MSAWs and healthcare providers.
- Educate MSAWs about prevention, detection, and treatment at their homes, workplaces, or community centers.
- Include migrant health care in medical, nursing, and dental school curricula (e.g., interactive lectures).
- Improve physician recognition, management, and reporting of pesticide-related illnesses.

Wrap-Up

Chapter Summary

These are serious problems that contribute to the health status gap of rural communities as compared to the rest of the U.S. population, based on key factors. One specific factor, that is key to the overall problem, is lack of access to care. Additionally, there are risky behaviors that must be considered that impact rural health, including smoking, heavy alcohol consumption, and lack of regular exercise. Stress and lack of funds and access to productive, positive exercise facilities are the primary reasons for such behaviors. MSAWs have particular health concerns due to their lack of access to care. Specific solutions must be considered to address this population's myriad health problems.

Chapter Problems

1. List three specific factors that contribute to poor health conditions for people in rural communities.
2. Compare life expectancies for three racial groups in rural versus urban groups. What are the differences?
3. What is the estimated number of migrant farmworkers in the United States?
4. What do you think are the best solutions for improving the health status of MSAWs? Why?

References

Colt, J., Stallones, L., Cameron, L., Dosemeci, M., & Zahm, S. H. (2001). Proportionate mortality among U.S. migrant and seasonal farmworkers in twenty-four states. *American Journal of Industrial Medicine, 40*(5), 604–611.

De la Torre, A., & Rush, L. (1989). The effects of health care access on maternal and infant health among migrant and seasonal farmworker women in California. *Migrant Health Newsline, 6*(1), 1–2.

Georgetown University Health Policy Institute. (2003). Rural and urban health. Retrieved from https://hpi.georgetown.edu/agingsociety/pubhtml/rural/rural.html

Hansen, E., & Donohoe, M. (2003). Health issues of migrant and seasonal farm workers. *Journal of Health Care for the Poor and Underserved, 14*(2), 153–164.

Kandel, W. (2008). Profile of migrant farmworkers. Economic Research Report No. (ERR-60). U.S. Department of Agriculture. Retrieved from http://www.ers.usda.gov/publications/err-economic-research-report/err60.aspx

Larson, A. (2013). Oregon update: Migrant and seasonal farmworker enumeration profiles study. Retrieved from https://www.oregon.gov/oha/oei/reports/Migrant%20and%20Seasonal%20Farmworker%20Enumeration%20Profiles%20Study.pdf

Mobed, K., Gold, E. B., & Schenker, M. (1992). Occupational health problems among migrant and seasonal farm workers. *Western Journal of Medicine, 147*(3), 367–373.

Mehta, K., Gabbard, S. M., Barrat, V., Lewis, M., Carroll, D., & Mines, R. (2000). *Findings from the National Agricultural Workers Survey (NAWS) 1997–1998: A demographic and employment profile of United States farmworkers.* Washington, DC: U.S. Department of Labor.

Rural Health Information Hub. (2014). Rural health disparities. Retrieved from https://www.ruralhealthinfo.org/topics/rural-health-disparities

Rural Health Information Hub. (2015). Rural migrant health. Retrieved from https://www.ruralhealthinfo.org/topics/migrant-health

Slesinger, D. P., Christenson, B. A., & Cautley, E. (1986). Health and mortality of migrant farm children. *Social Science and Medicine, 23*(1), 65–74.

U.S. Department of Agriculture. (2016). Rural America at a glance (2015 ed.). Retrieved from http://www.ers.usda.gov/media/1952235/eib145.pdf

U.S. Department of Health and Human Services. (2002). *Strategic research plan and budget to reduce and ultimately eliminate health disparities, volume I, fiscal years 2002–2006.* Washington, DC: National Institutes of Health.

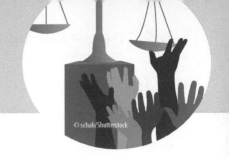

CHAPTER 8

Women and Health Disparities: Specific Issues, Concerns, and Solutions

A woman's health is her capital

—**Harriet Beecher Stowe**

KEY TERMS

Aid to Families With Dependent Children (AFDC)
diabetes
family wage
hypertension
infant mortality rate (IMR)

low birth weight (LBW)
mass incarceration
maternal mortality rate (MMR)
morbidity rates
Temporary Assistance for Needy Families (TANF)

LEARNING OBJECTIVES

After reading this chapter, you should be able to do the following:

1. Discuss key factors that impact the health status of women.
2. Identify specific illnesses that are more prevalent in women.
3. Explain potential solutions for closing the health status gap between emerging majority women and White women.

▶ Introduction

In considering the health status of women in the United States, key factors that must be taken into consideration include race/ethnicity and socioeconomic status. These factors are quite complex, relating to neonatal care, birth outcomes, and increased prevalence of certain diseases. Moreover, the quality and accessibility of care to women vary drastically from one social setting to another, with particular hardship experienced by women in low-income areas and incarcerated women.

▶ Race

In exploring race in terms of women's health, cultural norms are significant. Often, Black women, for example, are burdened by poverty, lack of access to care, and limited education. Poor diet is also a critical factor for some. However, it is important to recognize that not all Black people, including Black women, are poor. Recently, Senator Bernie Sanders, a candidate in the U.S. presidential primary race of 2016, was chided for making this generalization. He stated at the Democratic debate in Flint, Michigan, on March 16, "When you're white … you don't know what it's like to be poor." He later corrected this statement, as the reality is that in terms of sheer numbers, there are more poor White people than poor Black people in the United States. In a 2013 article, Yen helps identify the "face" of poverty in the United States:

> While poverty rates for blacks and Hispanics are nearly three times higher, by absolute numbers the predominant face of the poor is white. More than 19 million whites fall below the poverty line of $23,021 for a family of four, accounting for more than 41% of the nation's destitute, nearly double the number of poor blacks. Sometimes termed "the invisible poor" by demographers, lower-income whites generally are dispersed in suburbs as well as small rural towns, where more than 60% are white. Concentrated in Appalachia in the East, they are numerous in the industrial Midwest and spread across America's heartland, from Missouri, Arkansas and Oklahoma up through the Great Plains.

Hence, poverty is not limited to emerging majorities of any race or ethnicity, although there is disproportionality, which lends to the health status gap. This insight can be applied to women, as a specific group.

For women who live in low-income communities, there is an increased risk of poor health conditions. Women generally experience illnesses such as cancer, heart disease, stroke, and diabetes, particularly when their income and access to care are limited. Black women are disproportionately impacted. Nevertheless, a report released by the Kaiser Family Foundation (2009) offers the following insight:

> In states where disparities appeared to be smaller, this difference was often due to the fact that both white women and women of color were doing poorly. It is important to also recognize that in many states (e.g., West Virginia and Kentucky) all women, including white women, faced significant challenges and may need assistance (p. 2).

According to the Kaiser Family Foundation's report (2009), as indicated by **TABLE 8-1**, "American Indian and Alaska Native women had higher rates of health

TABLE 8-1 U.S. Women's Health Indicators by Race/Ethnicity (National Averages and Rates)

Health Status	All Women	White	Emerging Majorities	Black	Hispanic	Asian and Pacific Islander	American Indian and Alaska Native
Fair or poor health	12.8%	9.5%	19.7%	16.9%	26.9%	7.9%	22.1%
Diabetes	4.2%	3.3%	6.2%	7.5%	6.1%	3.2%	8.6%
Heart disease	3.2%	2.7%	3.9%	4.8%	4.0%	1.2%	8.7%
Obesity	22.7%	20.1%	28.4%	37.8%	27.3%	8.4%	30.4%
Cancer mortality per 100,000 women	162.2	161.4	—	189.3	106.7	96.7	112.0
Serious psychological distress	15.7%	16.7%	13.8%	13.5%	14.1%	9.6%	26.1%

Note: All emerging majority women includes Black, Hispanic, Asian American and Native Hawaiian/Pacific Islander, American Indian/Alaska Native women, and women of two or more races.
Data from The Kaiser Family Foundation. (2009). Putting women's health care disparities on the map: Examining racial and ethnic disparities at the state level. Retrieved from https://kaiserfamilyfoundation.files.wordpress.com/2013/01/7886es.pdf

and access challenges than women in other racial and ethnic groups on several indicators, often twice as high as White women (p. 3)." This finding has implications not just for the women in these populations, but for the whole family, as the women often oversee the family's health, and their poor health can directly impact their children's health. To the contrary, "White women fared better than minority [emerging majority] women on most indicators, but had higher rates of some health and access problems than women of color (Kaiser Family Foundation, 2009, p. 3). White women experience poverty and in rural areas often experience health and access to care issues.

▶ Socioeconomic Status and Women's Health

In exploring the socioeconomic status of women, a specific example that is very relevant to the health status gap is African American women who experience mental health issues. Low income and educational levels are associated with lower socioeconomic status overall and correlate with low self-esteem and poor self-concept (Murthy & Smith, 2010). The poor mental health status of some Black women is a reflection of their low socioeconomic status, and racism is also a contributing factor (Murthy & Smith, 2010). Depression must also be considered in exploring mental health because of its direct correlation with low self-esteem and low socioeconomic status (Munford, 1994). In caring for mental health issues, there is limited help that would be culturally supportive in terms of same-race practitioners, as there is a lack of significant numbers of Black medical practitioners, particularly in relevant disciplines. Furthermore, in Black communities in general, mental health is stigmatized for Black women, who are seen as the "rock" of the family—essentially the strength and caretaker of pressing issues, including health. Hence, seeking treatment for mental health issues is not the norm.

Additionally, Black women are often at risk for obesity and overweight (Braithwaite, Taylor, & Treadwell, 1992). There are a number of reasons for this outcome, but the key issues are soul food, which is often prepared with pride and satisfaction for the immediate and extended family (Counihan & Esterik, 1997). Soul food is prepared with a great deal of seasoning, especially salt, with numerous fried dishes and is not a healthy approach to eating. As discussed previously, soul food emerged from slavery as the refuse from the White slave masters and was often the only sustenance available to the slaves. This type of food contributes to obesity for Black women and their families. Additionally, there are social constructs among various racial and ethnic groups. For Black women, specifically, often strength and resilience can be attributed to a larger size, with dieting sometimes considered a "White thing" (Hill, 2009).

Diabetes and Hypertension

In continuing to explore the health status of Black women, as an example, there are particular diseases that are quite prevalent among this group. Black women have higher rates of **hypertension**, as compared to other groups, and the onset is early on in their lives. Critical factors may include racism (Braithwaite et al., 1992). Discrimination and racism are known to cause anger, frustration, and psychosocial stress. These problems can lead to elevated blood pressure with the ensuing result of hypertension.

Another factor that must be considered is socioeconomic status, as financial stress leads to hypertension (Braithwaite et al., 1992). One relief for stress is exercise. Unfortunately, Black women have the highest rate of physical inactivity when compared to other racial groups (Eyler et al., 1998). One of the reasons for lack of exercise is time limitation, as many are single parents. Hence, physical activity is a low priority. Another health outcome is disproportionately high rates of cardiovascular disease, including hypertension, but also heart disease and stroke (Braithwaite et al., 1992). Lack of exercise and diet-related issues (poor diet or food that should be prepared more healthfully, namely soul food) are contributing factors to obesity and **diabetes**.

Cancer

Cancer is a major issue for the Black population in the United States, in terms of survival rates. African American/Black people experience the lowest survival rate and highest death rate from cancer as compared to any other racial/ethnic group. The main reasons are lack of access to care, mistrust of providers, and cultural barriers. The mistrust stems from numerous scenarios in which Black people were mistreated and abused in the United States by healthcare providers and used as guinea pigs for research and beyond (Spencer, 2010). Indignities such as the Tuskegee experiment have deeply damaged Black people's faith in the medical establishment. Many Black people in the United States are aware of these atrocities and, consequently, will not go to the doctor for preventive care (Braithwaite et al., 1992). Therefore, Black women are less apt to undergo mammograms and other types of screenings because of distrust of healthcare providers (Musa, Schulz, Harris, Silverman, & Thomas, 2009). Given the racial discrimination discussed here and the low socioeconomic status and related financial stress, the resulting psychological duress leads to increased incidence of breast cancer (Taylor et al., 2007).

Although the emphasis of the preceding discussion is on Black women, there is no doubt that emerging majority women in general, beyond Black women, who are also poor, experience serious health issues that contribute to the health status gap between emerging majorities, poor people in general, and the White population in the United States.

Birth Outcomes

To help ensure that women experience healthy birth outcomes, the Centers for Disease Control and Prevention (CDC) recommends certain protocols for pregnant women. However, socioeconomic status may impact their ability to adhere to such guidelines for the following reasons:

- *Health literacy.* Women of low socioeconomic status may not have access to, or understand, the information provided by the CDC and beyond regarding important steps toward a healthy pregnancy and delivery.
- *Socioeconomic status.* Poor women may not have access to healthy food to meet the needs of the mother and child during pregnancy.
- *Lack of access to care.* Low-income mothers may not have insurance to see an obstetrician throughout their pregnancy. Even though Medicaid may be available, these women may not know how to access the program or may access it very late in the pregnancy, precluding an opportunity to get proper medical guidance.

There are key health indices relevant to birth outcomes, which are low birth weight (less than 2500 grams), **infant mortality rate (IMR)**, and **maternal mortality rate (MMR)**. **Low birth weight (LBW)** refers to the weight of the baby at the time of birth and determines if the baby has a healthy start to life. This measure offers some predictability regarding future **morbidity rates** (incidence of disease) and health outcome relative to maternal risk. The infant mortality rate indicates the number of infants who die during their first year of life. The IMR is based on the number of infant deaths per 1,000 live births. It is an extremely important measure, as it is commonly used as an indicator of the general health of a population. Per the Central Intelligence Agency (2009), the maternal mortality rate refers to the annual number of female deaths per 100,000 from any cause aggravated by pregnancy or its management, excluding accidental or incidental causes. The rates of these indicators are higher for emerging majority women and White women of low socioeconomic status.

However, Dr. Michael Lu, obstetrician and gynecologist at UCLA and Associate Administrator of the Maternal and Child Health Bureau of the Health Resources and Services Administration (HRSA), believes that for many women of color, racism over a life time, not just during the 9 months of pregnancy, increases the risk of preterm delivery. To improve birth outcomes, Lu argues, "we must address the conditions that impact women's health not just when they become pregnant but from childhood, adolescence and into adulthood" (*Unnatural Causes*, 2008). He also points out that racism is stressful and that stress is impactful to health on many levels, producing wear and tear on the body systems, including hormonal, metabolic, and inflammatory functions, and over time, this damage may create an overload on the organs and systems, disabling optimal functionality (*Unnatural Causes*, 2008).

Unfortunately, women will carry these burdens into their pregnancy, impacting the physiology of the pregnant mother and the unborn child. Steps that have been taken thus far to increase healthcare accessibility for low-income women, particularly those of color, have done very little to decrease prematurity, low birth weight, infant mortality, and morbidity rates. Dr. Lu points out further that trying to cram the positive aspects of care (nutrients and vitamins) into less than 9 months of prenatal care does not reverse all of the cumulative shortcomings and inequities throughout one's life before pregnancy. This is expecting too much of health care in a short time (*Unnatural Causes*, 2008).

Potential Causes Impacting Overall Socioeconomic Status of Women

Recently, in a radio interview with Dr. Richard Wolff, who hosts *Economic Update* on a listener-supported radio station in New York City, WBAI, Dr. Harriet Fraad was interviewed by Dr. Wolff. Dr. Wolff is Professor Emeritus of Economics at the University of Massachusetts, Amherst, where he taught economics from 1973 to 2008. He is currently a visiting professor in the Graduate Program in International Affairs at The New School in New York City. He also teaches classes regularly at the Brecht Forum in Manhattan. Previously, he taught economics at Yale University (1967–1969) and at the City College of the City University of New York (1969–1973).

In 1994, he was a visiting professor of economics at the University of Paris, France, at the Sorbonne. Dr. Fraad, a graduate of Teachers College, Columbia University, is a mental health counselor/psychotherapist with a practice in New York City and a frequent collaborator with Dr. Wolff. She is also Dr. Wolff's wife.

Dr. Fraad's (2016) analysis of the current status of women in the United States is intriguing and provides insight regarding the current socioeconomic status of some women. In her discussion on air with Dr. Wolff, which took place on March 25 (WBAI, 2016), she explains that there are a significant number of unmarried women in the United States and attributes this situation largely to the decline of the family wage. The **family wage** is deemed as the amount of income for a family to live on, in terms of meeting basic needs. She attributes the loss of the family wage in the United States to the outsourcing of jobs to other nations, where U.S. corporations may pay workers lower wages. These outsourced jobs were primarily, before outsourcing, designated for U.S. men. Industry, including heavy machinery work and factory jobs, she points out, were the main jobs lost. Consequently, the concept of a man and woman marrying, moving to the suburbs, having a family, and him supporting them (the family wage) while the wife stayed home and took care of the kids, was also lost.

Additionally, Fraad (2016) notes that due to the feminist movement, prior to outsourcing, and the need for women to work to supplement the family income as a result of outsourcing and women's desire to work outside of the home, there are many women in the workforce. Her perspective is that, with other factors withstanding, outsourcing led to unemployment and lower-wage jobs, particularly for men who were formerly blue-collar workers. Also, for those men and women who went to college, it is often necessary to factor in student loan debt and the impact repayment has had on the socioeconomic status of young people. Additionally, she emphasizes that many families moved to, or are considering moving to, the city, due to loss of wages and their homes, in many cases with renting as their only option, which is often expensive.

Ultimately, Fraad's point is that this change in, or loss of, the family wage has gravely impacted women, as now the option of working is no longer a choice, but a must. Lower-wage jobs are now more commonplace and, consequently, women and men who choose not to marry, which is often the case, currently are choosing to cohabitate. Many women also find themselves, by choice or circumstances, single mothers. This situation has resulted, per Fraad, in the transformation of children's lives. Single mothers end up with only one income. There is a need to be home with children, but if mothers are working, they cannot be. Finding appropriate people to watch their children is a challenge for single mothers with low income. Hence, many children are "latchkeyed" (left home alone when they return home from school, unsupervised by parents/adults). Fraad (2016) points out that as an unfortunate result, children may become victims or abused.

This is an interesting and controversial analysis presented by Fraad (2016), and leaves out some key points that may necessitate deeper consideration from the vantage point of many single mothers who vehemently disagree that raising their children alone places them at a disadvantage. Nevertheless, the issue is somewhat different for emerging majority women, particularly those who are Black and poor. For the purposes of this chapter, it is worth pointing out that Fraad does not discuss race in her analysis.

▶ Welfare and Welfare Reform

The family wage has always been a difficult scenario for Black women, as under the **Aid to Families With Dependent Children (AFDC)** welfare program, Black men were not permitted to live in the homes of Black women and their children or they would lose their benefits. Cummings (1983) considers the effects of this policy:

> For many years, the nation's primary welfare program, Aid to Families with Dependent Children (AFDC), denied benefits to families if an adult male was in the house. That bar was stricken in 1968, and states were permitted, but not required, to cover two-parent families in which the would-be breadwinner was unemployed or underemployed. Some people believe that the man-in-the-house rule has contributed to family breakup by forcing fathers to leave the home. Others disagree.

Often, Black men and women would not be able to find work, so social services/welfare benefits were the only option, although it must be clear that Black people were not the sole recipients of welfare at any time in the U.S. history. As Kindred (2003) explains, "More white women of childbearing age received AFDC than Black or Hispanic women, but Black and Hispanic women received AFDC in disproportionate numbers." Marchevsky and Theoharis (2000, p432) provide further insight into the AFDC program: Programs existed to keep women working in the home rather than in the workplace–in domesticity. One such program was AFDC which emerged from state level pension programs (1910's and 1920's). These state level pension programs were for White married or widowed women, who it was deemed needed protecting, were termed "deserving mothers" and who were White, were provided with a small subsidy.

Initially known as ADC (Aid for Dependent Children), its name was changed to AFDC in 1950. The purpose was to allow mothers to stay home with their children, and indeed, they were required to do so (Marchevsky & Theoharis, 2000). Kindred (2003) explains the workings of the program:

> AFDC, as a federally mandated program, was designed to be a federal–state partnership, intended to provide cash assistance to needy children. The federal law required states to provide cash assistance to all eligible families. Each state administered the program and established the income eligibility level and the benefit level available to families within the state, in keeping with federal limitations. The federal government monitored the states' administration of the program and matched the state funds provided (p. 431).

Further, Kindred (2003) explains the program's outcomes:

> According to the Census Bureau, about 14 million people were receiving AFDC in 1995. This included 3.8 million mothers ages of 15 to 44 years; 500,000 mothers age 45 and over; 300,000 fathers living with dependent children; and 9.7 million children. Nearly half of women on AFDC have

never been married. The average mother on AFDC gave birth at age 20, compared to age 23 for women not on AFDC. The average AFDC family has 2.6 children, compared to 2.1 children for families not on AFDC…. More white women of childbearing age receive AFDC than black or Hispanic women, but black and Hispanic women received AFDC in disproportionate numbers. About 63.5 percent of AFDC recipients lived in private-market housing; only about 9 percent lived in public housing. (p. 432)

The AFDC would eventually evolve into the **Temporary Assistance for Needy Families (TANF)**. As described by Marchevsky and Theoharis (2000), Temporary Assistance for Needy Families (TANF) was a state program, which fell under the auspices of welfare reform (1955). Congress passed a law entitled the Personal Responsibility and Work Opportunity Reconciliation Act (PRA, Public Law 104-193). This eliminated Aid to Families with Dependent Children (AFDC), which was a cash assistance program. TANF followed shortly after as a temporary measure with the aim of moving those who had been receiving welfare to work. It also had the added component of 'family values' in that one of its aims was to encourage poor people to marry.

This reform is considered controversial. Those who were against it deemed it punitive for the poor, while others found it a necessary measure to stop dependency. No matter one's perspective, the reality is that it did not respond to "the real demographics of poverty—the inadequate labor market, a lack of childcare and health benefits, urban divestment from social services and poor communities" (Marchevsky & Theoharis, 2000). Welfare rolls had to be decreased by at least 50 percent by the year 2000 with a 5-year limit on cash benefits. Also, 80 percent of states' welfare recipients were required to find work within 2 years. The options were find a job, work for the public sector (workfare), or lose their benefits (Marchevsky & Theoharis, 2000).

The bottom line is that programs to assist the poor, particularly poor women and their children, are based on the poverty level. Kindred (2003), citing researchers in the field, explains how the government goes about defining poverty:

> To assess the number of persons living in poverty, the government uses a poverty index by which it sets thresholds that take into account total family income and family size; the thresholds are adjusted annually for inflation. According to this measure, "for example, the 1995 poverty threshold for a single individual was $7,929, while for a family of four (two adults, two children), the threshold was $15,455, and for a family of six (two adults, four children) the threshold was $20,364." In 1998, the official poverty threshold for a family of four was $16,660. According to the official poverty measure "more than 20% of the nation's 67 million children are poor (p. 421)."

Women and children are severely impacted by poverty in the United States. Until this problem is addressed health disparities will persist. As welfare reform has caused a grave impact, further problems have ensued that are specifically impacting emerging majorities, particularly Black women. One specific example is mass incarceration.

▶ Mass Incarceration and Black Women

Mass incarceration is a serious issue in the Black community. It is a contributing factor to the disruption/destruction of the Black family, leading to the lack of availability of Black men for Black women to marry and leaving Black women alone to raise their children. Wolfers, Leondhart, and Quealy (2015) explain the effects of this problem on the family:

> The disappearance of these men has far-reaching implications. Their absence disrupts family formation, leading both to lower marriage rates and higher rates of childbirth outside marriage, as research by Kerwin Charles, an economist at the University of Chicago, with Ming-Ching Luoh, has shown...black women...find that potential partners of the same race are scarce, while men...don't need to compete as hard. ...The imbalance has also forced women to rely on themselves...to support a household.

However, the mass incarceration of Black people does not pose a problem to the Black family solely in regard to Black women being left to raise children alone. The reality is that Black women are also disproportionately imprisoned. The American Civil Liberties Union (n.d.) provides the following insights:

> Women of color are significantly overrepresented in the criminal justice system. Black women represent 30% of all incarcerated women in the U.S., although they represent 13% of the female population generally. Hispanic women represent 16% of incarcerated women, although they make up only 11% of all women in the U.S.

Mass incarceration is an atrocity beyond belief. Often, there is lack of consideration regarding how such a process of imprisoning people, in vast numbers, impacts health. However, when families are destroyed, under such tragic circumstances, the stress related to the loss of loved ones and the economic fallout of such is beyond comprehension in terms of family devastation. Mass incarceration has been likened to a public health epidemic. *The New York Times* Editorial Board (2014) offers the following thoughts:

> When swaths of young, mostly minority men are put behind bars, families are ripped apart, children grow up fatherless, and poverty and homelessness increase. Today 2.7 million children have a parent in prison, which increases their own risk of incarceration down the road.

Failure to deal with the debilitating effects of poverty as well as the implementation of practices that contribute to it, such as mass incarceration, will not serve to close the health status gap but to widen it, particularly for emerging majority women.

▶ Emerging Majority Providers

Unfortunately, on July 1, 2012, the government disallowed the option of federal subsidized loans for graduate students. Essentially, this means that interest accrues on student loans while individuals are pursuing graduate/professional studies, including medicine. This course was deemed necessary as the Congressional Budget Office indicated it was either the end of subsidized loans or the end of the Pell Grant. Pell Grants are funds that are made available to low-income students for colleges (Hopkins, 2012). The Pell Grant time frame was also reduced from 9 to 6 years, which means less availability of those funds to graduate students. Hence, the outcome is insurmountable debt for future physicians and other healthcare professionals and the need to take out unsubsidized loans to fund their studies, as the options for merit scholarships and other competitive funds are limited.

To make matters worse, the interest rates on the loans are very high, at 7.9 percent for Grad Plus Loans. Hence, individuals, particularly those most in need of funding to pursue their education—emerging majorities—may opt out of pursuing degrees in the health professions, due to the high cost and tremendous debt for doing so.

Overall, there is a projected shortage of 45,000 primary care doctors and 46,000 specialists by 2020 (Ollove, 2014). This is clearly a problem given the increase in the number of people with health insurance resulting from passage of the Affordable Care Act (ACA) in March of 2010, as millions of Americans are now required to get health insurance or pay a fine. Although more access to care is positive, there must be a sufficient number of culturally competent healthcare providers to meet the demand. The ACA also includes the addition of extra fees and equipment for private practicing physicians. This expense has driven many out of private practice and into hospitals as employees (Gottlieb, 2013), contributing still further to the physician shortage.

The impact of this scenario on the overall population, and women in particular, is dreadful. To improve the health status of low socioeconomic status women of color, who are not at parity in terms of health with their White affluent counterparts, preventive care is essential. Preventive care involves lifestyle changes, good diets, exercise regimens, and optimal health care. One of the prime goals of the ACA is to focus on preventive care. However, given the shortage of physicians and the pressures, timewise, associated with seeing more patients, how will that goal be accomplished? Patients now have less time with their providers, and preventive care requires significant time, effort, and information distribution through effective communication.

Many physicians, and other healthcare providers in the United States, have major concerns about income, paperwork associated with ACA requirements, repayment of student loans, mass patient influxes, and other woes that occur in such a strenuous environment. These pressures lead to a bottom-line approach rather than an approach focused on reducing health disparities. For poor, emerging majority women in particular, who are in dire need of optimal health care before, during, and after pregnancy (if they have children), this is a major problem that must be resolved. There is no doubt that the patient–doctor relationship has an impact on disparities in medical care (Street, O'Malley, Cooper, & Haidet, 2008).

▶ Solutions

The primary issues that contribute to health disparities in regard to women are race and ethnicity, culture, and low socioeconomic status. The convergence of these factors leads to a multitude of issues, including lack of access to optimal health care, lack of sufficient education, lack of access to healthy/quality foods, low self-esteem, stress, racism, discrimination, and lack of trust of the medical establishment.

Some of the solutions, broadly speaking, to close the health status gap for women include the following:

- Establishing economic parity between men and women in the United States
- Ensuring access to optimal care for poor people
- Improving the educational system in low-income communities in the United States
- Eliminating racism and discrimination in the United States, specifically as directed toward emerging majority women
- Verifying, communicating, and establishing, in an effort to gain trust toward the medical establishment, that medical experimentation and mistreatment is not currently occurring and will not in the future occur against emerging majorities in the United States
- Recognizing and understanding cultural norms and the need to modify diet (e.g., soul food) and exercise regimens
- Ensuring that women are taken care of before pregnancy, throughout the duration of their lives, not just during pregnancy
- Educating healthcare providers and researchers about the culture, history, and socioeconomic status of women in an effort to improve birth outcomes for all
- Providing culturally competent care for diverse groups, recognizing that these groups have diverse histories, languages, cultures, religions, beliefs, and traditions that impact women's health outcomes
- Recognizing the importance of health literacy in improving the health status of women and their families, as women are usually the caretakers of health for their households/families
- Educating and placing more physicians and other healthcare providers of color in low-income communities
- Improving the U.S. poverty crisis and unemployment concerns in terms of women's health overall, ensuring access to health care and other necessary resources
- Ending mass incarceration in the United States, thus enabling the rebuilding of families of color, particularly Black families, and the elimination of significant stress on low-income communities related to such

Ultimately, the U.S. medical system must be willing to tailor its efforts to meet the needs of emerging majority women, women of low socioeconomic status and poor White women and to ensure them access to care in culturally competent environments to offer a comfort level, culturally and beyond. One step toward this outcome would be ensuring more emerging majority participants in their workforces, from staff to clinicians. Furthermore, there must be recognition of the myriad problems impacting all women, beginning with poverty and the impact of these conditions on women's overall health and the health of their children and their families at large. Issues of racism and discrimination must not be ignored as a factor contributing to the poor health of emerging majority women, particularly of Black women, who are impacted disproportionately. It must be clear that Hispanic is not a race but rather an ethnicity; thus, Black Hispanic (Spanish-speaking) women must be included in the category with Black women in general when considering the numbers related to health, or lack thereof, of Hispanic people.

Wrap-Up

Chapter Summary

Race, ethnicity, socioeconomic status, and diet are some of the factors associated with health disparities and women. Some key health issues to focus on in regard to women are diabetes, hypertension, cancer, and birth outcomes. Poverty must be emphasized in exploring the health status of women, along with issues that contribute to the problem, such as loss of the family wage and mass incarceration. Solutions toward closing the health status gap for women, particularly emerging majority women and all women experiencing poverty, must be sought.

Chapter Problems

1. Explain the difference between Temporary Assistance for Needy Families (TANF), Aid for Dependent Children (ADC), and Aid to Families With Dependent Children (AFDC).
2. How are student loans contributing to the shortage of healthcare practitioners?
3. What is mass incarceration, and what is its relevance to some emerging majority communities and their health status?
4. List and explain three potential solutions that may positively impact the goal of closing the health status gap for women in the United States.
5. What is the family wage?

References

American Civil Liberties Union. (n.d.). Facts about the over-incarceration of women in the United States. Retrieved from https://www.aclu.org/facts-about-over-incarceration-women-united-states

Braithwaite, R., Taylor, S., & Treadwell, H. (1992). *Health issues in the Black community (p. 55)*. San Francisco, CA: Jossey Bass.

Central Intelligence Agency. (2009). *The world factbook*. Retrieved from https://www.cia.gov/library/publications/the-world-factbook/docs/profileguide.html

Counihan, C., & Esterik, P. (1997). *Food and culture: A reader (p. 272)*. New York, NY: Routledge.

Cummings, N. (1983, November 20). Breakup of Black family imperils gains of decades. *The New York Times*. Retrieved from http://www.nytimes.com/1983/11/20/us/breakup-of-black-family-imperils-gains-of-decades.html?pagewanted=all

Eyler, A., Baker, E., Cromer, L., King, A., Brownson, R., & Donatelle, R. (1998). Physical activity and minority Women: A qualitative study. *Health Education and Behavior, 25*(5), 640–652.

Fraad, H. (2016, March 25). Economic update: How capitalism changes intimacy and family. *Economic Update [radio broadcast]*. New York, NY: WBAS.

Gottlieb, S. (2013). The doctor won't see you now. He's clocked out. *The Wall Street Journal*, Retrieved from http://www.lucasgeorgandellis.com/Documents/OPINION.pdf

Hill, S. (2009). Cultural images and the health of African American women. *Gender and Society, 23*(6), 733–746.

Hope, Y. (2013, September 17). Four in five in USA face near-poverty, no work. *USA Today*. Retrieved from http://www.usatoday.com/story/money/business/2013/07/28/americans-poverty-no-work/2594203/

Hopkins, K. (2012, March 13). Grad students to lose federal loan subsidy. *U.S. News*. Retrieved from http://www.usnews.com/education/best-graduate-schools/paying/articles/2012/03/13/grad-students-to-lose-federal-loan-subsidy

Kaiser Family Foundation. (2009). Putting women's health care disparities on the map: Examining racial and ethnic disparities at the state level. Retrieved from https://kaiserfamilyfoundation .files.wordpress.com/2013/01/7886es.pdf

Kindred, K. P. (2003). Of child welfare and welfare reform: The implications for children when contradictory policies collide. *William and Mary Journal of Women and the Law, 9*(3). Retrieved from http://scholarship.law.wm.edu/cgi/viewcontent.cgi?article=1169&context=wmjowl

Marchevsky, A., & Theoharis, J. (2000). "Welfare reform, globalization and the racialization of entitlement". *American Studies, 41*(2/3), 235–265.

Munford, M. B. (1994). Relationship of gender, self-esteem, social class and racial identity to depression in Blacks. *Journal of Black Psychology, 20*(2), 157–174.

Murthy, P., & Smith, C. (2010). *Women's global health and human rights* (p. 148). Sudbury, MA: Jones and Bartlett Learning.

Musa, D., Schulz, R., Harris, R., Silverman, M., & Thomas, S. (2009). Trust in the health care system and the use of preventive health services by older Black and White adults. *American Journal of Public Health, 99*(7), 1293–1299.

The New York Times Editorial Board. (2014, November 26). Mass imprisonment and public health. The opinion pages. *The New York Times*. Retrieved from http://www.nytimes.com/2014/11/27 /opinion/mass-imprisonment-and-public-health.html?_r=0

Ollove, M. (2014). Are there enough doctors for the newly insured? Kaiser Health News. Retrieved from http://khn.org/news/doctor-shortage-primary-care-specialist/

Spencer, D. (2010). The legacy of Tuskegee: Investigating trust in medical research and health disparities. *Journal of the Student National Medical Association*. Retrieved from http://jsnma .org/2010/09/the-legacy-of-tuskegee-investigating-trust-in-medical-research-and-health -disparities/

Street, R., O'Malley, K. J., Cooper, L. A., & Haidet, R. (2008). Understanding concordance in patient–physician relationships. *Annals of Family medicine, 6*(3), 198–205.

Taylor, T., Williams, C., Makambi, H., Mouton, C., Harrell, J., Cozier, Y., ... Adams-Campbell, L. (2007). Racial discrimination and breast cancer incidence in U.S. Black women: The Black Women's Health Study. *American Journal of Epidemiology, 166*(1), 46–54.

Strain, T. H. (Director). (2008). When the bough breaks [Video documentary episode]. In T. H. Strain, R. MacLowry, & E. Stange (Producers), *Unnatural Causes: Is Inequality Making Us Sick?* San Francisco, CA: Newsreel With Vital Pictures.

Wolfers, J., Leonhardt, D., & Quealy, K. (2015, April 20). 1.5 million missing Black men. *The New York Times*. Retrieved from http://www.nytimes.com/interactive/2015/04/20/upshot/missing -black-men.html?_r=0

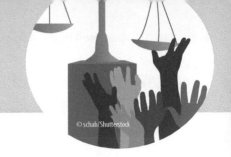

CHAPTER 9

Health Disparities and the Impact on the Lives of Children: Issues, Concerns, and Solutions

Clarence Cryer, Jr., MPH

Health disparities are differences in the incidence, prevalence, mortality and burden of disease and other adverse health conditions that exist among specific groups in the United States.

—**The National Institutes of Health**

KEY TERMS

Agency for Healthcare Research and
   Quality (AHRQ)
asthma
childhood obesity
discrimination

Healthy People 2010 and 2020
National Healthcare Disparities Report
   (NHDR)
social determinant of health

LEARNING OBJECTIVES

After reading this chapter, you should be able to do the following:

1. Identify health conditions with a disproportionate representation of traditional minority and poor children.
2. Discuss viable solutions and potential barriers to achieving health equity.
3. Understand the relationship between socioeconomic status/race and health status of the nation's children.
4. Explain the potential impact of changing demographics on the overall health status of the nation's children.

▶ Introduction

The dawn of the 21st century, the United States is marked by renewed and continued interest in longstanding inequities in the nation's health status. This reaffirmed allegiance to social justice is coupled with deliberate action to illuminate and purge historical imbalances characterized by significant differences in illness and mortality between population subgroups. In 2000, the National Institutes of Health founded the National Center on Minority Health and Health Disparities (NCMHD, 2016). The mission of the NCMHD is to lead scientific research to improve minority health and eliminate inequalities. In 2003, the **Agency for Healthcare Research and Quality (AHRQ)** issued its first annual *National Healthcare Disparities Report (NHDR)* (AHRQ, 2003). The *NHDR* was the first national comprehensive effort to measure differences in the quality of, and access to, healthcare services overall and by various populations. The same year, a milestone study of disparities, *Unequal Treatment: Confronting Racial and Ethnic Disparities in Health Care*, was released by the Institute of Medicine (Smedley, Stith, & Nelson, 2003). The Department of Health and Human Services (DHHS) included the reduction of disparities as a primary goal in its initial **Healthy People** initiative, Healthy People 2000. This publication of national initiatives for improving the health of all Americans is updated every 10 years. For the next two decades, overarching goals of the program have included health disparities: Healthy People 2010 focused on the elimination and, not just the reduction of, health disparities (DHHS, 2000b). In Healthy People 2020, the goal was expanded even further: to achieve health equity, eliminate disparities, and improve the health of all groups (DHHS, 2000b). The elimination of health inequities is also a strategic imperative of the Centers for Disease Control and Prevention (CDC, 2010b). In 2006, a federal bipartisan bill (the Minority Health Improvement and Health Disparity Elimination Act) targeting healthcare disparities was introduced (govtrack.us, 2006). These initiatives invoked the anticipation of equity in the new era.

A review of strategic plans for the Eunice Kennedy Shriver National Institute of Child Health and Human Development (National Institute of Child Health and Human Development, 2000) confirms that the new millennium zeal for achieving parity in health did not discount our nation's youth. Consistent with this trend, the elimination of health disparities appeared as the first of three Maternal and Child Health Bureau goals in 2003 (Van Dyck, 2003). In a 2006 report (*Improving Children's Health*), the Children's Defense Fund advised that reducing health disparities among children is an important aspect of improving the well-being of all children and, by extension, the nation as a whole (Children's Defense Fund, 2006). Despite numerous efforts at the turn of the century, disparities in illness and death experienced by traditional minorities (people of color) and the poor, including their children, remain a major obstacle to improving national health.

Disparate health remains at the forefront of the nation's priorities. It is a reality confirmed and supported by the review, analysis, and summary of currently available data. Decades of empirical research demonstrate the persistent (longstanding), extensive (across racial/ethnic and sociodemographic groups), and profuse (including a litany of health conditions) nature of this national tragedy. Understanding the impact on the lives of children is the goal of this chapter, which reviews the related issues, concerns, and solutions.

▶ The Health of U.S. Children: Historical Perspective

Compared to their peers in earlier times, the health status of America's nearly 80 million children has generally improved. Collectively, they have a much brighter outlook than did people 18 years and younger during the 19th and 20th centuries. In the 1800s, many children were undernourished, and many did not survive to adulthood, often dying of diseases that are now easily cured or prevented.

At the beginning of the 20th century, infectious diseases, including diarrheal diseases, diphtheria, measles, pneumonia and influenza, scarlet fever, tuberculosis, typhoid and paratyphoid fevers, and whooping cough remained leading causes of child mortality (Guyer, Freedman, Strobino, & Sondik, 2000). Toward the end of the 1900s, the percentage of child deaths attributable to infectious diseases declined from 61.6 percent in 1900 to 2 percent by 1998 (Guyer et al., 2000).

During the first decade of the 21st century, there was a shift from infectious disease to unintentional injuries and homicide as the first and second leading causes of death. These causes jointly accounted for 47.0 percent of all deaths of children and adolescents in 2011 (Hamilton, Hoyert, Martin, Strobino, & Guyer, 2013). Today, prevention efforts have led to the elimination/reduction of previously fatal or disabling conditions. Twenty-first-century survival rates for major childhood diseases are high. There have been remarkable declines in mortality from pneumonia and influenza, birth defects, prematurity and low birth weight, respiratory distress syndrome, sudden infant death syndrome, and unintentional injuries (Hamilton et al., 2013).

Since the 19th century, overall life expectancy (see **FIGURE 9-1**) has increased from just under 50 years of age to nearly 80 years in the current century. Infant mortality (deaths to infants during the first year of life, measured as the rate of infant deaths per 1,000 live births) has decreased consistently over the past several decades (see **FIGURE 9-2**). Improvements in living conditions, advances in medicine and

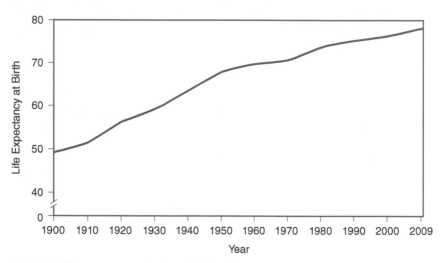

FIGURE 9-1 Life expectancy at birth in the United States, 1900–2009.

National Institutes of Health. (n.d.). *The NIH Almanac: National Center on Minority Health and Health Disparities.* Retrieved from https://www.nih.gov/about-nih/what-we -do/nih-almanac/nih-organization

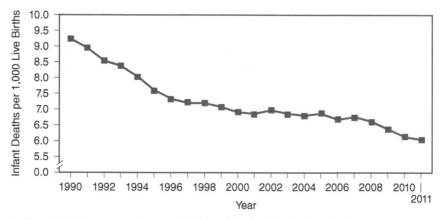

FIGURE 9-2 U.S. infant mortality rates, 1990–2010, final and preliminary, 2011.

Agency for Healthcare Research and Quality. (2003). *National Healthcare Disparities Report.* Rockville, MD: U.S. Department of Health and Human Services, Agency for Healthcare Research and Quality.

health care, reductions in smoking during pregnancy, and increased access to, and use of, prenatal care have all been suggested as responsible factors (National Center for Health Statistics, 2010; Singh & Kogan, 2007; Singh & Yu, 1995).

Life expectancy and infant mortality are vital statistics generally regarded as key indicators of the nation's health. These factors influence policy development as well as research and program funding. In conjunction with better public policies, the nation's rising standard of living, improving nutrition, and income support, pro- grams have also improved circumstances (DHHS, CDC, 2012). This information is critical to measuring health-related quality improvement and progress toward pub- lic health goals for our nation's children.

▶ Issues Relating to Health Disparities

Many dimensions of disparity exist in the United States, particularly in health. If a health outcome is seen to a greater or lesser extent between populations, there is disparity. Despite remarkable improvements in the national health status of children, undeniable challenges remain. The gains have not been evenly distributed. Inequalities have endured for prolonged periods. In fact, the persistence of disparities over time is one of the most arresting features in the history of U.S. health (Satcher et al., 2005). Inequalities have continued (often worsening) despite programs targeting elimination. Over the past several decades, there have been many policy agendas to improve access to societal resources, including medical care. Special initiatives that began in the 1960s, such as the War on Poverty, civil rights legislation, and Medicaid and Medicare have essentially failed. The lack of parity in health for affected groups (including children) has not improved in over 50 years (Williams & Jackson, 2005).

Some children continue to have higher rates of unfortunate health conditions. They also tend to have more barriers to care, poorer quality of care, and unfavorable health outcomes. These differences are best understood within the context of the **social determinants of health**. The World Health Organization (WHO) defines social determinant of health as the conditions in which people are born, grow, live, work, and age. It is the distribution of money, power, and resources at global, national, and local levels that shapes these unfortunate circumstances (National Rural Health Alliance, 2016).

Likewise, the pervasive (ubiquitous and unwelcomed) influence and effect of disparate health are spread widely throughout various groups of children defined by race and ethnicity. A number of studies reinforcing the impact of race and ethnicity on the health of children indicate that children of color (African Americans, Native Americans/Alaska Natives, Latinos/Hispanics, and Asian Americans/Pacific Islanders) or traditional minorities are more likely than are White children to experience adverse health, growth, and development from birth through adolescence and into adulthood (Children's Defense Fund, 2006).

The disparate issues tied to race not only exist but continue to flourish, owing in part to the conditions from which they emerge: geographic location, education, income, and other sociodemographic variables. Public health research increasingly recognizes that racial/ethnic disparities in health are rooted in these and other social issues (Williams & Jackson, 2005). It follows that disparity in socioeconomic status is a fundamental cause of health inequity in the United States and that health disparities among children are best understood as a combination of the effects of race, ethnicity, and socioeconomic status.

To reiterate, children in Non-White or low socioeconomic status families are prone to poorer health than are children in White or higher socioeconomic status homes across profuse conditions. The profusion of adverse health among poor children and children of color is enumerated in a litany of inequities in morbidity and mortality. This list includes, but is not limited to, incidence, prevalence, and outcomes in infant mortality (Kung et al., 2008), oral health (Paradise, 2012), pediatric asthma (McDaniel, Paxon, & Waldfogel, 2006), childhood obesity (Federal Interagency Forum, 2015; Wang & Beydoun, 2007), and juvenile diabetes (CDC, 2014). A closer look at some of these conditions provides a better understanding of the impact of disparate health on the lives of children.

The Impact of Infant Mortality

Infant mortality is one of the health statistics most frequently used to compare national healthcare systems. It has long been understood as a reflection of how well a society takes care of its most vulnerable citizens and demonstrates the level of commitment to preventing potential adverse consequences of low socioeconomic status.

Dramatic declines among all demographic groups represent a major public health success. The preliminary infant mortality rate for 2011 was 6.05 infant deaths per 1,000 live births—not significantly different from the 2010 rate of 6.15 deaths per 1,000 live births. When viewed over time, however, a clear trend emerges: between 1990 and 2011, infant mortality in the United States dropped 34 percent. Although the national rate has exponentially declined, disparities in infant mortality remain marked (National Center for Health Statistics, 2010; Singh & Yu, 1995).

In a 2010 publication, the Health Resources and Services Administration, Maternal and Child Health Bureau, reported that during 1935–2007, the infant mortality rate for White infants declined by 3.2 percent per year, while the rate for Black infants declined by 2.6 percent annually. As a result of the slower decline in mortality for Black infants, the racial disparity in the infant mortality rate increased between 1935 and 2007 (Singh & van Dyck, 2010). In 1935, the rate for Black infants was 81.9 deaths per 1,000 live births, 58 percent higher than the rate for White infants (51.9). In 2007, the Black infant mortality rate of 13.2 was 135 percent higher than the White infant mortality rate of 5.6 (see **FIGURE 9-3**).

The U.S. infant mortality rate is consistently ranked among the bottom when compared internationally. According to the CDC, the United States has higher

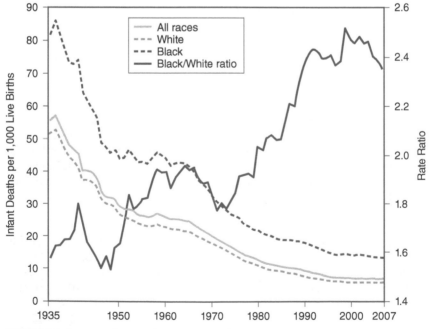

FIGURE 9-3 Infant mortality rates by race—United States, 1935–2007.

Singh, G. K., & van Dyck, P. C. (2010). *Infant mortality in the United States, 1935–2007: Over seven decades of progress and disparities. A 75th anniversary publication.* Rockville, MD: U.S. Department of Health and Human Services, Health Resources and Services Administration, Maternal and Child Health Bureau.

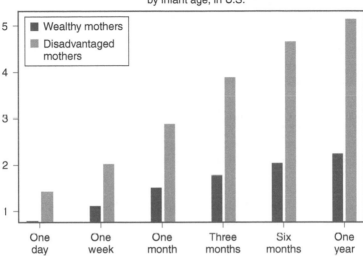

Cumulative probability of infant death per 1,000 live births, by infant age, in U.S.

FIGURE 9-4 A growing income gap in infant mortality.

Data from Chen, A., Oster, E., & Williams, H. (2014, September). Why is infant mortality higher in the U.S. than in Europe? NBER Working Paper No. 20525. Retrieved from http://www.eccbouldercounty.org/wp-content/uploads/2016/07/Infant-Mortality-Brown-University.pdf

rates of infant mortality than any of the other 27 wealthy countries. In 2014, Chen, Oster, and Williams reported that higher infant mortality in the United States is due "entirely, or almost entirely, to high mortality among less advantaged groups" (Chen, Oster, & Williams, 2014). In other words, babies born to poor mothers in the United States are significantly more likely to die in their first year than are babies born to wealthier mothers (see **FIGURE 9-4**).

While considerable data imply a significant portion of the financial burden is owed to traditional minorities and the poor, there are no current estimates of the total cost or economic effect of infant mortality at the national level. The bulk of associated costs stems from treating the individual and collective impact of preterm and low-weight births. In 2007, the Institute of Medicine found that annual expenses associated with premature birth in the United States totaled $26.2 billion, broken down as follows: $16.9 billion in medical and healthcare costs for the baby, $1.9 billion in labor and delivery costs, $611 million for early intervention services, $1.1 billion for special education services, and $5.7 billion in lost work and pay for people born prematurely (Behrman & Butler, 2007).

In terms of fiscal demands, direct costs of preterm and low-weight births have been clearly quantified. The emotional toll of these precursors to infant mortality is undeniable but less tangible. A negative impact on the quality of life for children and their families is certain.

The Impact of Oral Health

Childhood tooth decay (dental cavities and caries) is one of the most common chronic infectious diseases for children in the United States (Dye, Xianfen, & Beltrán-Aguilar, 2012). The epidemic affects about 1 of 5 (20%) children aged 5 to 11 years who have at least one untreated decayed tooth and 1 of 7 (13%) adolescents aged 12 to 19 years with at least one untreated decayed tooth (Dye, Thornton-Evans, Li, & Iafolla, 2015). It is a public health crisis that poses immediate and long-term threats, not just to the teeth of young children but to their overall health and development.

Despite major improvements for the population as a whole, profound disparities persist in children from some races and ethnic groups. In March 2015, the National Center for Health Statistics reported that Black and Latino children are about twice as likely as White children to have untreated tooth decay in primary teeth (Dye et al., 2015). Association between tooth decay and socioeconomic status has been well documented. Studies suggest that it is more commonly found in children who live in poverty or in poor economic conditions (Colak, Dülgergil, Dalli, & Hamidi, 2013). Furthermore, the burden of untreated dental caries is also concentrated among low-income children (see **FIGURE 9-5**). The percentage of children and adolescents aged 5 to 19 years with untreated tooth decay is twice as high for those from low-income families (25%) as compared with children from higher-income households (11%) (Dye et al., 2015).

Understanding the relationship between oral health and general health underscores the consequences of oral health disparities for children. These inequities are due wholly and in part to complex social and behavioral determinants. Many children, especially those from low-income and traditional minority families, lack basic dental care. The economic factors that often relate to poor oral health include lack of access to health services and an individual's ability to get and keep dental insurance. Oral health has been well established as a fundamental component of general health. Many systemic diseases and conditions have oral manifestations. These manifestations may be the initial sign of clinical disease and, as such, serve to inform clinicians and individuals of the need for further assessment (DHHS, 2000b). Children without regular dental care forfeit this residual benefit. Other consequences of oral

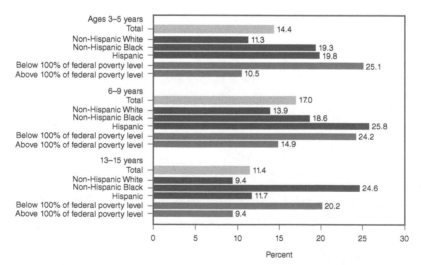

FIGURE 9-5 Prevalence of untreated dental caries among children and adolescents, by age, race and ethnicity, and poverty level: United States, 2009–2010.

Dye, B. A., Li, X., & Thornton-Evans, G. (2012). *Oral health disparities as determined by selected Healthy People 2020 oral health objectives for the United States, 2009–2010.* NCHS data brief, no 104. Hyattsville, MD: National Center for Health Statistics.

health disparities among children include, but are not limited to, the following: Children with dental problems are three times more likely to experience pain and to miss school than are children with no oral health problems, and poorer oral health status leads to a greater likelihood of reduced academic performance (Jackson, Vann, Kotch, Pahel, & Lee 2011).

Evidence that not all children have achieved the same level of oral health and well-being presents a major challenge. These facts demand the best efforts to address inequities in pediatric oral health.

The Impact of Childhood Obesity

Childhood obesity, which is defined as a body mass index greater than 30 kg/m² and relative to age and gender, has become a serious public health problem in the United States. Changes in obesity prevalence from the 1970s show a rapid increase in the 1980s and 1990s, when obesity prevalence among children and teens tripled, from nearly 5 percent to approximately 15 percent (see **FIGURE 9·6**). The **Healthy People 2020** program identifies obesity as a leading health indicator. The federal initiative calls for significant reduction among children and adolescents, but the nation has made little progress toward the target goal (10%) (DHHS, n.d.). In fact, childhood obesity in the United States affects approximately 12.5 million children and teens. The prevalence of obesity is monitored using data from the National Health and Nutrition Examination Survey (NHANES). Results from the 2011–2012 NHANES indicate that an estimated 16.9 percent of U.S. children and adolescents aged 2 to 19 years are obese, and another 14.9 percent are overweight (Ogden, Carroll, Curtin, Lamb, & Flegal, 2010).

The available data also show disparities between sociodemographic groups (Wang & Beydoun, 2007; Wang & Lobstein, 2006; Wang & Zhang, 2006; WHO,

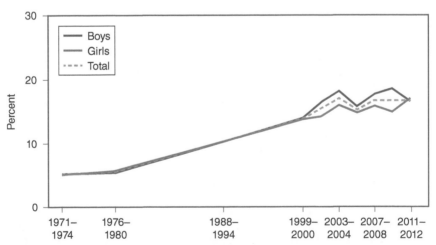

FIGURE 9·6 Trends in obesity among children and adolescents aged 2–19 years, by sex: United States, selected years 1971–1974 through 2011–2012.

CDC/NCHS. National Health and Nutrition Examination Surveys 1971–1974, 1976–1980, 1988–1994, 1999–2000, 2001–2002, 2003–2004, 2005–2006, 2007–2008, 2009–2010, and 2011–2012; Ogden, C. L., Carroll, M. D., Curtin, L. R., Lamb, M. M., & Flegal, K. M. (2010). Prevalence of high body mass index in U.S. children and adolescents, 2007–2008. *JAMA, 303*, 242–249.

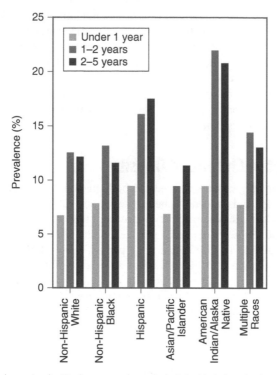

FIGURE 9-7 Prevalence in obesity, by age and race/ethnicity. Variations in the prevalence of childhood obesity in the United States among different races.

Data from Institute of Medicine. (2015). *Examining a developmental approach to childhood obesity: The fetal and early childhood years: Workshop summary*. Washington, DC: The National Academies Press.

2000). The 2015 Institute of Medicine workshop summary *Examining a Developmental Approach to Childhood Obesity* scrutinizes disparities in the prevalence of obesity by age and race/ethnicity (see **FIGURE 9-7**). The recent study shows higher rates of obesity during the fetal and early childhood years among Hispanics and Native Americans. These groups exceed the average rate for all races/ethnicities. Non-Hispanic African Americans and Non-Hispanic Whites have comparatively lower rates, while prevalence among Asian American/Pacific Islanders is lowest in these age groups.

Low-income status (below 130% of the poverty level) is also highly associated with overweight/obese status. This finding is confirmed in a recent summary of data from 68 Massachusetts school districts involving 111,799 students in grades 1, 4, 7, and 10. In the 2015 study on the relationship between childhood obesity, low socioeconomic status, and race/ethnicity, researchers found that low socioeconomic status plays a more significant role in the childhood obesity epidemic than does race/ethnicity. In fact, for every 1 percent increase in low-income status, there was a 1.17 percent increase in overweight/obese status (Rogers et al., 2015). This pattern was observed across all African American and Hispanic rates in the communities studied.

In the short run, obesity can lead to psychosocial problems (Freedman, Mei, Srinivasan, Berenson, & Dietz, 2007). In the long term, it often tracks to adulthood.

The epidemic has also been associated with other consequences: diabetes, asthma, cardiovascular disease, and cancer. In a 2014 study, the best current estimate of the incremental lifetime per capita medical cost of an obese child in the United States relative to a normal-weight child ranged from $12,660 to $19,630 (Finkelstein, Graham, & Malhotra, 2014). In addition to health costs, there is the social stigma associated with being overweight. It is often as damaging to a child as the physical conditions that often accompany obesity.

The Impact of Childhood Asthma

Asthma, a respiratory condition that causes difficulty breathing, is one of the most common chronic disorders affecting children (American Lung Association, 2014). It can be a life-threatening disease if not properly managed. In 2014, an estimated 7 million children under the age of 18 years had asthma in the United States (American Lung Association, 2014). The Child Trends Databank (2015) reports the following trends in asthma prevalence (see **FIGURE 9-8**):

> After a period of fairly steady increase from the 1980s to the mid-1990s the proportion of children with current asthma has remained steady over the past decade, remaining between eight and ten percent. Eight percent of children currently had asthma in 2013.

Not all things are equal when it comes to the burden of asthma. The weight is heavier for children than for the rest of the population (Grant, Wagener, & Weiss, 1999; Mannino et al., 2002). They have two times the rate of emergency department visits and hospitalizations for asthma as compared to adults (Akinbami, 2003). Moreover, it is most common among African American (Black) children, who suffer higher morbidity and mortality. Research also shows that Black children have a higher prevalence of asthma than do White children at all income levels. Even after controlling for numerous factors, studies show that Black children are 20 percent more likely than are White children to be diagnosed with asthma and to have had an attack in the prior year (McDaniel et al., 2006). The Child

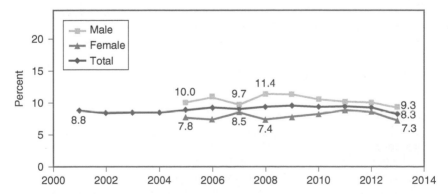

FIGURE 9-8 Percentage of children ages 0–17 reported to have current asthma. Total by gender, 2001–2013.

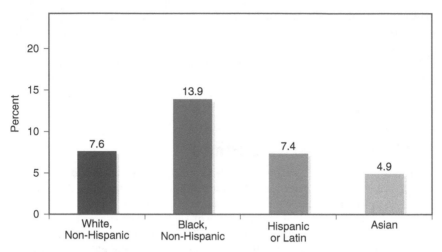

FIGURE 9-9 Percentage of children reported to currently have asthma, by race and Hispanic origin, 2013.

Reproduced from Child Trends Databank. (2015, March). Indicators on children and youth. Retrieved from http://www.childtrends.org/wp-content/uploads/2012/07/43_Asthma.pdf

Trends Databank (2015) explains that Black children are most affected by this disease (see **FIGURE 9-9**):

> Asthma is most common among black children, followed by white and Hispanic children. Asian children are the least likely to currently have asthma. About one in seven (14 percent) of black children had asthma in 2013, compared to eight and seven percent of Hispanic and white children, respectively. Five percent of Asian children were diagnosed with asthma in 2013.

The Child Trends Databank (2015) also notes the correlation between prevalence and income level:

> Asthma is reportedly more common among children living in families with incomes below the federal poverty level. In 2013, 12 percent of children in poor families had asthma, compared with eight percent of children in families that were near-poor and seven percent of children in families that had incomes of at least twice the federal poverty level.)

Living with asthma is fraught with unpopular consequences. It is one of the leading causes of school absenteeism. In 2008, it was associated with an estimated 10.5 million missed school days and was the third leading cause of hospitalization among children under age 15 years (Akinbami, Moorman, & Lui, 2011). The combination of illness-related absence (due to doctors' visits as well as to illness) and potential asthma emergencies in the classroom reduces student and teacher productivity (American Lung Association, 2016) and can negatively affect children's academic performance. While deaths due to asthma are rare among children, the number increases with age. In 2011, asthma claimed the lives of

169 children under the age of 15 years (CDC, National Center for Health Statistics, 2010). According to CDC estimates in 2008, the annual direct healthcare cost of asthma was approximately $50.1 billion. Adding another $5.9 billion for indirect costs (e.g., lost productivity), the total was $56.0 billion (CDC, National Center for Health Statistics, 2008).

▶ Concerns

Despite ongoing efforts to eliminate disproportionate health among children in the United States, the amalgamation of public health data confirms the persistence and often worsening of this national tragedy. Time and again it is the children of the low-income populations and people of color who continue to bear an inferior health status when compared to more affluent and White peers. This imbalance is exaggerated by the ever-widening income gap between the wealthy and the poor (see **FIGURE 9-10**) and the exponential growth of traditional minorities (see **FIGURE 9-11**).

As racial and ethnic demographics in the United States approach an explosion of diversity, this transformative period is also witnessed in the differences between the rich and poor. As divides continue to widen faster than ever, ramifications remain unclear. However, without systemic changes, implications for the improved health status of children are bleak. Existing nationwide trends, along with aggravating and mitigating factors, are of primary concern regarding the impact of health disparities on children.

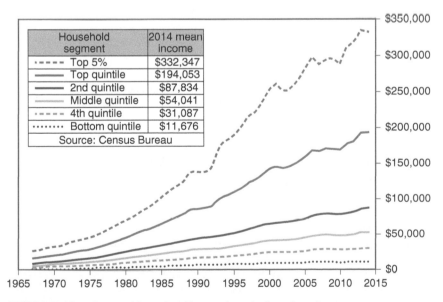

Household segment	2014 mean income
Top 5%	$332,347
Top quintile	$194,053
2nd quintile	$87,834
Middle quintile	$54,041
4th quintile	$31,087
Bottom quintile	$11,676
Source: Census Bureau	

FIGURE 9-10 Mean (average) household income by quintile and top 5 percent.

Reproduced from Short, D. (2015, September 17). U.S. household incomes: A 47-year perspective. Retrieved from http://www.advisorperspectives.com/dshort/updates/2016/09/15/u-s-household-incomes-a-49-year-perspective

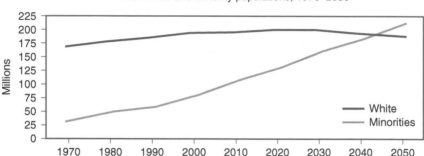

FIGURE 9-11 White and minority populations, 1970–2050.

Reproduced from Frey, W. H. (2015). *Diversity explosion: How new racial demographics are remaking America.* Washington, DC: The Brookings Institution Press.

Widening Income Gap

Wealth inequality (the gap between rich and poor) in the United States has dramatically increased over time. According to the 2013 Survey of Consumer Finances performed by the Board of Governors of the Federal Reserve System, the top 3 percent of income earners held 54.4 percent of all wealth in 2013. This number is up by nearly 10 percent from 44.8 percent in 1989. Conversely, the bottom 90 percent held 24.7 percent of wealth, down from 33.2 percent in 1989. The top 10 percent held 75 percent of wealth.

The Federal Reserve System's triennial survey also indicates that average, or mean, pretax income for the wealthiest 10 percent of U.S. families rose 10 percent in 2013 from 2010, but families in the bottom 40 percent saw their average inflation-adjusted income decline over the same period (Leubsdorf, 2014).

In the last 50 years, real income growth occurred for a small portion of families. Over the last couple of decades, the top quintile of household incomes saw true income growth. The top 5 percent (a tiny portion of the U.S. population) have done exceptionally well. In the remaining 80 percent of households, income growth has been marginal (see Figure 9-10) (Short, 2015). In short, the rich have gotten richer while the poor remain poor.

Growth of Traditional Minority Groups

According to U.S. Census data, the nation reached a demographic milestone in July 2011. For the first time, the majority of new members of society (children younger than 1 year) were Non-White. These traditional minority populations constituted 50.4 percent of babies born in American society during that period. A year prior, this figure was 49 percent. In total, 36.6 percent of the U.S. population were minorities in 2011 (some 114 million people), up from 36.1 percent in 2010 (Wihbey, 2012).

In 2012, the U.S. Census Bureau compiled updated statistics on changing demographic patterns across the United States. The Bureau's findings included the following, as reported by Wihbey (2012):

(1) There are now five "majority-minority" states/districts: California, Texas, Hawaii, New Mexico and the District of Columbia. Additionally,

"more than 11% (348) of the nation's 3,143 counties were majority-minority as of July 1, 2011, with nine of these counties achieving this status since April 1, 2010." (2) "Nationally, the most populous minority group remains Hispanics, who numbered 52 million in 2011; they also were the fastest growing, with their population increasing by 3.1% since 2010. This boosted the Hispanic share of the nation's total population to 16.7% in 2011, up from 16.3% in 2010." (3) "African-Americans were the second largest minority group in the United States, at 43.9 million in 2011 (up 1.6% from 2010)." (4) "Asians, who numbered 18.2 million nationally in 2011, were the second fastest-growing minority group, growing by 3% since 2010." (5) "The nation's American Indian and Alaska Native population was an estimated 6.3 million in 2011, up 2.1% from 2010."

In *Diversity Explosion: How New Racial Demographics Are Remaking America* (2015), author William Frey comments (see Figure 9-11), "I think the big thing in the first half of this century will be the diversity boom that we're seeing in this country. It's the part of the population that's going to change everything." Frey explains that the rapid growth of minorities—Hispanics, Asian Americans, and multiracial people—combined with the slow growth and aging of the White population means that Whites will no longer be a majority of the U.S. population. Moreover, "in about ten years we'll have an absolute decline in the nation's White population" (Frey, 2015). With this new generation of young minorities, who are having children at a faster rate than Whites are, the U.S. Census Bureau projects more minorities than Whites in the United States by 2044.

National Health Status

According to the CDC's Office of Minority Health and Health Equity official website, "minority health determines the health of the nation." In other words, all members of a community are affected by the poor health status of its least healthy members. Infectious diseases, for example, know no racial/ethnic or socioeconomic boundaries (Smedley, Stith, & Nelson, 2003).

The health of the country's most socially advantaged group indicates a level of health that should be possible for everyone. However, studies have shown that children of color have persistently higher adjusted odds of fair or poor health and lower odds of excellent or very good health when compared to White children (Flores & Committee on Pediatric Research, 2010). As currently available data confirm the proliferation of traditional minority populations, if trends in disparate health continue, a decline in the overall health status of the nation is certain. Due to the long-lasting impact of childhood conditions, reducing health disparities among children is vital to improving the well-being of all children and, by extension, the nation as a whole.

Financial Impact

As previously discussed, poor health (e.g., asthma, obesity, oral decay) is costly. It increases direct medical costs (such as emergency department visits and hospitalizations) and indirect costs (lost productivity due to absenteeism). These costs have rapidly increased over time. In fact, as the California Department of Public Health

(2013) reports, "People with chronic conditions account for approximately 80 per-cent of health care costs, 80 percent of hospital admissions, 90 percent of all pre-scriptions filled, and 75 percent of all doctor's visits." Health disparities add to these costs. One study found that disproportionate rates of several common preventable chronic diseases among African Americans and Latinos cost the nation's healthcare system $23.9 billion in 2009 (Waidmann, 2009). The indirect cost of disparities is even higher—an estimated $1 trillion in lost work time and lower productivity from 2003 to 2006 (LaVeist, Gaskin, Richard, 2009). These numbers do not include the personal toll on individuals.

Implications

From a data-informed perspective, the nation is experiencing a surge in its most vul-nerable populations. The association between income, race/ethnicity, and persistent disparities in health, as related to children in the United States, is well documented. These phenomena continue to evolve in environments not only burdened with explosive costs but proven ill-equipped to manage existing challenges. As current trends continue, so does the need for comprehensive interventions that acknowl-edge and appropriately respond to the inequities confronting children's health. Until then, concern for widening income gaps and the growth of traditional minorities is not only valid but fraught with discouraging implications.

Race and Ethnicity

Race and ethnicity continue to play a major role relative to health disparities in the United States. This fact underscores a need for closer attention to the next gener-ation's "minorities." As seen earlier, children of color have fared worse than have White children with respect to various indicators (oral health, obesity, asthma, infant mortality). As the nation's populace becomes more ethnically and racially diverse and less affluent (as patterns imply), its children will potentially become more susceptible to many health conditions and show higher rates of mortality.

Poverty

Disparities in wealth correlate to disparities in children's health. Poverty, like race and ethnicity, is linked to sustained health disparities. It is also strongly associated with multiple risk factors (e.g., education, housing, access to care) for poor health. Children who are lower on the socioeconomic hierarchy suffer disproportionately from almost every disease and show higher rates of mortality than those above them. Low-income children are more likely to be in fair or poor health than are their White contemporaries (Hughes, Kreger, Kushner, Pirani, & Surie, 2007).

When combined, race and poverty have more severe implications. Poverty factors among the full range of social inequalities to which children in communi-ties of color in the United States are often exposed. Inequalities in income contrib-ute significantly to disparities in health for children, particularly children of color (Sanders-Phillips, Settles-Reaves, Walker, & Brownlow, 2009). Poverty and race each involves a myriad of core dynamics. Each has a unique relationship to health outcomes. They are both subject to the positive or negative influence of additional factors critical to the impact of health disparities on children. Two of those factors are *cultural competence* and *discrimination*.

Cultural Competence

The evolving national landscape challenges contemporary mainstream systems to understand and accept differences, engage in self-assessments at individual and organizational levels, and make necessary adaptations to respond effectively. In the face of ongoing change, cultural competence is a major priority. It has been defined as "the ability to [value] understand, appreciate, and interact with persons from cultures and/or belief systems other than one's own, based on various factors" (*Modern Medical Dictionary*, 2015). It has long been recognized as a "prerequisite to achieving equity in health status" (van Dyck, 2003). This prerequisite is worthy of emphasis. It is an essential ingredient in the recipe for responding to actual and projected demographic changes in the United States. One strategy is to ensure a diverse workforce of public health professionals in the most affected communities. (See Appendices II, III, and IV for cultural competence assessment surveys.)

In recognition of the underrepresentation of racial and ethnic minorities in the public health professions, researchers have concluded that a workforce resembling the society it serves is likely to be more effective in improving health equity in the United States (Duffus et al., 2014). Without a culturally competent infrastructure to appropriately address health disparities among emerging populations, elimination of the problem is unlikely.

Discrimination

It is a basic principle of public health that all people, including children, have a right to reach their full health potential. The existence of disparities, particularly among children separated by race and income, is compelling evidence that realization of this right is without equity. Whether requisite and necessary environmental changes, such as social and political policy and supportive behaviors, will keep pace with the changing demography remains to be seen.

Historically, **discrimination**, defined as unjust or prejudicial treatment, has played a significant, if not deliberate, role in establishing and maintaining social imbalances in employment, income, housing, education, and health status. In a 2010 study on child and adolescent health, researchers described racial/ethnic discrimination as the foundation for the proximate causes of the social determinants of racial/ethnic disparities in health (Price, McKinney, & Braun, 2010). Given current demographic changes, implications for the future impact of health disparities on children of color suggest uncertainty. Despite the proliferation of traditional minority children, an optimistic outlook may be premature. History has shown that neither discrimination nor its consequences are easily eliminated. While the Civil Rights Act of 1964 prohibited discrimination, it did not eliminate discriminatory practices already embedded in the nation's structures and institutions. Subsequent court rulings and changes in statutes have continued for more than 50 years in response to sustained discriminatory treatment.

How these and other compelling implications are confronted and managed will prove essential to addressing the impact of health disparities on children. Their resolution is key to successful implementation of comprehensive solutions.

▶ Solutions

Stratospherically high, continually rising healthcare costs and preponderance of evidence will eventually force us to make a core re-evaluation of our healthcare system. We think we're working on radical change, but we're not. We are only making tweaks to our current schema, which is simply unsustainable and completely unable to provide an effective foundation to address our nation's many needs. I predict that constrained by politics and lack of true leadership, our federal partners challenged with the task of architecting change will remain unable to develop the necessary framework to make the changes needed in time to prevent catastrophe. We will instead first have to endure national devastation before doing what we seem to do best: implement patchwork solutions just in the nick of time to stave off death.

—**Raul Recarey**, Office of Health Equity Advisory Committee (former member)
California Department of Public Health, 2016
(Original quote sent via email on May 27, 2016)

The nation's anticipation of health equity for children found tremendous support in the new millennium. Federal agencies, national and local coalitions, and other groups came together in support of this cause. One highlight included the Affordable Care Act (ACA) of 2010. The progress of these efforts is routinely monitored and evaluated. Early reports revealed substantial gaps. More recent data continue to suggest failure and a need for reevaluation and overhaul of our current system. The preponderance of evidence has served to heighten awareness of issues, validate concerns, and inspire commitment to permanent solutions.

In the United States, the elimination of health disparities in children has been historically addressed by a fragmented network, characterized by a series of knee-jerk reactions often referred to as action plans, initiatives, strategies, programs, interventions, or similar buzzwords. Collective stopgap measures have typically been adopted by the federal or state public health authorities in conjunction with local partners to include, among other parties, community health centers and grassroots organizations. Agencies often operate on short-term, shoestring budgets acquired via intense competition for limited funding. Typically, program longevity is highly dependent upon the availability of financial support. Features have included behavioral interventions (focusing on diet and exercise), screenings (for asthma, oral health, and obesity), and public awareness campaigns (such as immunization and fluoride treatment). This list of popular strategies is not exhaustive but includes common public health promotion and health education programs introduced to priority populations. Various health status analyses suggest that continuing the patchwork methodology is not likely to support the federal vision for health care. Leading performance indicators have demonstrated little improvement over the past several decades. The DHHS vision to eliminate health disparities will remain elusive within the current dystopia.

The present model for elimination of this nationwide catastrophe is unsustainable due to ongoing challenges. There is a lack of foundation to tackle and overcome aggravating factors. Health disparities occur across a broad range of dimensions, including poverty, discrimination, and other national crises. Reliance on myopic interventions has consistently proven ineffective. In the absence of a magic bullet, a more systemic resolution is in order. It should include the following essential components.

Transformation

A strong and supportive infrastructure of communities and public health systems is essential to the success of any proposed solution to the national crisis: *health disparities and the impact on the lives of children*. Continued adjustments to our current (failed) system don't work. Starting anew with the development of an overall (all-encompassing) framework is promising. It is a solution that will require cooperation across industry sectors and governments, and thereby challenge the current boundaries and established norms of operation.

Transforming the current system into one of greater value and functionality will require abandonment of the traditional practices that created barriers to advancing the health of racial and ethnic minorities and the poor. These efforts include unconventional linkages between health care and social service agencies that promote health and well-being within specific geographic areas and among specific populations.

Infrastructure

One integrated/interagency, generalized action plan with individual agency responsibilities centered on shared goals and objectives is in order. Without appropriate physical and organizational composition, sustainability is unlikely. It requires effective, accountable, and inclusive participation at all levels. At times, the United States is one country. Other times it is a collection of states. For example, every state has its own version of privacy and security. Even some municipalities have weighed in and created their own unique framework. Each framework is the same as a unique language. When one group does not understand the other, communication is impossible. A transformed infrastructure free of fragmentation would provide assistance to patients and families across providers and care settings.

Funding

Most communities and public health systems are committed to doing the right thing, but the finances are not aligned. Public health systems across the country have wonderful plans, all showing positive returns on investment, yet they cannot get the needed funding to see them through.

The Impact of Social Determinants of Health

Social determinants of health significantly affect health status and are at the core of racial and ethnic disparities. For example, education and income impact access to the resources necessary for health maintenance. Proactively addressing the social determinants of health must be part of any proposed solutions. A participatory approach (buy-in) to understanding and addressing the issues increases the chances of resolving them over the long term. At the local level, community health assessments (CDC, 2010a) have helped to articulate what the social determinants are in a particular geographic area. Such a strategy can identify the need for specific community-based actions. A comprehensive system that identifies these issues would be equipped to readily address and resolve them.

Since discrimination (and its side effects) has been described as the foundation for proximate causes of the social determinants of racial ethnic disparities (Price et al., 2010), a broad-based strategy for the elimination of health disparities in children must include advocacy for necessary changes or implementations in law, policy, and practices relative to discrimination. Addressing determinants of health related to personal choices/behavior and the social environment is a solution requiring continued emphasis.

Cultural Sensitivity

With growing national diversity, the disparity between the racial and ethnic composition of the healthcare workforce and that of U.S. children widens as well. A system that incorporates and promotes awareness of cultural differences without assigning positive or negative values will be better enabled to serve the diverse patient population.

Data Management System

Oversight of data is essential to ensure system effectiveness and should include monitoring and evaluating results over time and the ongoing use of data to develop, implement, and refine solutions. The use of collected information will lead the transformation from documenting health disparities toward eliminating them. Monitoring key performance indicators should occur at regularly scheduled intervals and be reported annually.

Sustainability

Broad-based (comprehensive) strategies for a sustainable system must be implemented in conjunction with appropriate public policy modifications to address social issues that lie at the root of disparities. Effective broad-based systems manage and integrate controlling factors in such a way that optimum health is realized regardless of race, ethnicity, or socioeconomic status. Maximizing quality of care and emphasizing prevention, screening, routine care, and chronic disease management help to cut direct and indirect healthcare costs and reduce financial drains on the system that threaten sustainability.

Education/Awareness and Access

A renewed commitment to prevention, with an emphasis on strengthening community-based approaches to reduce high-risk behaviors, will include creating environments that promote wellness and healthy behaviors to prevent and control chronic diseases and their risk factors. Efforts toward improving access to care are also in progress (e.g., the ACA).

Wrap-Up

Chapter Summary

The harsh reality of health disparities among children remains a persistent problem in the United States. It has led to certain groups experiencing worse health outcomes. While these imbalances are commonly viewed through the lens of race and ethnicity, they occur across a broad range of dimensions (such as poverty and education) and reflect a complex set of individual, social, and environmental factors. These disparities limit continued improvement in the nation's overall health status and result in diminished quality of life, loss of income, and other unnecessary costs.

The issue becomes increasingly important to address as the nation's children become more economically divided and racially diverse. After decades of increased federal, state, and local focus and initiatives to reduce and/or eliminate health disparities, significant barriers to progress remain.

The increasingly diverse population calls for broad and integrated efforts. Solutions must address the wide range of implications that contribute to disparities, including social and environmental factors that extend beyond the healthcare system.

Chapter Problems

1. Compared to the health status of children in the 1800s, has the health status of today's children improved or declined? If it has improved, what are the reasons? If not, why not?
2. What role has discrimination played in social imbalance in U.S. society?
3. Explain the problems associated with childhood obesity.
4. Is the infant mortality rate in the United States high or low? Which racial groups are impacted most severely by infant mortality? Why does this disparity exist?
5. What role does poverty play in the health status of children?

References

Agency for Healthcare Research and Quality. (2003). *National healthcare disparities report*. Rockville, MD: U.S. Department of Health and Human Services, Agency for Healthcare Research and Quality. Retrieved from http://archive.ahrq.gov/qual/nhdr03/nhdr2003.pdf

Akinbami, L. (2003). *Asthma prevalence, health care use and mortality: United States, 2003–05. Centers for Disease Control and Prevention*. Retrieved from http://www.cdc.gov/nchs/data/hestat/asthma03-05/asthma03-05.htm

Akinbami, L. J., Moorman, J. E., & Lui, X. (2011). *Asthma prevalence, health care use, and mortality: United States, 2005–2009. National Health Statistics Reports, 32*. Hyattsville, MD: National Center for Health Statistics.

American Lung Association. (2014). Asthma and children fact sheet. Retrieved from http://www.lung.org/lung-health-and-diseases/lung-disease-lookup/asthma/learn-about-asthma/asthma-children-facts-sheet.html

American Lung Association. (2016). *Why use the asthma friendly schools initiative?* Retrieved from http://www.lung.org/lung-health-and-diseases/lung-disease-lookup/asthma/asthma-education-advocacy/asthma-friendly-schools-initiative/why-use-the-asthma-friendly.html

California Department of Public Health. (2013). *The burden of chronic disease and injury: California, 2013*. Retrieved from http://www.cdph.ca.gov/programs/Documents/Burden%20Report%20 Online%2003-20-13.pdf

Centers for Disease Control and Prevention, National Center for Health Statistics. (2008). *National health interview survey raw data analysis by the American Lung Association Research and Health Education Division using SPSS and SUDAAN software*. Washington, DC: Department of Health and Human Services.

Centers for Disease Control and Prevention, National Center for Health Statistics. (2010). *National hospital ambulatory medical care survey. Analysis by the American Lung Association Research and Health Education Division using SPSS software*. Washington, DC: Department of Health and Human Services.

Centers for Disease Control and Prevention. (2010a). *Community Health Assessment and Group Evaluation (CHANGE) action guide: Building a foundation of knowledge to prioritize community needs*. Atlanta, GA: U.S. Department of Health and Human Services.

Centers for Disease Control and Prevention. (2010b). *Strategic Realignment of Funding to Support Priorities in Sexual Health and STD Disparities Among Racial and Ethnic Minorities July 8, 2010* (Record of the proceedings). Retrieved from https://www.cdc.gov/std/health-disparities /strategic-funding-realignment-report-july-8-2010.pdf

Centers for Disease Control and Prevention. (2014). *National diabetes statistics report: Estimates of diabetes and its burden in the United States, 2014*. Atlanta, GA: U.S. Department of Health and Human Services.

Chen, A., Oster, E., & Williams, H. (2014, September). Why is infant mortality higher in the U.S. than in Europe? NBER Working Paper No. 20525. Retrieved from http://www.eccbouldercounty.org /wp-content/uploads/2016/07/Infant-Mortality-Brown-University.pdf

Child Trends Databank. (2015). *Asthma*. Retrieved from http://www.childtrends.org/?indicators =asthma

Children's Defense Fund. (2006). *Improving children's health: Understanding children's health disparities and promising approaches to address them*. Washington, DC: Author.

Çolak, H., Dülgergil, Ç. T., Dalli, M., & Hamidi, M. M. (2013). Early childhood caries update: A review of causes, diagnoses, and treatments. *Journal of Natural Science Biology and Medicine, 4*(1), 29–38.

Duffus, W. A., Trawick, C., Moonesinghe, R., Tola, J., Truman, B., & Dean, H. D. (2014). Training racial and ethnic minority students for careers in public health sciences. *American Journal of Preventive Medicine, 47*(5), S368–S375.

Dye, B. A., Thornton-Evans, G., Li, X., & Iafolla, T. J. (2015). *Dental caries and sealant prevalence in children and adolescents in the United States, 2011–2012. NCHS data brief, no. 191*. Hyattsville, MD: National Center for Health Statistics.

Dye, B. A., Xianfen, L., & Beltrán-Aguilar, E. D. (2012). *Selected oral health indicators in the United States, 2005–2008*. NCHS data brief, no. 96. Hyattsville, MD: National Center for Health Statistics, Centers for Disease Control and Prevention.

Federal Interagency Forum on Child and Family Statistics. (2015). *America's children: Key national indicators of well-being, 2015*. Washington, DC: U.S. Government Printing Office.

Finkelstein, E. A., Graham, W. C. K., & Malhotra, R. (2014). Lifetime direct medical costs of childhood obesity. *Pediatrics, 133*, 854.

Flores, G., & Committee on Pediatric Research. (2010, April). Racial and ethnic disparities in the health and health care of children. From the American Academy of Pediatrics Technical Report. *Pediatrics, 125*(4).

Freedman, D. S., Mei, Z., Srinivasan, S. R., Berenson, G. S., & Dietz, W. H. (2007). Cardiovascular risk factors and excess adiposity among overweight children and adolescents: The Bogalusa Heart Study. *Journal of Pediatrics, 150*, 12–17.

Freedman, M. A., Strobino, D. M., & Sondik, E. J. (2000). Annual summary of vital statistics: Trends in the health of Americans during the 20th century. *Pediatrics, 106*(6), 1307–1317.

Frey, W. H. (2015). *Diversity explosion: How new racial demographics are remaking America*. Washington, DC: The Brookings Institution Press.

Grant, E. N., Wagener, R., & Weiss, K. B. (1999). Observations on emerging patterns of asthma in our society. *Journal of Allergy Clinical Immunology, 104*, S1–S9.

govtrack.us. (2006). S 4024: Minority Health Improvement and Health Disparity Elimination Act. Retrieved from https://www.govtrack.us/congress/bill.xpd?bill=s109-4024

Guyer, B., Freedman, M. A., Strobino, D. M., & Sondik, E. J. (2000). "Annual summary of vital statistics: Trends in the health of Americans during the 20th century". *Pediatrics, 106*(6), 1307–1317.

Hamilton, B. E., Hoyert, D. L., Martin, J. A., Strobino, D. M., & Guyer, B. (2013). Annual summary of vital statistics: 2010–2011. *Pediatrics, 131*(3). doi:10.1542/peds.2012-3769

Hughes, D., Kreger, M., Kushner, K., Pirani, H., & Surie, D. (2007, February). *Reducing health disparities among children: Strategies and programs for health plans.* San Francisco, CA: NIHCM Foundation.

Institute of Medicine. (2015). *Examining a developmental approach to childhood obesity: The fetal and early childhood years: Workshop summary.* Washington, DC: The National Academies Press.

Jackson, S. L., Vann, Jr., W. F., Kotch, J. B., Pahel, B. T., & Lee, J. Y. (2011). Impact of poor oral health on children's school attendance and performance. *American Journal of Public Health, 101*(10), 1900–1906.

Kung, H. S., Hoyert, D. L., Xu, J., & Murphy, S. L. (2008, January). Deaths: Final data for 2005. Division of Vital Statistics. U.S. Department of Health and Human Services, National Center for Health Statistics. *National Vital Statistics Report, 56*(10), Table 30.

LaVeist, T. A., Gaskin, D. K., & Richard, P. (2009, September). *The economic burden of health inequalities in the United States. Joint Center for Political and Economic Studies.* Retrieved from http://jointcenter.org/sites/default/files/Economic%20Burden%20of%20Health%20Inequalities%20Fact%20Sheet.pdf

Leubsdorf, B. (2014, September 4). Fed: Gap between rich, poor Americans widened during recovery. *The Wall Street Journal.* Retrieved from http://www.wsj.com/articles/fed-gap-between-rich-poor-americans-widened-during-recovery-1409853628

Mannino, D. M., Homa, D. M., Akinbami, L. J., Moorman, J. E., Gwynn, C., & Redd, S. C. (2002). Surveillance for asthma–United States, 1980–1999. *Morbidity and Mortality Weekly Report, 51*(SS-1), 1–13.

McDaniel, M., Paxon, C., & Waldfogel, J. (2006). Racial disparities in childhood asthma in the United States: Evidence from the National Health Interview Survey, 1997 to 2003. *Pediatrics, 117*(5), e868–e877.

Modern Medical Dictionary. (2015). Cultural competence. Retrieved from https://www.modernmedicaldictionary.com/?s=cultural+competence

National Center for Health Statistics. (2010). *Health, United States, 2009 with special feature on medical technology.* Hyattsville, MD: U.S. Department of Health and Human Services.

National Institute of Child Health and Human Development, National Institutes of Health, Department of Health and Human Services. (2000). *Health disparities: Bridging the gap.* Washington, DC: U.S. Government Printing Office.

National Institutes of Health, National Center on Minority Health and Health Disparities. (2016). *The NIH almanac.* Retrieved from https://www.nih.gov/about-nih/what-we-do/nih-almanac/national-institute-minority-health-health-disparities-nimhd

National Rural Health Alliance. (2016). Social determinants of health. Retrieved from http://ruralhealth.org.au/advocacy/current-focus-areas/social-determinants-health

Ogden, C. L., Carroll, M. D., Curtin, L. R., Lamb, M. M., & Flegal, K. M. (2010). Prevalence of high body mass index in U.S. children and adolescents, 2007–2008. *JAMA, 303*, 242–249.

Paradise, J. (2012, June). Children and oral health: Assessing needs, coverage, and access. Kaiser Family Foundation's Commission on Medicaid and the Uninsured. Retrieved from https://kaiserfamilyfoundation.files.wordpress.com/2013/01/7681-04.pdf

Price, J. H., McKinney, M. A., & Braun, R. E. (2010). Social determinants of racial/ethnic health disparities in children and adolescents. Retrieved from http://www.hcno.org/community/Social%20Determinants%20of%20Racial-Ethinic%20Health%20Disparities%20in%20Children%20&%20Adolescents.pdf

Rogers, R., Eagle, T. F., Sheetz, A., Woodward, A., Leibowitz, R., Song, M. K., ... Eagle, K. A. (2015). The relationship between childhood obesity, low socioeconomic status, and race/ethnicity: Lessons from Massachusetts. *Childhood Obesity, 11*(6), 691–695.

Sanders-Phillips, K., Settles-Reaves, B., Walker, D., & Brownlow, J. (2009). Social inequality and racial discrimination: Risk factors for health disparities in children of color. *Pediatrics, 124*(suppl 3).

Satcher, D., Fryer, Jr., G. E., McCann, J., Troutman, A., Woolf, S. H., & Rust, G. (2005). What if we were equal? A comparison of the Black-White mortality gap in 1960 and 2000. *Health Affairs, 24*(2), 459–464.

Short, D. (2015, September 17). *U.S. household incomes: A 47-year perspective.* Retrieved from http://www.advisorperspectives.com/dshort/updates/2016/09/15/u-s-household-incomes-a-49-year-perspective

Singh, G. K., & Kogan, M. D. (2007). Persistent socioeconomic disparities in infant, neonatal, and postneonatal mortality in the United States, 1969–2001. *Pediatrics, 119*(4), e928–e939.

Singh, G. K., & van Dyck, P. C. (2010). *Infant mortality in the United States, 1935–2007: Over seven decades of progress and disparities.* A 75th Anniversary Publication. Health Resources and Services Administration, Maternal and Child Health Bureau. Rockville, MD: U.S. Department of Health and Human Services.

Singh, G. K., & Yu, S. M. (1995). Infant mortality in the United States: Trends, differentials, and projections, 1950 through 2010. *American Journal of Public Health, 85*(7), 957–964.

Smedley, B. D., Stith, A. Y., Nelson, A. R. (Eds.). (2003). *Unequal treatment: Confronting racial and ethnic disparities in health care.* Washington, DC: National Academies Press.

U.S. Department of Health and Human Services. (2000a). *Healthy People 2010: Understanding and improving health.* Washington, DC: Author.

U.S. Department of Health and Human Services. (2000b). *Oral health in America: A report of the Surgeon General—executive summary.* Rockville, MD: U.S. Department of Health and Human Services, National Institute of Dental and Craniofacial Research, National Institutes of Health.

U.S. Department of Health and Human Services. (n.d.). Nutrition and weight status. Healthy People 2020. Retrieved from https://www.healthypeople.gov/2020/topics-objectives/topic/nutrition-and-weight-status/objectives

U.S. Department of Health and Human Services, Centers for Disease Control and Prevention. (2012, September 7). National, state, and local area vaccination coverage among children aged 19–35 Months: United States, 2011. *Morbidity and Mortality Weekly Report, 61*(35), 689–696.

van Dyck, P. C. (2003). A History of child health equity legislation in the United States. *Pediatrics, 112*(suppl 3). Retrieved from http://pediatrics.aappublications.org/content/112/Supplement_3/727

Waidmann, T. (2009, September 22). Estimating the cost of racial and ethnic health disparities. The Urban Institute. Retrieved from http://www.urban.org/UploadedPDF/411962_health_disparities.pdf

Wang, Y., & Beydoun, M. A. (2007). The obesity epidemic in the United States: Gender, age, socioeconomic, racial/ethnic, and geographic characteristics: A systematic review and meta-regression analysis. *Epidemiologic Reviews, 29*, 6–28.

Wang, Y., & Lobstein, T. (2006). Worldwide trends in childhood overweight and obesity. *International Journal of Pediatric Obesity, 1*, 11–25.

Wang, Y., & Zhang, Q. (2006). Are American children and adolescents of low socioeconomic status at increased risk of obesity? Changes in the association between overweight and family income between 1971 and 2002. *American Journal of Clinical Nutrition, 84*, 707–716.

Wihbey, J. (2012, October 25). Census Bureau: Minorities in U.S. growing toward a majority. Retrieved from http://journalistsresource.org/studies/society/race-society/minorities-in-us-growing-toward-majority-census-bureau#sthash.DN3I4ZHV.dpuf

Williams, D. R., & Jackson, P. B. (2005). Social sources of racial disparities in health. *Health Affairs, 24*(2), 325–324.

World Health Organization. (2000). *Obesity: Preventing and managing the global epidemic: Report of a WHO consultation. Technical report series 894.* Geneva, Switzerland: Author.

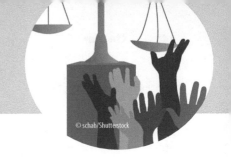

CHAPTER 10

The Elderly and Health Equity

Patti R. Rose, MPH, EdD

Older persons should be able to live in dignity and security and to be free of exploitation and physical and mental abuse.

—From the United Nations Principles for Older Persons

LEARNING OBJECTIVES

After reading this chapter, you should be able to do the following:

1. Understand selected key issues relevant to health disparities/inequities and the elderly population.
2. List chronic diseases that impact the elderly population.
3. Discuss the impact of mass incarceration of the elderly for incarcerated individuals and their families.
4. Explain the term filial piety and its relevance to health equity for the elderly population.

▶ **Introduction**

Respect, obedience, and caring for parents are all key aspects of a concept known as **filial piety**, based on notion of **Confucianism**. This notion of providing the utmost care for the **elderly**, is not such a familiar concept in the United States. This is traditionally a Chinese concept, and relevant to other cultures, but it is definitely one which warrants serious consideration. In terms of care of the elderly, the recent atrocity, in 2017, pertaining to patients in Texas during hurricane Harvey, provides a concrete example of problems that must be considered. In this case, elderly patients, in two **nursing homes**, were left wallowing and suffering in murky, dirty flood waters when the state did not provide evacuation orders for the facilities (Emily, & Branham, n.d.). Additionally, in a nursing home in Florida, 11 elderly people died when they were left in sweltering heat due to the lack of air conditioning in their facility, after Hurricane Irma, in 2018. Apparently, a tree fell, knocking out the power to the air conditioner and the facility did not have a generator (Kennedy & Slotkin, 2017).

The treatment of the elderly, in these seemingly extreme examples, is woefully inadequate. However, it not uncommon, for elderly people to experience myriad problems. Overall, life for the elderly in the United States may involve estrangement from their loved ones, isolation, abuse, **over-medication**, too many surgical procedures and more. In fact, abuse of the elderly is so pervasive that per Bryant, 2019:

> June 15 is recognized internationally as World Elder Abuse Awareness Day, and by wearing Purple on June 15, you show your recognitions of the importance of ending elder abuse. Why purple? Purple represents royalty, a position of respect, and a dignified personage (pg. 24).

Furthermore, in terms of estrangement, many elderly people in the United States live alone. According to (Robnet, Brossoie, & Chop, 2018):

> Older persons of color are more apt to live alone than older White adults. Specifically, 46% of older Black women lived alone, and older Black men live alone three times more often than older Asian men. However, older men of color were more apt to live with relatives than their white counter parts. Approximately 14% of Black and Hispanic men of color lived with a relative other than a spouse compared to only 4 % of white men doing the same. Older people living alone are three times as likely to live in poverty and less likely to view their economic status as "living comfortably." (p. 11).

Further consideration of the health status of the elderly in the United States, per Healthy People 2020, namely those individuals 65 and over, yields a very disconcerting picture as many are plagued by **chronic diseases**. Some of the most prevalent are:

- Heart Disease
- Cancer
- Chronic bronchitis or emphysema
- Stroke

- Diabetes mellitus
- Alzheimer's disease
- Arthritis

Additionally, per Healthy People 2020, falls, the leading cause of injury among older adults, are treated in emergency departments every 13 seconds and claim a life every 20 minutes. Every year, one out of three older adults fall, yet less than half tell their doctor (CDC, 2015).

Greater efforts are needed to assist the elderly to prevent these chronic issues, rather than just treating them after the fact, as they are more apt to use prescription drug treatments, compared to other age groups, to treat chronic problems. Treatment currently outweighs efforts to prevent chronic diseases.

▶ Prescription Drugs

According to the National Center for Health Statistics (NCHS) (2018) "…more than 90% of older people use at least one prescription and more than 66% use three or more in any given month." As a specific example, the *New York Times* recently published an article entitled "Older Americans Are Awash in **Antibiotics**." As stated by Span (2019) in this piece:

> "The drugs are not just overprescribed. They often pose special risks to older patients, including tendon problems, nerve damage and mental health issues."

He further states:

> Patients over age 65 have the highest rate of outpatient prescribing of any age group. A new CDC study, published in the *Journal of the American Geriatrics Society* (AGS), points out that doctors write enough antibiotic prescriptions annually — nearly 52 million in 2014 — for every older person to get at least one.

Additionally, according to a brief report published by the American Geriatric Society

> From 2011 to 2014, outpatient antibiotic prescribing rates remained stable in older U.S. adults (P = .89). In 2014, older adults were dispensed 51.6 million prescriptions (1,115 prescriptions/1,000 persons). Persons aged 75 and older had a higher prescribing rate (1,157 prescriptions/1,000 persons) than those aged 65 to 74 (1,084 prescriptions/1,000 persons). … Azithromycin was the most commonly prescribed drug, followed by amoxicillin and ciprofloxacin. Internists and family physicians prescribed 43% of antibiotic courses (Kabbani, Palms, & Bartoces, 2018).

According to Robnett, Brossoie, and Chop (2020) "advances in medicine and technology have extended life expectancy, and with that, the numbers of drugs used by the average older patient has increased dramatically (pg. 58)." Due to the many chronic diseases experienced by the elderly population as mentioned above, there is a great deal of pain that needs to be quelled, which is quite problematic as this too leads to significant concerns, including misuse and drug dependence/addiction. In short, Robnet, Brossoie and Chop (2020) further state:

> Pharmacotherapeutics in the older adult is complicated. This may be the most challenging area of geriatric medicine. The physiologic changes that occur with aging lead to significant changes in both **pharmacokinetics** (i.e., what the body does to a drug) and **pharmacodynamics** (i.e., what the drug does to the body). The variability of these changes relating to chronologic aging adds to the challenge. The need for multiple medications to treat multiple chronic diseases over long periods of time can lead to even more potential complications (pg. 272).

▶ Mass Incarceration and the Elderly

According to Gibson (2019), historian Elizabeth Hinton, in her book, *From the War on Poverty to the War on Crime: The Making of Mass Incarceration in America*, states that the "The War on Crime and the War on Drugs are two of the largest policy failures in the History of the United States." Hinton also points that "A total of 184,901 Americans entered state and federal prisons. Between 1965 and the War on Drugs less than 20 years later, state and federal prisons added another 251,107 inmates."

The numbers of people incarcerated today, in the United States are staggering and the racial and ethnic disparity is glaring. Gibson (2019) states:

> Today, roughly 2 million people are incarcerated in this country, 66% of them African American or Latino. The United States, with 5 percent of the global population but 25 percent of its prisoners, is home to the largest prison system in the world, with an incarceration rate that is five to 10 times that of peer nations.

This unfortunate situation of **mass incarceration** has also impacted the elderly in the United States. In general, when one thinks of the elderly population, imprisonment is not necessarily what comes to mind, in mass numbers. Based on the above, as one ages, there is a tendency toward chronic diseases and other concerns that would seemingly suggest that alternatives should be considered before warehousing the elderly behind prison bars, in confinement. This is particularly true if they are not in a physical/mental condition to commit further crimes. The reality is that the opposite is occurring. Per the American Civil Liberties Union (ACLU) (2012):

> In 1981, there were 8,853 state and federal prisoners age 55 and older. Today, that number stands at 124,900, and experts project that by 2030 this number will be over 400,000, amounting to over one-third of prisoners in the United states. In other words, the elderly prison population is expected to increase by 4,400% over this fifty-year time span. This astronomical projection does not even include prisoners ages 50–54, for which data over time is harder to access." (Introduction)

This warrants consideration of the types of crimes that the elderly have a propensity to commit. Chettiar (2012) states the following regarding the types of crimes the elderly are likely to commit:

"Further, most aging prisoners are not incarcerated for murder, but are in prison for low-level crimes. For example, in Texas, 65% of prisoners age 50 and older are incarcerated for nonviolent drug, property, and other nonviolent crimes."

The reality is that if a person commits a crime, there are laws that require his/her imprisonment, if he/she is found guilty of doing so, but perhaps the frailty of age should be taken into consideration, particularly if he/she is unable to commit the crime he/she was accused of or any other crimes as the progression of age takes place. Furthermore, "As is the case with the overall American prison population, America's elderly prisoners are overwhelmingly male. Women make up a mere 6% of aging prisoners." (Chettier, 2012)."

This means that many of the women are left without their spouses and children and grandchildren lose their grandfathers, in significant numbers, relative to women in the United States, which is similar to the loss that young families experience when men are incarcerated in mass. Since most of the elderly prisoners who are incarcerated are men, this creates an imbalance in society and an undeniable dismantling of the family, particularly when individuals are supposed to be experiencing their golden years and a sense of respect from society for their wisdom, including mistakes, that others can learn from. This is especially true if there were alternative options for the elderly who commit non-violent crimes, rather than mass incarceration. Some may argue that if one commits a crime he/she must do the time, which is one way of looking at this problem. However, besides the fact that consideration should seriously be given to age and the impact that it has on the body and the minds of individuals, it is a tremendously costly endeavor as many will need special care to tend to their healthcare needs and daily living activities as they age further. This reverts to a consideration of filial piety in regard to the elderly. To what extent, based on the nature of the crime, should elderly people be forgiven, paroled or afforded some other options, which take into consideration that they are nearing the end of life? Should they, perhaps, be given the opportunity to impart wisdom, based on their mistakes, rather than languish in prison cells for extended periods of time, including until death? These questions are worthy of consideration in terms of compassion for the elderly and ultimately costs to society in a number of ways.

▶ Nursing Homes

Although elderly people in the United States have often lived full lives and have made it to their golden years, it is unfortunate that many are relegated to experiences in which they are not dwelling with their loved ones, but rather in nursing homes. Oftentimes there may not be a choice as perhaps they are experiencing non-health issues that do not necessitate hospitalization but are beyond the care that can be provided for them at home in terms of their activities of daily living (ADL). Nursing homes generally have skilled nurses, occupational and physical therapy and other services that may be helpful in meeting their needs. In general, the average stay is less than 100 days as elderly individuals may merely need rehabilitation and when they improve, home may be better for them. Nursing homes are not free so in addition to the need for care, there is an affordability factor that includes determining if a patient has long term insurance, Medicaid, Medicare, veteran's insurance or can afford to pay out-of-pocket. There are assessments and requirements to determine one's eligibility for assistance.

▶ Insight From a Licensed Nursing Home Administrator and Deputy Commissioner of Health for the State of Connecticut

In exploring potential solutions to the problems specific to nursing homes in the United states, input from Nursing Home Administrators and public health practitioners is imperative. In the following interview, conducted with Ms. Heather Aaron, she offers insight regarding Nursing Homes in the United States. This interview has been condensed and edited. Heather Aaron has served in the Healthcare Industry for 35 years. She completed her undergraduate studies at Quinnipiac University in Hamden, Connecticut where she received a Baccalaureate of Science Degree in Health Services Administration and a Baccalaureate of Arts in Psychology. Ms. Aaron subsequently completed her graduate studies at the Yale School of Medicine, Department of Epidemiology and Public Health, where she received her Master's in Public Health Administration. Ms. Aaron's experience is very diverse, including hospital administration, nursing home administration and the development of Independent Housing and Residential facilities. She has served as a Chief Executive Officer (CEO), Chief Operations Officer (COO) and Chief Financial Officer (CFO) in Hospital Systems and in the nursing home industry. Ms. Aaron started as an Analyst for Harlem Hospital and Bellevue Hospital in New York City, learning from the trenches, while developing a strong knowledge base of Healthcare systems.

In 2010 Ms. Aaron relocated to Connecticut and has spent the last nine years as a Nursing Home Administrator, ensuring innovative methods in the quality delivery of care for the poor, elderly, and other marginalized individuals. Her service included the development and implementation of Independent housing and residential care housing for nursing home residents.

Ms. Aaron's focus continues to be the social determinants that affect the delivery of quality care and the steps necessary to continue to improve the standards of care for all. She currently serves as a Deputy Commissioner for the Department of Health for the State of Connecticut.

▶ Interview

Dr. Rose: What is the essential role of nursing homes for the elderly?

Ms. Aaron: The essential role of Nursing Homes is to provide a loving supportive environment for the elderly. As I describe the nursing environment you will discover that the definition of nursing homes only for the elderly is not an absolute today. In many nursing homes the average age is 65. In some chronic care facilities residents can be as young as 18 years of age. All nursing homes are regulated by the state and federal government to follow standards of care and are surveyed by the state and federal government to ensure that standards are met. Over the last 12 years nursing home guidelines have been enhanced by trainings for staff on Person Centered Care to improve the standards of care. The theory behind Person Centered Care is that residents should have a personalized care plan that is specific to the residents likes and dislikes. For example, residents take part in their meals and have a variety of choices. Residents rooms can be personalized. Visiting hours can be extended. Families can stay in the resident's rooms during the end of life stage. Residents can have their choice of music and many more resident centered choices.

Additionally, nursing homes have varying levels of care. A typical elderly nursing home is for someone who can no longer take care of themselves without assistance. The residents require assistance with ADL. If the individual cannot be assisted at home, then they have an opportunity for care in a nursing home. Many of the elderly may have chronic conditions such as coronary heart disease, diabetes, high blood pressure and are in a variety of stages of care.

The nursing home will provide the medical care needed. The medical care is led by a medical doctor who is typically a primary care physician. Specialist are called in as necessary or appointments are made to transport a resident for specialist care as needed. The nursing homes are staffed for 24/7 care and staffing is regulated by the state department of public health under the umbrella of state and federal regulation. Many nursing homes are short term rehabilitation facilities. These are typically for those individuals who have had surgery and require rehab services then return to their homes.

There are many programs with states to assist the elderly to stay in their homes with support. Data must be collected and reviewed to validate outcomes. In a perfect world all should be able to live out their last years with family around for care as we pass along the stories of our life for the next generation. It is my hope that we will get back to basics and take the responsibility of caring for our elderly in a loving home and a gentle environment.

Dr. Rose: Sometimes, there is significant harm that comes to elderly individuals in nursing homes in the U.S. Why do you think this occurs?

Ms. Aaron: Yes, there have been reports of elderly abuse and it is indeed unacceptable and should not be tolerated. All offenders should be prosecuted to the highest extent of the law. There are several reasons why this happens including depraved indifference, power, and control. Some would say that is harsh but taking advantage of someone who cannot fight back is a cowardly, sick act of violence. To address this in the work place, supervisors must be diligent in their duties and monitor the floor staff and residents' rooms. The facilities must train staff based on proper standards to enable them to be deployed in the most effective and caring manner.

For example, double shifts are not good because when humans are overly tired, bad care is inevitable. Unfortunately, not all nursing homes follow the standards of care to the letter and not all state public health departments follow federal guidance for oversight. Backgrounds checks are of the utmost importance to secure the appropriate safe staffing. Supervisors are to work with residents every day and find out their concerns. Lack of complete appropriate training of staff is a primary variable in the abusive care of the elderly. More training and proper supervision will decrease the incidence of inappropriate care.

Dr. Rose: Describe what you believe is an optimal nursing home setting, in an ideal scenario.

Ms. Aaron: The optimal nursing home would have joy, beauty and tranquility.

- The staffing would be 5 C.N.A.'s Certified Nursing Assistants for every 30 residents for each 8-hour shift
- Three (3) Registered nurses for every 30 residents for each 8-hour shift
- All staff would have the same residents assigned
- Staff will work (4) 8 hours shifts and rotate
- Week days Shift (Monday, Tuesday, Wednesday and Thursday)
- Weekend Shift (Friday, Saturday and Sunday)
- Rotating Weekends
- All state and Federal guidelines of care and standards are strictly enforced
- Poetry readings
- Recreation would be staffed to personalize what residents enjoy
- Weekly trips to museums, parks, theatres, and movies
- Art classes and art work
- Music and memory programs
- Elementary school choirs visit to sing to the residents
- A robust volunteer program where every resident's room has a buddy assigned that they can rely upon to always visit regularly and consistently
- Keep the environment alive

Dr. Rose: That seems that it would be a very viable and comforting environment. Is there a shortcoming of funding for nursing homes in the U.S.? How can this be alleviated?

Ms. Aaron: This is a very complicated reimbursement system. The system has private for-profit nursing homes and non-for-profit nursing homes. Many for profit have a targeted bottom line and projected profits. Sometimes care suffers because of profit margins. Many not-for-profit rates are enough to provide the bare minimum but cannot afford to provide the quality of life amenities that make life enjoyable. The reimbursement only covers medical care. Therefore, things like theatre and the arts are not included. Many facilities don't have enough funding in the rate to upgrade facilities. To alleviate the identified issues, I recommend a commission on nursing homes to evaluate the future of nursing home care and decide, as a country, how we want to support our elderly as we all have that road to travel.

Dr. Rose: How are nursing homes for the elderly funded in the U. S.?

Ms. Aaron: Nursing Homes are funded by Medicaid, Medicare, Private Insurance and self-pay.

Dr. Rose: Is there a racial disparity/inequity in terms of nursing homes for the elderly?

Ms. Aaron: The research would need to be done but from my experience the nursing homes with the primary payor as Medicaid have some significant negative outcomes and are filled with those who cannot afford private insurance and don't have Medicare as a secondary.

Dr. Rose: What are the training requirements for staff/clinicians that work in Nursing homes for the elderly?

Ms. Aaron: Nursing home staff comprise the following:

1. Licensed Nursing Home Administrator
2. Medical Director who must be a licensed MD and have admitting privileges to an accredited hospital.

3. Director of Nurses who must be a licensed registered nurse with an active license in good standing
4. Licensed nursing staff, Registered Nurses and Licensed Nurse Practitioners
5. C.N.A.'s (Certified Nurse Assistants)
6. Licensed Social Worker or an MSW (Mastered Prepared Social Worker)
7. Licensed Dietician
8. Dietary Department Director
9. Certified Recreation Therapist
10. Physical Therapist
11. Speech Therapist
12. Occupational Therapist
13. Plant and Maintenance Staff
14. Housekeeping staff
15. Internal and External Laundry Service
16. Oxygen Company and Oxygen Tank room specified by state standards
17. Biomedical Waste disposal company and process
18. Admissions Leaders
19. Discharges Leader
20. Business office providing banking service to residents 24/7
21. 24/7 Security staff and protocol
22. Grounds Keeper
23. Resident Council run by the residents with staff support as requested by the residents

Dr. Rose: What are three main problems nursing homes for the elderly face, along with a solution for each problem identified in your opinion?

Ms. Aaron: The three main problems are loneliness/boredom, disrespect, and the high risk of abuse and neglect. Loneliness and boredom are the result of leaving your home, after 50 years, for example, and moving to a new environment with no family. This is a gut-wrenching event. Residents become depressed. Some get introverted while others become verbally abusive. Some experience health deterioration quickly, and they are no more.

The solutions are to train staff to understand the issues and be more supportive along with:

- locating family to visit often
- Identifying a care plan that would include the resident interests
- Enhancing activities, internal and external
- Developing caring teams with staff and volunteers
- Being consistent in delivering high-quality person-centered care

Disrespect occurs as we lose full capacity of our senses with aging and others in our environment tend to see no value in our input to our daily lives. The nursing home is set up to deliver quality care. To do so the staff must follow protocol in delivering medication, food and daily hygienist care. All of these are done on a schedule including the fun things such as art work and music. This routine life may sometimes lead to neglect in terms of checking with the resident for input, hence the feeling of disrespect. It is important to remember that these individuals have made all their decisions in life and at one time may have been a professional who was part of the decision-making process.

The solution entails understanding that many Nursing Homes have acquired funding from the federal government on Person Centered Care Initiatives. If done correctly this program includes trained staff to involve residents in their care and decisions about their life at the nursing home. By listening to the residents and working with them instead of dictating all elements of care, respect is rebuilt over time.

Lastly, in terms of the high risk of abuse and neglect, all nursing homes across the country must offer the highest quality of delivery of care. A major part of the delivery of care is the appropriate staffing levels of the nursing home and the appropriate training of staff members. For example, if a resident is unable to help support his or her daily hygiene care, and a Hoyer lift must be used, there will be risk of injury if the staff has not been trained within proper guidelines of the use of a Hoyer lift. A Hoyer lift helps elevate the resident so care can be delivered. If a resident has urinary incontinence and is unable to call to be changed and the staff has not monitored to change the resident as often as required, this resident will be at risk for skin breakage. If a resident is not eating meals and staff does not monitor their intake, that resident is at risk. If the facility does not properly staff and staff is not observing every resident, then that resident is at risk. Every year there are hundreds of elderly nursing home patients admitted to hospitals for dehydration. This means the resident fluid intake was not monitored putting the resident at risk for hospitalization. Also, every year there are hundreds of residents admitted to hospitals for Urinary Tract Infections. Again, this is closely related to insufficient hydration. There are many other risk factors that have been studied.

The solution is based on the fact that the Centers for Medicare and Medicaid have been developing a measurement for payment directly correlating quality of care for hospitals. I hope to see a similar structure for nursing homes. State survey processes for nursing homes should make better efforts to enforce the standards on substandard nursing homes. More effort and dollars should be put into additional state monitors providing hands on care. The current monitoring process should be studied and evaluated for effectiveness. Closing the nursing homes is not the solution. Correcting the delivery of safe care is better especially in underserved neighborhoods. Ongoing training and competencies testing for all staff delivering direct and indirect care is a must.

Dr. Rose: Thank you Ms. Aaron for this thorough and comprehensive detail. The solutions are especially appreciated.

▶ Ageism

Jackson, et. Al (2019) ask a very important question regarding health systems, which is: Are existing arrangements institutionally ageist? One item in a survey by Jackson and colleagues concerned elderly people receiving "poorer service or treatment than other people from doctors or hospitals." The ageism question is very interesting as some have the belief that once an individual lives beyond the life expectancy of their nation or what may be considered a normal lifespan, healthcare entitlement should be reduced.

When considering health inequity and the elderly, it is important to determine whether discrimination is a factor. Per Enright (1994) if we consider the term coined by Dr. Robert Butler in 1969:

> Ageism can be seen as a systematic stereotyping of and discrimination against people because they are old, just as racism and sexism accomplish this with skin color and gender. Old people are categorized as senile, rigid in thought and manner, old fashioned in morality and skills…Ageism allows the younger generation to see older people as different from themselves; thus, they subtly cease to identify with their elders as human beings.

According to Vespa (2018), per U.S. Census data, by 2035 it is expected that there will be 78.0 million people over 65. This is because the baby boomer generation will reach the ages of over 65 and it was the one of the largest generations in the United States (Census, 2018). There are currently more than 46 million people age 65 and older living in the United States. With this swelling number of older adults, the country could see greater demands for health care, in-home caregiving and assisted living facilities. It could also affect Social Security. The U.S. census projects three-and-a-half working-age adults for every older person eligible for Social Security in 2020. By 2060, that number is expected to fall to two-and-a-half working-age adults for every older person.

Wrap Up

In general, there are a myriad of problems impacting the elderly population in the United States. This problem is exceedingly worse for those who are in the lower socioeconomic status as well as those who are members of certain emerging majority groups. Therefore, solutions are needed to try and resolve some of these issues and ensure a better quality of life for the elderly. Some suggestions are indicated here:

Solutions

- Societal emphasis on filial piety to endear greater respect and appreciation of elderly people, amongst all generations in the U.S.

As suggested by Wedmedyk (2015):

- Remove financial barriers to care by supporting expanded insurance coverage and free clinical services, such as screening programs
- Work to strengthen safety nets and supports for caregivers to ensure long-term care, safe housing, and retirement security
- Increase access to healthcare services and recreation by improving public transportation and promoting safe, livable communities
- Develop community education programs led by culturally-sensitive community health workers that reach targeted populations
- Support policies that ensure livable minimum wages, equal hiring, and fair firing, especially as it relates to older adults
- Engage with academic researchers and organizations that highlight issues facing the aging poor, such as the American Society on Aging, Justice in Aging, and the National Association of Social Workers

- Implement research or utilize existing data sources that measure health disparities, such as the Elder Economic Security Index, to raise awareness and drive action. To motivate stakeholders and legislatures, Mullen suggests enacting actuarial analyses of Medicaid enrollment projections based on current poverty levels
- Educate others and broaden the conversation on health disparities to include healthy aging to influence systems-level change
- Implement policies or programs that fight income inequality and the effects of poverty
- Re-evaluate and tailor existing policies and programs according to what barriers may exist for reaching marginalized groups

Furthermore, to reduce health inequalities that adversely affect older persons and to promote their social inclusion, the following policy suggestions are proposed per the United Nations Department of Economic and Social Affairs (UNDESA) (N.D.):

- Ensure affordable, quality and accessible social services, including health care and long-term care, to all older persons, and increase support to education and training in geriatrics and gerontology;
- Introduce/enhance legislation to promote equality and non-discrimination on the basis of age in the provision of health and health insurance services and
- Improve the collection, analysis and use of health and other data by age, across the life course, including through upper age bands to age 100;

Finally, Medical schools must teach students the specifics in caring for the elderly in terms of pharmacokinetics and pharmacodynamics (Robnet, Brossoie, & Chop, 2020).

Wrap-Up

Chapter Summary

It is quite a challenging experience to be an elderly person in the United States. Health-wise, there are significant issues, and although quantity of life exists in terms of longevity, quality of life, in the latter years of one's existence, becomes a problem. Some of the concerns mentioned are chronic illnesses (which the elderly suffer from disproportionately relative to younger members of the U.S. population), overuse of pharmaceuticals and the ensuing problems associated with these drugs, nursing homes and the poor treatment received by the elderly in many of them, and finally, the mass incarceration of the elderly. This, by no means, is an exhaustive list, since there are a vast number of problems that the elderly experience in the United States. But, it is an opportunity to think about their quality of life. If one does not die prematurely, to be an elder is what every person will experience. It is a frightening prospect for many, particularly for those individuals who are poor and from certain racial and ethnic groups in the United States who experience lack of health equity throughout in terms of chronic illness. There should be prevention, not only treatment, which in turn would reduce the overuse of pharmaceuticals.

Additionally, as discussed by Ms. Heather Aaron, in the earlier interview, oversight is the key for nursing homes. It would be best if the elders in the United States were taken care of, with love and compassion by their family members. However, when this is not possible and nursing homes are needed, care for the elderly must be done with respect and the preservation of their dignity. Family members must visit their elderly relatives, on an impromptu basis, with regularity, to ensure that all of their needs are met. Nursing homes must be monitored to ensure that no elderly person is harmed, during their greatest time of need. Furthermore, mass incarceration of the elderly must end. Medical and general parole must be a serious consideration for each elder in prison along with compassionate release and community service as priority options. If elders have committed non-violent crimes in their golden years, perhaps it would be best to have them provide lectures at schools to younger people about mistakes/crimes and consequences.

The solutions mentioned here are merely ideas towards solving big problems specifically pertaining to the elderly in the United States. Health equity must be in place from the cradle to the grave, without exception, for all members of the population in the United States. Elderly people must be given the utmost respect, with an emphasis on maintaining their dignity, within the context of valuing and appreciating all that they have contributed to society throughout their lives. The latter years of life are the periods of time where wisdom must be shared and stored by and from the elderly, so that future generations will have the opportunity to learn from the lives of individuals who preceded them and sit with them, whenever possible, to garner wisdom and insight.

Chapter Problems

1. List five chronic illnesses that the elderly experience in the United States.
2. Identify key factors associated with mass incarceration of the elderly and list two solutions.
3. What are the most overly prescribed drugs provided to members of the elderly population?
4. There are important steps that can be taken to improve nursing homes. Why is oversight one of the most important?
5. Explain the concept entitled filial piety and how it can be used as an effective approach to care for the elderly in the U.S.?

References

American Civil Liberties Union. At America's expense: The mass incarceration of the elderly. Available at https://www.aclu.org/files/assets/elderlyprisonreport_20120613_1.pdf

Bryant, A. (2019). Wear purple, show the world your heart! *Elder-Update*. The Department of Elder Affairs.,30(3) 24.

Chettiar, I. (2012). At America's Expense: The mass incarceration of the elderly. NELLCO Legal Scholarship Repository. New York University Public Law and Legal Theory: New York University School of Law.

Emily, J. and Branham, D. (N.D.) Nursing homes that didn't evacuate as Harvey flooding rose now remain closed as state reopens investigation. Available at: https://www.dallasnews.com /news/investigations/2018/08/23/nursing-homes-enough-save-patients-hurricane-harvey-hit -widow-wants-answers. Accessed on April, 25 2019.

Enright, R. B. Jr. (Ed.). (1994). *Perspectives in social gerontology. Needham Heights, MA: Allyn and Bacon; p.3.*

Flechas, J. (2018, March 26). Florida Nursing Homes now permanently required to have generators to power A/C. *The Miami Herald*, Retrieved from https://www.miamiherald.com/news/state/florida/article206911334.html

Gibson, L. (2019). Color and Incarceration. *Harvard Magazine, 122 (1), pgs. 40-45*

Guilliford, M. (2019). *Discrimination and Public Health.* Available at: https://doi.org/10.1016/S2468-2667(19)30044-1. Accessed on June 15, 2019.

Healthy People 2020. Available at: https://www.healthypeople.gov/2020/topics-objectives/topic/older-adults. Accessed on June 10, 2019.

Jackson, S., Hackett, R and Steptoe, A. (2019). Associations between age discrimination and health and well-being: Cross sectional and prospective analysis of the English longitudinal study of aging. *The Lancet, 4*(4). Available at: https://www.thelancet.com/journals/lanpub/article/PIIS2468-2667(19)30035-0/fulltext. Accessed on July 8, 2019.

Kabbani S., Palms, D. and Bartoces, M. (2018). Outpatient antibiotic prescribing for older adults in the United States: 2011 to 2014. *Journal of the American Geriatrics Society*, Retrieved. From https://onlinelibrary.wiley.com/doi/abs/10.1111/jgs.15518. Accessed on May 14, 2019.

Kennedy, M. and Slotkin, J. (2017). At Least 8 dead at Florida Nursing Home after Irma. NPR. Available at: https://www.npr.org/sections/thetwo-way/2017/09/13/550695498/at-least-6-dead-at-florida-nursing-home-without-power-after-irma. Accessed on April 16, 2019.

Robnet, R., Brossoie, N., and Chop, W. C. (2018). *Gerontology for the health care professional.* Burlington, MA: Jones and Bartlett Learning.

Span, P. (2019, March 15). Older Americans are awash in antibiotics. *The New York Times*. Retrieved from https://www.nytimes.com/2019/03/15/health/antibiotics-elderly-risks.html. Accessed June 15, 2019.

UNDESA (N.D.) Health inequalities exist in access to health care as well as health outcomes Department of Economic and Social Affairs programme on ageing. The focal point on ageing in the United Nations system Retrieved from: https://www.un.org/development/desa/ageing/wp-content/uploads/sites/24/2018/04/Health-Inequalities-in-Old-Age.pdf. Accessed on June 20, 2019.

Vespa, J. (2018). The U.S. joins other countries with large aging population the graying of America: More older adults than kids by 2035. Retrieved from: https://www.census.gov/library/stories/2018/03/graying-america.html. Accessed June 21, 2019.

Wedmedyk, S. (2015). Older adults in poverty face compounded health inequities. Association of State and Territorial Health Officials. [Web blog post]. Retrieved from http://www.astho.org/StatePublicHealth/Older-Adults-in-Poverty-Face-Compounded-Health-Inequities/8-25-15.

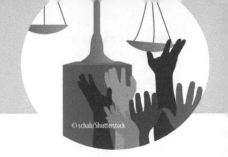

CHAPTER 11

The Future of Health Disparities and Diversity: Recommendations Toward Solutions

We pledge ourselves to liberate all our people from the continuing bondage of poverty, deprivation, suffering, gender and other discrimination.

—**Nelson Mandela**

KEY TERMS

criminalization in the classroom   tolerance
inclusiveness

LEARNING OBJECTIVES

After reading this chapter, you should be able to do the following:

1. Discuss the key elements of a diversity plan.
2. Explain the concept of tolerance and its relevance to diversity.
3. Understand the health disparity implications of the school-to-prison pipeline.
4. List the contributing factors associated with health illiteracy.

▶ Introduction

In an attempt to resolve the most salient issues impacting health disparities in the United States and enhance diversity in health care and academic institutions, there are two key approaches/steps that may prove instrumental. The first is the development of a diversity plan by all health-related entities, including academic institutions and care providers. The second is the review of existing recommendations that are worthy and doable but that have yet to be implemented.

Often, diversity initiatives consist of taking head counts of the numbers of emerging majority individuals providing services in healthcare clinical settings and teaching and learning in health and medical academic institutions. Additionally, there may be multicultural events and efforts toward tolerance without the necessary commitment to diversity in terms of policy and practice. There is also a tendency to continually broaden the term diversity by including multiple elements in its definition beyond racial and ethnic categories, which is the focus of this text. Using a wide net—applying a broad definition, that is—results in the appearance of diversity while simultaneously watering down the concept. Healthcare organizations must go beyond these cursory steps and make serious efforts toward change.

Use of terminology that is well meaning but negatively impacts the problem of diversity is also an issue. A key example is the term *tolerance*, as explained next.

▶ Tolerance

Imagine a person of color, at a predominantly White healthcare institution, starting a new position and attending orientation. Within the context of the orientation, a representative of the organization announces with pride that the organization has a tolerance program as part of its diversity initiatives. Tolerance? How is that appropriate within the context of any organization? **Tolerance** refers to acceptance, which may seem admirable, but usually the connotation is that the thing being "tolerated" is something that one really disagrees with. John Achrazoglou (2016) considers the implications of this term:

> Diversity needs to go beyond tolerance. Tolerance is a first step. It is much better than conflict. But tolerance is a somewhat negative word, according to David See-Chai Lam, former lieutenant governor of British Columbia. To "tolerate" and to be "tolerated" involves an unequal relationship. Tolerance implies that the tolerator has the power to not tolerate.

Often, in the United States, people of color find themselves as part of a very small group or as the only person of color in an organization of predominantly White people. No one wants to be merely tolerated at such organizations that choose to move forward with diversity initiatives and inclusive hiring practices. Diversity is an effort of **inclusiveness**, to ensure that the workforce is not homogeneous. Homogeneity is not reflective of the U.S. population as a whole. A U.S. Census Bureau report shows that by 2044, Whites will no longer comprise a racial majority in the United States (Frey, 2015). Hence, when an organization decides to ensure that diversity happens, it should not be within the context of tolerating people of color, but of valuing and appreciating individuals who will add to a vibrant milieu.

If an organization chooses to have a tolerance program, the term must be clearly defined from a positive vantage point. Unesco (n.d.) offers an excellent definition of tolerance:

> Tolerance is respect, acceptance and appreciation of the rich diversity of our world's cultures, our forms of expression and ways of being human. It is fostered by knowledge, openness, communication, and freedom of thought, conscience and belief. Tolerance is harmony in difference.

However, tolerance, if not properly defined, is limiting and demeaning. Valuing and appreciating is a better place to begin.

Furthermore, in an effort to close the health status gap between emerging majorities and the White population, healthcare organizations (academic and clinical) must develop a diversity plan. The purpose of said plan is not only to diversify organizations but also to move healthcare organizations toward the ultimate goal, which is to resolve the problem of health disparities. Ensuring access to quality health care is the primary goal, but who will implement such a process? Diversity is needed so that there is a multicultural approach to doing so.

▶ Diversity Plan

A diversity plan must be a living, breathing document that sets forth strategic goals toward ensuring a diverse environment to meet the growing demographic changes in the United States in terms of the provision of health care. It must focus on incorporating the reality of diversity into the full milieu of the health care or academic organization, including human resources policies, the mission and vision statements, values, and practice.

The first step in developing such a plan is a thorough review to determine the status of the healthcare organization's current diversity initiatives, beginning with these key questions:

- Does the institutional mission statement of the organization include an emphasis/focus on diversity?
- Are the marketing materials reflective of a commitment to serve diverse populations? Will patients/students find this commitment visually affirmed by the materials?
- Is there a dedicated staff with a focus on implementing diversity policies and practices to ensure the existence of a culturally competent environment?
- Does the healthcare organization make efforts to recruit diverse students and faculty and to create a diverse workforce overall?
- How does the organization define diversity? Is the definition too broad, which ultimately waters down the notion of diversity merely to make the organization appear diverse?
- Is the faculty's makeup in the healthcare programs/departments/schools reflective of the student population in terms of demographics?
- Is the clinical workforce reflective of the patients/clients served in terms of demographics?
- Does the healthcare organization/academic institution have mechanisms in place to ensure the avoidance of racial stereotypes, the promotion of cultural

and linguistic competence, and the valuing and appreciation of a diverse workforce/student body, rather than mere tolerance?

■ Is part of the mission of the healthcare organization/academic institution to reduce the health disparity that exists between the White population and emerging majority populations?

A critical element of the diversity plan is a set of achievable objectives. Members of the healthcare/academic institution must be aware of these objectives and must participate in achieving them. Examples of specific objectives relevant to diversity and health disparities include the following:

1. Developing an effective mission statement that reflects the organization's commitment to diversity and closing the health status gap between emerging majorities and the White population
2. Defining the term diversity so that it is clear to all members of the organization at every level
3. Identifying strong leadership for diversity at all levels of the organization
4. Illustrating the healthcare/academic institution's commitment to diversity by establishing an office of diversity and multicultural affairs with the sole responsibility of fostering a climate of diversity at the organization
5. Recruiting a diverse workforce based on the organization's clearly indicated definition of diversity
6. Retaining diverse members of the workforce by ensuring that they are valued and appreciated at every level of the organization
7. Incorporating cultural competence in all aspects of the organization as stated in the mission statement
8. Examining health disparities and facilitating efforts to focus on this issue with specific goals to eliminate the problem
9. Identifying and acquiring funding through grants and other efforts to conduct relevant research and projects to reduce health disparities

Beyond these sample objectives, healthcare organizations and academic programs, departments, and schools focused on health must explore current recommendations that often emerge regarding closing the health status gap. There must be openness to understanding the issues associated with social injustice, the impact of poverty, racial discrimination, and other factors that impact health, both directly and indirectly.

▶ Data and Statistics

Organizations in the field of health must be committed to maintaining a database, which ensures an understanding of diversity progress. Specifically, health administration, both in academic and non-academic settings, should keep tabs on the numbers of various racial groups and the Hispanic ethnic group. Specifically, in healthcare organizations, data on White (Non-Hispanic), Black/African American, Native American/Alaska Native, Native Hawaiian/Pacific Islander/Asian American, and Hispanic (ethnic group) populations should be collected continuously to determine the numbers/percentages for each group, including board members, administrators, providers, and patients. Academic institutions that have health programs/departments/schools must collect diversity data for the same racial and ethnic categories relating to boards of trustees, faculty, staff, and students. These statistics will ensure that entities are meeting necessary diversity benchmarks and moving toward solutions for areas of identified weakness through recruitment efforts. Each year, data should be reviewed to see where there are increases toward diversity in an effort to maintain or enhance successful approaches.

A diversity advisory board is also necessary, comprised of representatives of all of the racial/ethnic groups, to ensure that diversity goals are set and met. The advisory board must consist of national health industry leaders with a broad array of talents, capabilities, and expertise. The goal of such an advisory board is to advocate for diversity in the institution where they are serving, foster diversity and inclusion, and ensure that efforts toward diversity, through the mission of the organization, are always active and solution oriented. In addition, the advisory board must bring funding recommendations for consideration by administration and ultimately the board of directors or trustees, as diversity efforts must be amply funded. Often, recommendations must be focused and targeted toward a problem or concern that is particularly disheartening and severe. An example of such a scenario is the United Nations recently sought recommendations from the Working Group of Experts on People of African Descent in the United States. The outcome of said recommendations is discussed in the following section. Although this example is on a much broader scale than the situation encountered in most healthcare/academic institutions, specific to one group but varied in focus, it is an excellent example of the depth that is needed to resolve problems associated with health disparity and lack of diversity, as the two issues are interrelated.

▶ Recommendations Toward Solutions— Example: Black/African American People in the United States

The following discussion centers on the statement to the media made by the United Nations' Working Group of Experts on People of African Descent upon the conclusion of its official visit to the United States from January 19 to 29, 2016. In its statement, the Working Group recommends various measures to improve racial/ethnic conditions in the United States. Excerpts are presented here based on their relevance to this text, followed by commentary by this author regarding specific recommendations as they impact health disparities and diversity. This practice of reviewing recommendations, understanding them, and implementing change as a result, where appropriate, will be very useful in the United States by health care and academic institutions that are committed to closing the health status gap and moving toward diversified work forces in the health industry. The focus of this report is African Americans, which is useful, as the major health disparity (i.e., most significant health status gap) is between Black/African American people and White people in the United States.

The following recommendations are intended to assist the United States in its efforts to combat all forms of racism, racial discrimination, Afrophobia, xenophobia, and related intolerance (United Nations High Commissioner for Human Rights, 2016):

> *Recommendation:* Establish a national human rights commission, in accordance with the Paris Principles. The Government should establish within this body a specific division to monitor the human rights of African Americans.

Commentary: Looking at this from a health vantage point, a starting point would be health disparities, as the health status of African American/Black people is poor overall in comparison to that of the White population in the United States, particularly for African Americans with a low socioeconomic status.

> Reparatory justice is needed subsequent to the acknowledgement that a crime against humanity took place, namely the transatlantic slave trade. People of African descent are the victims of the consequences of racism, racial discrimination, xenophobia and related intolerance. This victimization continues.

Commentary: Until it is understood and acknowledged that a grave injustice was committed against people of African descent (and Native Americans) and that there has not been a level playing field for these groups in terms of health (and other aspects of life) in the United States, the prospect of actually closing the health status gap remains slim. Slavery was not merely an act of social injustice, but true crimes were committed against a group of people, including rape, murder, and neglect in terms of health care and overall quality of life, inhumane brutality, and cultural genocide. Reparatory justice is a controversial matter of serious debate because to place a monetary figure on such atrocities is essentially impossible.

However, perhaps the assurance of health care for all who are descendants of slavery, regardless of their ability to pay, may be a point to begin such a discussion. This provision may seem far-fetched to some, raising many difficult questions: Who would pay for this? Would this be a tax on the rest of society, and if so, who would support that? Although the answers to these questions may not be apparent, exploration of the matter by the federal and state governments, followed by implementation, is surely achievable. It would seem that the government would place significant emphasis on some type of reparatory justice, as thus far there has merely been paltry apologies for the atrocity of slavery and its horrific long-term ramifications, which is clearly not enough.

> The government (federal and state) is urged to further implement policies, which focus on disparities.

Commentary: Racial disparities exist in the United States as evidenced by apparent health disparities, as one significant example. However, the key and overarching factor is socioeconomic status. The issue of poverty must be addressed in the

United States, for all people, which will assist with closing the health status gap. Most African Americans are not immigrants living in the United States. Native Americans are also not immigrants living in the United States. People of African descent were brought to what we know as the United States, against their will, to work without pay, and hence without legacy opportunities, financial or otherwise, for future generations. Native Americans had their land and all that they held dear taken from them. As this was happening, the White population was ensuring a society to meet their needs, reaping the benefits of forced labor, taking land inhabited by others (Native Americans), passing wealth and prosperity from one generation of White people to the next, and creating political, monetary, health, and other systems to largely meet their needs without the inclusion of people who currently comprise the emerging majority groups. This kind of approach has contributed significantly to racial and health disparities that must be addressed if parity among the races is ever to be established in the United States.

> All criminal justice reform bills that are pending are under consideration for reform. Congress is urged to do so by The Working Group regarding the End Racial Profiling Act and the Second Chance Reauthorization Act. In terms of drastically reducing mandatory minimum sentencing, The Working Group is encouraging bi-partisan support.

Commentary: Mass incarceration is a problem that is dramatically and devastatingly impacting Black/African American families in the United States. There are pending criminal justice reform bills in the works to end the injustice that is taking place related to over-incarcerating predominantly poor, emerging majority people for low-level drug offenses and other nonviolent offenses with inordinate lengths of time in prison, including life sentences. The United States has more people in prison than any other industrialized nation (Alexander, 2012). This over-incarceration of Black men and women is leading to the inability to create families, and existing families are being ripped apart, leaving children without parents, devastated and traumatized. This is causing a tremendous strain on grandparents and other family members, who must rear children that should be raised by their parents. The children are devastated as they are being forced to live in a world where their parents are locked away in cages, unable to be with them to offer them the love and guidance they deserve. It is obvious that this kind of stress and duress is a contributing factor to the problems of health disparities, as there is neglect from a parenting vantage point and overall quality of life as the children and their families are severely impacted.

> Review and revisit school security policies along with the abolishment of school policing.

Commentary: The notion of policing in schools is bizarre, as K-12 schools are buildings where children are housed. The reality is that in many public schools in America, children are required to enter through metal detectors and police are placed inside of the schools, or summoned to the schools, to arrest children for minor infractions normally handled by teachers, a trip to the principal's office, contacting parents, or in-school detention. Emerging majority children, particularly

Black children, are becoming part of an awful process known as the school-to-prison pipeline. This development is indeed an atrocity. Failures related to school systems must be rectified, as education is a key aspect of resolving health disparities. Health illiteracy is an outcome of poor education and combining this problem with incarceration of emerging majority children is certain disaster for future generations.

> Mental health issues should be handled with counseling. There should be no use of restraint along with the prohibition of seclusion. In terms of children with autism, ADHD (Attention deficit hyperactivity disorder) and other disabilities, students should be afforded focused attention and their protection should be ensured.

Commentary: Autism, ADHD, and other disabilities experienced by children in the K-12 system are part of the spectrum of illnesses that are contributing to health disparities of emerging majority populations. Acts such as restraining, medicating and secluding children who experience mental health issues are not solutions but rather contribute to the problem. Seemingly, common sense dictates that we take care of the needs of children with the goal being to protect them and keep them healthy, with their well-being always at the forefront. When society fails its children, there is little hope. We must begin to close the health disparity gap to ensure our children's health and therein ensure that future generations will not suffer. Meeting this recommendation of the Working Group is an excellent way to begin the process of closing the health status gap.

> Guidelines should be developed to ensure compliance in terms of human rights in terms of school discipline policies and practices, based on human rights standards. These guidelines should be developed by the government. To reduce incidents involving discipline particular methods should be used such as positive behavior intervention and support and restorative practices specific to school discipline. The goal is learning improvement in schools.

Commentary: Although this recommendation seems obvious, there seems to be an overriding consensus that the school-to-prison pipeline must end. The recidivism rate for prisoners is high. Children who are imprisoned do not have the opportunity to develop the necessary skill sets (technology or otherwise) to function in society. Self-esteem and other concerns arise, placing the child in a position to develop in an unhealthy way. There must be an end to **criminalization in the classroom**, with a reemphasis on teaching and learning as the only focus. The classroom must include culturally and linguistically competent interactive activities that engage students, while simultaneously ensuring compassion and responsiveness to the needs of the children.

> Quality and affordable health care, with a target of reducing maternal mortality of African American women as a priority, is the recommendation per the working group.

Commentary: Although the Affordable Care Act (ACA) is focused on increasing access to care for all—and indeed requires that all people have health care—there are significant shortcomings. The options are Medicaid (for the poor), Medicare (for the elderly), or private insurance, usually offered through a person's workplace. Besides these categories, people in the United States are required to locate insurance and pay the monthly premiums and their deductibles. Meeting this demand is very difficult for many people, and failure to do so results in a penalty, administered by the Internal Revenue Service. So although maternal mortality rates are continuing to rise in the United States, particularly among Black women, having the ACA as a law does not necessarily rectify the problem. Other problems must also be addressed. For example, food injustice (generally associated with low socioeconomic status) leads people to eat poor-quality food, often a contributing factor to obesity, diabetes, hypertension, and other problems. Maternal mortality is a key health indicator, and as with other factors contributing to health disparity, a comprehensive approach is needed to address it.

> There are rights that are recommended which include food, water and adequate housing. This will ensure that living standards are adequate.

Commentary: It seems that the need to ensure these basic needs (food, water, and housing) for all human beings in a society would be common sense to anyone. Nevertheless, these basic needs are not always met, particularly for low-income people in the United States. According to the expanded version of Maslow's hierarchy of needs (McLeod, 2007), the following needs must be met by all people:

1. *Biologic and physiologic needs*—air, food, drink, shelter, warmth, sex, sleep, etc.
2. *Safety needs*—protection from elements, security, order, law, stability, etc.
3. *Love and belongingness needs*—friendship, intimacy, affection, and love (from coworkers, family, friends, romantic partners, etc.)
4. *Esteem needs*—self-esteem, achievement, mastery, independence, status, dominance, prestige, managerial responsibility, etc.
5. *Cognitive needs*—knowledge, meaning, etc.
6. *Aesthetic needs*—appreciation and search for beauty, balance, form, etc.
7. *Self-actualization needs*—realizing personal potential and self-fulfillment, seeking personal growth and peak experiences
8. *Transcendence needs*—helping others to achieve self-actualization.

It seems that ensuring that these needs are met will be very useful to the process of reducing maternal mortality rates and other indices that continue to contribute to the health status gap. Affordable, accessible care is a key aspect of resolving the problem.

▶ Solutions: A Voice From Academia Regarding Closing the Health Status Gap

In an effort to further explore solutions to the problems associated with health disparities and lack of diversity in health care, this author interviewed a leading African American figure in the academic community—Dr. Isiah M. Warner. The Department of Chemistry at Louisiana State University (LSU) is the number one producer of African American PhD chemists in the nation, a title long held, largely due to Dr. Warner's efforts. His suggestions and thoughts regarding "where do we go from here?" are reviewed in hopes of gathering ideas toward solutions.

Dr. Warner is a Boyd Professor in the LSU system. He has more than 340 scholarly publications in a variety of journals relevant to the general areas of analytical and materials chemistry. His expertise is in the area of fluorescence spectroscopy, where he has focused his research for more than 35 years. He is considered one of the world's experts in the analytical applications of fluorescence spectroscopy. He has chaired 59 doctoral theses. In addition to fundamental research, Dr. Warner has conducted educational research, which focuses on mechanisms for maintaining and enhancing student education in science, technology, engineering, and mathematics (STEM), with a particular focus on encouraging his students to pursue terminal degrees.

Many of his students have gone on to pursue PhDs and postdoctoral studies at some of this country's most prestigious institutions, including Harvard, the Massachusetts Institute of Technology (MIT), Georgia Tech, the University of Michigan, Rice University, and the University of Washington. His desire to be an educator has propelled him into an academic career. However, he is now considered more than an educator, as he is also a mentor to students all over the world. Mentoring is a mechanism by which he pays homage to those individuals who were mentors for him during his years of growth as an educator. He believes that teaching students how to do research is a form of education. In fact, he believes that it is the ultimate form of education since it involves the discovery of new knowledge—that is, knowledge not found in textbooks.

▶ Interview

DR. ROSE: What prompted your interest in studying science?

DR. WARNER: At 2 years old, I drank kerosene to figure out what that liquid was and ended up in the hospital. I tell people that was the start of my science career. I've always had this curious attitude about me. If something worked a certain way, I wanted to know why it worked that way. If something occurred, I wanted to know what's going on, why is it going on that way? I guess I didn't realize that it was an aptitude in science until later on when I was in high school and I was doing very well in the science courses and my teachers recognized that I was good in both mathematics and science.

DR. ROSE: Then I would presume that STEM is something that you support and believe in at this point in time?

DR. WARNER: Yes. I'm very much supportive of students pursuing STEM careers.

DR. ROSE: So you know that this book is about health disparities. I'm curious as to whether you think the issue of the health status gap between White and Black people can be closed by having more Black people studying science?

DR. WARNER: There is absolutely no doubt that is true. People tend to select subjects that are near and dear to their heart. I've heard of students who've come to me and say I want to study research on cancer because my grandmother died of cancer or my father has cancer or something like that. Those very personal issues really determine the kind of things that we focus on later on in life. If you have more minorities that are doing research, they will focus on those issues that are very much akin to the things that they have been exposed to. That happens naturally and anyone who denies that, they have a problem, not those who recognize that health disparity can be improved by having more minorities involved.

DR. ROSE: I definitely agree with that. I no longer use the term minority. The reason that I no longer use that term is because it has been projected by 2042, that's the last date I've seen, and already in some places, it has happened, that people of color in the United States will no longer be the minority but will be the majority. I use the term emerging majority. Based on that it seems clear to me that there seems to be another reason for us to make sure that we are training people of color to practice in the field of medicine and other areas of the health professions. Are you in tune with that demographic change that is happening, and what are your thoughts about that?

DR. WARNER: Yes, I am. It's clear. That is an issue that has to be addressed sometime soon. So-called minorities are indeed becoming the majority. You see that in elections right now. Minorities can sway the way the vote goes right now. I have an example as a matter fact. I have hypertension/high blood pressure, and just recently, I guess a couple of years ago, I was alerted to the fact that there are certain medications, a beta blocker, that seems to help high blood pressure in African Americans better than others. They just happened to stumble upon that and I'm on that medication now and it's working very effectively for me. But it seems to work better for African Americans than other kinds of hypertension medication. So that is just one example of the things that we assume. I mean for many years, men were used as the model for health care. There were issues that were addressing men that were used for women and we found out that obviously there are differences between men and women and so those issues have become apparent and it is going to become apparent that this emerging majority will have different issues than the current majority.

DR. ROSE: Now in Baton Rouge, I was there recently at LSU where I gave speeches/presentations; I was the keynote speaker at the School of Veterinary Medicine, and while I was there, I was told that in Baton Rouge, the demographic changes have already occurred such that people of color are the dominant group. Is that accurate?

DR. WARNER: I am positive that is true because I know that African Americans in East Baton Rouge Parish is 60 percent and we add the Hispanic population to that and they certainly are the majority.

DR. ROSE: Okay, then there is verification of what we've been talking about, at least in one location. So my understanding is that you are graduating more PhDs in chemistry than any other program similar to yours in the nation. Is that accurate?

DR. WARNER: It's the Chemistry Department, and we are graduating more African American PhDs than any other university in the country, and this was a study done on the top 50 universities in the country as reflected by the amount of National Science Foundation funding the university or the department has. We are also number one in the percentage of women that receive PhDs. We don't graduate the largest number of women, but we do graduate the largest number of underrepresented minorities. We graduate the largest percentage of women of the PhDs who graduate.

DR. ROSE: What is the impact, from your perspective, of graduating so many African Americans with PhDs in chemistry?

DR. WARNER: Well, first of all, I would say it doesn't have to be a whole lot in order to be effective because so many universities are graduating so few that even a small increase in our population … we're … at one point, I think in the year 2000, we graduated about 10 percent of African Americans receiving PhDs. I think maybe there were 50 or so and we graduated like 5 of the 50.

DR. ROSE: So even in small numbers, it's still very impactful because it's just happening in such small numbers all around. Is that what you are saying?

DR. WARNER: That's correct. Right.

DR. ROSE: Upon graduation with these PhDs in chemistry, what do they do next in terms of careers?

DR. WARNER: Most of our students tend to go out and take industrial positions. A lot of them work in the pharmaceutical industry. So they are having an impact. As a matter of fact, one of our graduates was back last week and she's head of the cosmetic area at Proctor and Gamble. She's an African American female, and she's on television a lot. She's representing them. She's a beautiful brown-skin young lady. She is African American, and she is the face of Proctor and Gamble in the cosmetic industry.

DR. ROSE: In terms of diversity, this seems to be an issue that universities still struggle with in terms of diversity of faculty, students, and so forth. I'm looking for solutions. We have a history of touting the problems and we don't necessarily get to solutions, which is why I was so excited to speak to you, because you are doing something that is solution oriented. So from the vantage point of diversity, what do you think are some techniques that you recommend—at least two or three that you can recommend for diversifying faculty and then diversifying students?

DR. WARNER: I can tell you what the problem is. We need to start at the grassroots level and move students—for example, make sure that minority students get the best education at the elementary school level. Make sure they get the best education in high school and at the undergraduate level. There are lots of bright minds that are going to waste. There are some incredibly bright people that … I just happen to find a few of them because people know about me and they send students to me. There was a young woman who graduated from Grambling State University, and she'll readily admit this, that she came in and she struggled. The average professor would have given up on her. I didn't. I worked with her. She had financial problems and when she got a C in a course, which is failing in graduate school, I worked with her and turned her around. Now I've graduated 60 PhDs and I guarantee you that young woman is probably the best. She gave the best defense of any graduate student I've ever had and I've had lots of White students, some of whom were presidents of universities, CEOs of pharmaceutical companies, vice presidents of companies, and out of all of those 60 students, she gave the best thesis defense of any student I've ever had. She could have easily given up on graduate school. Just because someone didn't believe in her. I believed in her and she exceeded my expectations. I never expected her to be as good as she is.

DR. ROSE: Your recommendation then is to—

DR. WARNER: To not assume that because someone has deficiencies in their background, to not assume that is a sign of a lack of intelligence. In my opinion, it's simply a sign of someone who hasn't had all of the advantages that everyone else has had. That's the point that I think needs to be made. Sometimes there are students that can perform as bright as those that come from Georgia Tech, MIT, Harvard in graduate school, but they have not had the kind of training and background that those students that come from those institutions have had.

DR. ROSE: Now going back to what you said about education at the grassroots level, what can we do at the K-12 level, in terms of public schools, to identify those students who are in substandard schools, in many instances, that are excelling and get them into programs where they can ultimately help us reduce health disparities? What would you suggest?

DR. WARNER: There was a program that helped me out a lot. When I was going to attend Southern University, which was back when the schools were still segregated, Southern offered me a full scholarship and the way they did that was that they gave me an IQ test. An IQ test is more reflective of your ability than your current school is and so I received a full scholarship based on my IQ test. I think if people were to go to these schools and give kids some sort of aptitude test, whether they have high aptitude in the sciences or high IQs, and then get those students focused early on in an area where they can excel, then we can get these kids on track because that program has disappeared, but back in the day, that was a program that helped a lot of students move on to areas of science where they could excel.

DR. ROSE: Well, my doctoral dissertation was on development of an instrument to measure attitudes. Measurement and evaluation is a bit of my work and so one of the questions that comes to mind when I hear you say IQ tests is whether or not that rules out a bias that could be inherent in the tests and what about the young people that would have a lower IQ score based on those potentially biased tests? How would that be addressed?

DR. WARNER: There is no doubt that there are biases in those kind of tests, but if you compare them within an individual group it does tell you something. For example, if you want to know the brightest African American in a particular class and you compare the group of African Americans in terms of the test that they took within that group, that test is valid, even though there are biases. You know, I once told my son that there are biases in these kinds of tests and he didn't get it until one day he was taking one of these tests and he said, "Dad, I understand what you mean now." I said, "What do you mean?" He said, "There was a question on there that made a comparison about saddle oxfords to another kind of shoe and I was supposed to make a distinction." He said, "If you hadn't bought me a pair of saddle oxfords and told me what they were I would have never known how to make that comparison." This is my son who is an attorney now. He is a well-established attorney. He has a photographic memory and he's fluent in Spanish and English.

DR. ROSE: Well, I think that is a very good point, and you point that out because the testing is one of the areas where we get into controversy because you know we have the various tests that are administered now. We have the SATs, we have all kinds of issues with the Common Core with all of the testing and so forth—so when we begin to discuss testing, it brings up a myriad of issues. But I think beyond that, reducing health disparities is the key. I was an undergraduate biology student and I then received my master's degree in public health from Yale University. I focused on it more while pursuing my doctorate at Teachers College, Columbia University. When I worked on that degree, which was quite some time ago, I was talking about health disparities. That was my topic of interest. I am sad to say that today as I conduct this interview with you, I'm still talking about health disparities. In many areas, it is worse. From my vantage point, the reason that I feel that this work is so important is because we need to figure out how to resolve this. I'm beyond pointing out the data, the statistics, and proving that it is so. I'm trying to get to a point of answering the question of what shall we do to reduce health disparities? Do some of your students from your program go on to become medical doctors or practice in the clinical field at all?

DR. WARNER: No. With a PhD, typically they go on to industry or to do research. I have a number of my undergraduates who go on to become medical doctors.

DR. ROSE: Well, I ask because sometimes we find MD-PhDs, but that is a lot of work. So the bottom line is from what you are producing in terms of your graduates with PhDs, how do you feel that they will contribute directly to closing the health status gap?

DR. WARNER: They can go on to do research. I have a graduate that was working at a small company doing biomedical research up in Boston. There are students that are out there in companies, doing research that's relevant to biomedical research.

DR. ROSE: Do you think they have more of a propensity to target their research towards people of color because they are African American, or no?

DR. WARNER: When you are working for a company, quite often the company decides what the focus is and what you're going to work on, and that's the difference. Pretty much, you have to go into academia to work on the kind of problems you want to work on.

DR. ROSE: Okay. Well in closing, do you have any thoughts that you think are important to express in terms of the importance of diversity within academia and in the sciences and reducing health disparities?

DR. WARNER: One thing that I really want to say is that we talked about minorities being the majority in East Baton Rouge Parish. In fact, African Americans are 50 percent of the population. However, in the public schools African Americans are 94 percent. So most of the White students go to private or parochial schools. The public schools are still segregated, still poorly funded. So even though African Americans are a majority of the population, they still go to the worst schools within the city. Those kinds of problems have to be overcome in some way. I've had a program, which was funded by the National Science Foundation. It was focusing on STEM. It also focused on diversity. Diversity was a necessary component. So much so that, particularly the White students wanted to know, why are you always talking about diversity, because they had come from schools that didn't have diversity?

There is a young woman over at UCLA. Her name is Sylvia Hertado. She is a Hispanic woman. She has shown that students who come from a very diverse background tend to be better educated. The reason is that you are around people that think very differently from you and so you learn and gather information from them. In addition, you are able to articulate your opinion much better. So that is one of the reasons that I focus on diversity in my program. So, I've graduated something like 250 students, half of them who are probably getting MDs, some of whom are getting MD/PhDs but a good fraction of them are going on to get PhDs. Two of my students are getting PhDs from Georgia Tech.

and there have been other places too, but one was in chemical engineering and one was in engineering. The one in chemistry is definitely doing biomedical research. But I think that is where I will have more impact than the PhDs I'm graduating. These undergraduates have adapted my attitude. Many of them are talking about, they want to go out and do the kinds of things I've done. They want to form groups of students who will focus on the STEM area, and they want to include diversity and all of those things that I've done. They want to do the same thing. So those numbers can become magnified as these students go out and do their things.

DR. ROSE: That's fantastic. I agree with you because until we address the situation at the public school level, in lower income communities … because it is not necessarily race at all, it is the fact that the children are growing up in lower income communities and the schools are substandard and until that changes we remain in this struggle. It would then be your belief that, addressing this—how will this in your perspective reduce health disparities? What are your summarizing thoughts on that? How do we change this?

DR. WARNER: As I indicated, people tend to work on problems that are very familiar to them. If we have more minorities, or emerging majorities as you call them, going into fields that are relevant to health, as we learn more and more about the human genome, we're beginning to understand that there are factors, in addition to environmental factors, that determine our fate. Doing research in those areas is very important. There are a number of studies where they found certain genes that are particular to women that have breast cancer. I am positive that is going to happen in African Americans where we get, disproportionately, prostate cancer and diabetes. There is no doubt that those are genetic factors. Until someone starts to focus on those kinds of problems and working in those areas, you will not be able to advise that population appropriately.

DR. ROSE: I would like to focus here for a moment. There is a backlash to having the perspective that health disparities or illnesses are caused or are linked to genetics. For example, there was some indication in the literature, that Black people on the whole are sicker than other groups of people because of genetic factors. But if you do a comparative analysis of health issues of Black people in America and Black people in countries in Africa, you will find that connection, in terms of the same kinds of illnesses proportionately, doesn't really exist. So my position, very strongly is that it is not genes that we need to focus on but socioeconomic status.

DR. WARNER: I agree with that. You don't have a disagreement with me. I'm just saying that there is a combination of things. For example, Black people disproportionately have diabetes. Native Americans are number one and African Americans are number two, disproportionately. That is a genetic-based disease. There is the element that you speak of that people are poor, people are not eating properly and you have the onset of these diseases much earlier. So it is a combination of genetics as well as environmental issues.

DR. ROSE: Okay, so you feel it's a combination of the two. I'm really harping on this just for a moment because one of the things that requires caution is that the literature, that I think has evolved these days, used to argue to a certain degree that Black people are sicker because they are inherently, genetically, predisposed to illnesses. This seems to be problematic because if you look at diabetes, for those Black individuals that grew up in the same household as an example, where perhaps a member of the family grows up and moves on, becomes highly educated and changes his or her diet and no longer eats highly seasoned soul food, as an example, although he or she knows how to cook it based on family lineage from the South and enjoys it and knows what it is, but also understands the need to modify dramatically because it is salt and sugar laden, fried, etc.—when you look at such a family, you may find another member who may have a stressful job and living environment and continues to eat soul food, as an example, and becomes ill with diabetes and hypertension as for examples. The other, who works and lives in a less stressful environment and doesn't eat the heavily seasoned fried food, there is generally not a hint of the illness that the other experiences. Although this is merely a hypothetical, evidenced by real cases, it seems that diet and environment are serious factors.

DR. WARNER: You are exactly right. I have a brother who is military and he has always maintained his weight, whereas I have not maintained my weight. He has problems with more illnesses than I do because he has continued to eat those kinds of foods as you indicated, that we grew up with—chitterlings and barbeque and etc. I agree with you on that issue.

DR. ROSE: Well good. I'm glad we agree and I understand your point that perhaps it's a combination of things, but perhaps that is the case for every group because I just don't know if Black people are more predisposed. You know, I've traveled to Africa, North, South, East and West, and African Americans have an absolutely different diet. This soul food emerged out of slavery in America and it is not the food of African people. Not to say that there are not health issues in countries in Africa, but they are very dissimilar to what African Americans are experiencing. It is really about socioeconomic issues and colonization and all of those things in Africa. So if African Americans are descendants of West Africa, which is a fact for the most part, and genetic predisposition is the cause of illness, it would seem that African Americans and West Africans would have the same illnesses. It's multifactorial as opposed to pinpointing genes because that argument gives room to say Black people are genetically predisposed to illnesses that White people are not and that's why the health status of Black people is lower. That can create a tremendous bias.

DR. WARNER: Well, I've never heard that argument before, but I would totally disagree with it.

DR. ROSE: Thank you so much for this interview. I have really enjoyed our discussion.

Dr. Warner's insight regarding the importance of emerging majority students' participation in STEM is very compelling, as it provides a clear understanding as to why said students may participate in research that is akin to what they have been exposed to and increases the possibility of enhanced diversity in the healthcare field. The sheer fact that more emerging majorities are involved will help to reduce health disparities.

Wrap-Up

Chapter Summary

A diversity plan is an essential step toward enhancing diversity in health care and academic institutions. In developing a diversity plan, the term diversity must be defined. Per this text, the definition is confined to racial and ethnic characteristics. Additionally, review of recommendations toward closing the health status gap is a useful process. For example, the United Nations recently sought recommendations from the Working Group of Experts on People of African Descent in the United States. A review of some of these recommendations with commentary by this author is provided in this chapter. Furthermore, an interview is presented with insight from Dr. Isiah Warner regarding the inclusion of emerging majorities in STEM programs and other necessary steps, which will be useful in closing the health status gap.

Chapter Problems

1. What are the two key approaches/steps that have the potential to be useful in enhancing diversity and impacting health disparities in the United States?
2. Are there problems with the term *tolerance* as it is applied in diversity initiatives? Explain.
3. List three questions that should be considered to review an organization's current diversity initiatives.
4. What is the importance of data and statistics in regard to diversity?
5. What is STEM? Does it have relevance in the discussion of health disparities?

References

Achrazoglou, J. (2010, November 9). Perspectives: How diversity goes beyond tolerance. *Diverse*. Retrieved from http://diverseeducation.com/article/14369

Alexander, M. (2012). *The new Jim Crow: Mass incarceration in the age of colorblindness*. New York, NY: The New Press.

Frey, W. (2015, March 6). In the U.S., diversity is the new majority. *Los Angeles Times*. Retrieved from http://www.latimes.com/opinion/op-ed/la-oe-0310-frey-no-racial-majority-america-20150310-story.html

McLeod, S. (2007). Maslow's hierarchy of needs. Simply Psychology. Retrieved from http://www.simplypsychology.org/maslow.html

Unesco. (1995). Teaching tolerance. Learning to Give, Retrieved from http://portal.unesco.org/en/ev.php-URL_ID=13175&URL_DO=DO_TOPIC&URL_SECTION=201.html

United Nations High Commissioner for Human Rights. (2016). Statement to the media by the United Nations' Working Group of Experts on People of African Descent, on the conclusion of its official visit to USA, 19–29 January 2016. Retrieved from http://ohchr.org/EN/NewsEvents/Pages/DisplayNews.aspx?NewsID=17000

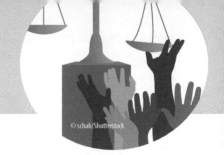
© schab/Shutterstock

CHAPTER 12
Case Studies and Health Disparities

The same things that lead to disparities in health in this country on a day-to-day basis led to disparities in the impact of Hurricane Katrina.

—**David Satcher**

▶ Introduction

The purpose of this chapter is to review 12 case studies relevant to U.S. health disparities. Many of the issues contributing to health disparities are not at the forefront of discussions toward solutions. These situations may quietly or overtly impact individuals without redress. Individuals who are not members of the mainstream American society often experience these scenarios with dire consequences. Concerns may arise in terms of understanding health issues, socioeconomic status, and lack of resolution, leading to ongoing health disparities. Although it is impossible to describe each and every scenario that contributes to health disparities, specific case studies, with commentary, will provide insight into the struggles of many members of the U.S. population, in hopes that a broader perspective may begin to take shape. As such, the following 10 examples will serve as a guide to help individuals approach similar situations in their own life experiences.

▶ Case Scenario 1: The Nail Salon

A Korean woman arrived in Manhattan and found a job working in a nail salon after looking through ads in the local Korean newspaper. As she got to know her coworkers on her first day of work, they began to warn her of the hazards of her new job. They explained how one of the manicurist's children was born "slow" and how another manicurist had had three miscarriages. They also pointed out that one of their coworkers who had worked there for many years had recently died of cancer. Upon the manicurists' asking her if she was married, she said yes and that she had recently become pregnant. An older manicurist who heard all of this warned her that she had made a bad work choice and should leave immediately. She advised her that she might lose her baby or have a baby with serious health problems. She noticed that the older woman had some difficulty breathing as she was speaking. "My breathing problems are from working here," the older woman stated as she noticed that the new, young manicurist was looking at her curiously every time she spoke.

The young manicurist, after doing a bit of reading from the material handed to her by the other ladies, in the form of articles and newspaper clippings about the health problems associated with nail salons and the chemicals used there and the resultant fumes, stood up, took her purse and waved to the other manicurists as she walked out the door. *I wonder why they didn't tell me this in training*, she thought. She never returned to the nail salon to work again.

Commentary

In the *New York Times* article "Perfect Nails, Poisoned Workers," which is part 2 of a series on the subject, the author, Nir (2015), describes an unfortunate situation that is having an impact primarily on women who choose to work as manicurists in nail salons. According to Nir, "A growing body of medical research shows a link between the chemicals that make nail and beauty products useful—the ingredients that make them chip-resistant and pliable, quick to dry and brightly colored, for example— and serious health problems." The research is still in progress, but essentially, this scenario is perhaps a contributing factor to growing health problems that exist primarily among Asian and Hispanic women working as manicurists. Most nail salons are located in New York City and the wages received by workers are generally low (Nir, 2015). The risks definitely do not seem to outweigh the benefits. So the young manicurist in this scenario made the right decision, in the best interest of her and her baby's health. This problem is perhaps another contributing factor to U.S. health disparities, primarily affecting people of color.

▶ Case Scenario 2: Hair Story

An African American woman, a graduate student in public health, decided that she wanted to launch a research project based on her interest in reducing health disparities. The focus of her project was the impact of the extensive use of hair products used by Black women to straighten and style their hair and the possibilities that these products with harsh chemicals may cause cancer and other problems. Her research inquiry was based on a literature review that raised speculation about these concerns. She received pushback from her faculty adviser, who indicated that such a study would not constitute a good research project because it was not a real public health issue. The student argued that her research was necessary and proceeded to find a collaborating organization to assist with her research project. Her adviser agreed that she should seek out a collaborator, if possible, and proceed accordingly. The student connected with a not for profit organization focused on health disparities, which agreed to explore her project with her and to seek funding to do so.

Commentary

Hair is a critical aspect of African American culture, particularly for women, as it has significant cultural and historical implications. During the atrocities of the slave trade, most Black people were brought to the Americas against their will, primarily from the West Coast of Africa. This brutal, inhumane process, known as chattel slavery, included removal of the identity of the individuals who were enslaved (cultural genocide). On the ships during the unsavory journey to the New World, slaves who spoke the same language or had the same markings of scarification were separated. Africans were no longer able to maintain elaborate hairstyles without their combs and herbal treatments used in Africa. White people looked upon Black people who learned to style their hair like White people as well adjusted.

Consequently, Black/African American women began to turn to products with harsh chemicals to straighten and style their hair. Currently, there is concern that these straightening products may be contributing to health disparities, as it is suspected that many may be carcinogenic and the cause of other health issues. The graduate student's project is warranted to investigate whether harsh chemicals found in the hair products used by African American women are a contributing factor to ill health and consequently health disparities.

▶ Case Scenario 3: The Meeting

An epidemiologist and a physician meet to discuss the focus of their presentation on health disparities at an upcoming health-related conference. The epidemiologist believes the focus of their discussion should be on what he believes are the causative factors associated with the health status gap between Black people and White people, namely with an emphasis on socioeconomic status. The physician argues that the focus of the presentation should be genetics, as it is his position that Black people are predisposed to those illnesses that are most prevalent among the Black population. The epidemiologist asks the physician if Black people in America suffer from the same illnesses as Black people in West Africa. The physician is unaware of the answer, so the epidemiologist informs him that the answer is no, which he argues diminishes the genetics perspective. That is, because most African Americans are descendants of West African people, brought over to the Americas as part of the slave trade, it would seem logical, from a genetics perspective, that the two groups would share the same health characteristics, including illness prevalence; yet, such similarities are not supported by scientific study, suggesting that an external variable is responsible for the poor health outcomes found in the Black/African American population. The physician concedes that the point made by the epidemiologist is an important one. However, unable to agree, they decide to proceed with separate presentations from their respective vantage points.

Commentary

There are varying perspectives on why the African American/Black community experiences poorer health, overall, than the White population. There are many factors, but the overriding issue is seemingly the difference in socioeconomic status between the two groups. Crimmins, Hayward, and Seeman (2004) offer the following insight into the role of socioeconomic status in health disparities:

> Mounting evidence indicates that racial/ethnic differences in morbidity and mortality are tied to socioeconomic resources. Largely because of data availability, most of this evidence is based on the health experiences of black and white people; with much less evidence on the role of socioeconomic factors in understanding racial/ethnic disparities when Americans of Asian or Pacific Island descent, Hispanics, and Native Americans are part of the picture. The potential power of the socioeconomic status (SES) paradigm in understanding health disparities—including racial/ethnic disparities—is evident in the fact that socioeconomic differences in health outcomes have been widely documented for most health conditions in most countries. People who are poorer and who have less education are more likely to suffer from diseases, to experience loss of functioning, to be cognitively and physically impaired, and to experience higher mortality rates. In the United States, few health problems are more likely to occur among those who are better off, and some health conditions are particularly sensitive to SES. In recent years socioeconomic differences in health also appear to be increasing in the United States and in other developed countries.

▶ Case Scenario 4: What's in the Water?

An African American woman wakes up in the morning in her Flint, Michigan, home in a low-income community. Like most people, the physical imperative of urinating is first, followed by a toilet flush. She sadly realizes that flushing the toilet is all that the water in Flint is good for. She walks over to brush her teeth and has to use bottled water, now donated to her after her fellow community members, who have been poisoned (based on decisions made by other fellow humans), expressed outrage when city management officials decided to use local water rather than water from Detroit, which had been the case previously. Proper research had not been done to determine if this was a healthy, appropriate choice.

After brushing her teeth and it's time to shower/bathe, how does she cope? Warm up bottled water and take a sponge bath every day? What about her two young children, her baby, and her elderly grandmother who lives with her? She wonders how she will explain this sudden use of only bottled water to her children.

She wonders about the homeless people who are already in a dire situation, often relying on water fountains or public bathrooms to take care of their hygienic and hydration needs. What about her dog? What about the stray animals? They drink water too. Bottled water only? Her pipes are ruined from the chemicals placed in the water, which caused corrosion of the pipes and ensuing lead poisoning. When will the pipes be replaced? What about the quality of life that water affords all living things? Her questions are endless and she is stressed. All she can do is weep as she goes to her stove and warms bottled water.

Commentary

Flint, Michigan is a predominantly Black community with socioeconomic characteristics, namely significant poverty, that have led some to believe that their lives are regarded as insignificant. However, people of all races in Flint are affected. As of 2016, a state of emergency has been declared in Flint, Michigan, which frees up $5 million in federal aid. The request was for a federal disaster declaration, which apparently is not available for man-made disasters. It seems, as of 2016, that $55 million is needed to actually assist with the contaminated water problem in the city, given the magnitude of it. While this disaster happened in Flint, it is important to understand that, from a low socioeconomic status vantage point and beyond, there are many more communities that may be at risk for such maltreatment or other types of man-made catastrophes. The what, when, where, and how for these catastrophes should be at the forefront of public health academia, given the knowledge within those walls, particularly in the area of environmental health.

Epidemiologists and many other experts in public health have the expertise not only to study this matter in Flint, but also to ensure that people of all walks of life understand how and why this happened. Water is essential to life and hence to the health of the public. The Federal Emergency Management Association (FEMA) sent water filter cartridges, bottled water, and water test kits. The actress Cher, in a partnership with Icelandic Glacial, donated 181,440 bottles of water. Other people and organizations also have donated water. This is a step in the right direction but is not enough. The fact is that this crisis is yet another contributing factor to health disparities.

▶ Case Scenario 5: The Spa Effect

In Miami, Florida, a young Hispanic woman and her husband, who is a prominent, well-paid attorney, join a country club at a local, luxury hotel near her community. Part of her membership includes use of the spa, where she has the opportunity to experience massages, hydrotherapy, a relaxation room, a sauna, a steam room, healthy snacks, soft soothing music, excellent fitness equipment, a swimming pool, yoga, cardio exercise classes, and beyond. She notices that whenever she goes to the club, there are only White Non-Hispanic and White Hispanic women present and no women of color.

As Director of Nursing at a public hospital in a low-income community where most of her patients are emerging majorities, she recognizes that such an environment would be extremely helpful to her clients but that such offerings are unavailable to them. She reflects on the fact that many of her patients/clients are stressed, overworked, overburdened, burnt out, and suffering from various illnesses that are stress and obesity related, including hypertension and diabetes. Each time she leaves the spa and fitness center of her club, approximately two or three times during the week and at least once on the weekend, she feels like a new person, leaving all of her stress on the massage table or in the Jacuzzi, the fitness center, the sauna, the steam room, etc., and she feels great as a result. She is grateful, but saddened that her clients cannot experience such tremendous stress relief and exercise, as she realizes that their being able to do so would be a positive contributing factor to their health.

Commentary

Stress is another reason that health disparities exist between some emerging majorities and the White population. Poverty exists in greater numbers among Black people, Non-White Hispanics, and Native Americans; there are also poor White people, but not to the same degree, on a percentage basis, as these emerging majority groups. Consequently, opportunities to find specialized sources of relaxation such as spas and fitness facilities are not available to the poor. The prices are exorbitant and often such resources are unknown to the poor. A parallel reality exists for the poor and middle classes when compared to the reality of the upper class and wealthy, for whom money translates not just to accessibility to health care but also to regimens that maintain and prevent health issues and provide opportunities for relaxation and destressing on a regular, consistent basis. These types of facilities are often not in the purview of the reality of poor people and are not discussed as possibilities for their participation. Hence, stress is often internalized without opportunities for release; moreover, these individuals often have very little opportunity to exercise and often consume poor-quality foods. Hidden, overlooked factors, such as the lack of access to healthy, stress-reducing facilities, contribute to health disparities. By considering such factors, they may be transformed into remedies for the problem. In this case, the task is making therapeutic facilities available to those who need them most.

▶ Case Scenario 6: Criminalization in the Classroom—The School-to-Prison Pipeline

A young Black Latino high school boy, who lives in a very poor area in the Bronx, New York, has found solace in his life through understanding the music and words of hip-hop artists who have successfully emerged from his community. He spends a significant portion of his life listening to their words and creating his own rhymes to try to express his dismay regarding the rampant poverty and violence in his community. He also uses his words to express his love for his family, his life goals, his desire to learn, and his hope for success through wealth and health in his life. His mother is a drug addict, his father is in jail, and his grandmother is raising him. She cares for him with love and he appreciates her, but she suffers from diabetes and hypertension and he is racked with fear regarding the possibility of her dying, as he has no idea how he will function and who will care for him if she becomes seriously ill. None of his teachers at school are Hispanic, and although many are kind to him and recognize his intelligence, they often chide him for not speaking up in class and for his many altercations with other students who tease him because his clothes are less than decent. As a result, he is often angry.

He gets into a fight in school and one of his teachers calls the school security officer (who is also a member of the county police force). The boy is taken out of the school in handcuffs, booked, and arrested. This incident ultimately leads to further arrests, as his time in jail enrages him and suppresses his ability to engage with others. He decides that there is no way out for him. His school progress declines and his teachers do not understand his problems, as he never shares them and they do not care to ask. The prospects of high school graduation diminish, and college is possibly not an option that he is able to explore because now he has a record and may not be eligible for financial aid. He feels that all he has left are his words, as he continues to write rhymes, which in his community is known as hip-hop. He shares this ability with no one, but he knows that this is the only medium that resonates with his voice.

Commentary

Often, young emerging majority boys and girls are criminalized in the classroom. Unfortunately, poverty often lends to a harsh environment that involves violence, drugs, lack of health care, and anger and rage, with few remedies for these myriad problems. Children must go to school, as education is compulsory, but teachers often come from communities outside of the environment where these children live and have no understanding of the realities of the lives of their students. They have no idea of what soothes them and how to be creative in helping them express their rage and intelligence. Children will often go inward, with pent-up voices, which can lead to lack of participation in standard, mainstream educational curricula and lashing out at their peers, who are having similar experiences. Hip-hop pedagogy has emerged as one approach to reach out to the children who find this form of expression useful. Ultimately, the role of the teacher is to find the voices of the children and to nurture them.

Criminalization of children via the school-to-prison pipeline—that is, carting them off to jail and entangling them in the snares of the criminal justice system—must not be the answer to environmental and social problems that manifest in adverse behavior at school. Hip-Hop pedagogy is being explored at Teachers College, Columbia University (Emdin, 2016), at the Hiphop Archive and Research Institute at Harvard University, and beyond. The bottom line is that children of low socioeconomic status must be reached. Otherwise, in terms of health, the outcome will be health illiteracy, as their continued opportunities to learn will be dismantled, leaving them with little understanding of what is necessary for them to lead healthy lives, to be carried forward from one generation to another. Lack of education, or poor-quality education, and the criminalization of K-12 children are contributing factors to health disparities for emerging majorities; the educational process is not leading to the stabilization and improvement of communities but rather the dismantling of them, which is unfavorably impacting the health and well-being of communities.

▶ Case Scenario 7: The Silent Epidemic

A bedridden 61-year-old African American man is in desperate need of a dentist because he has severe pain due to irritation of his gums as a result of ill-fitting dentures and tooth decay. He is unable to sit up after a severe back injury due to a fall. His only living relative, his adult son, has contacted several dentists in the community where he resides, only to be told that none of these offices in his area are able to accept bedridden patients. The man is also uninsured. He cannot afford to be seen in the emergency department, nor can he afford home dentistry, which uses mobile dental equipment. He is not eligible for Medicare because he is not yet 65 years old, he has not begun to collect Social Security yet, and he is not considered permanently disabled. His son does not have money to assist his father.

Eventually, his pain becomes unbearable. He is taken via ambulance to the hospital and receives a substantial bill for the emergency dental work and for the ambulance transportation cost. In a subsequent follow-up visit to the emergency department by ambulance, the dentist determines that because new dentures are unaffordable for him and his current ill-fitting set have caused substantial tooth decay, removing all of his remaining teeth would be the best option to resolve his problem. The patient and his son agree, as they see no alternative.

Commentary

Oral health has been defined by the World Health Organization as a state of being free from chronic mouth and/or facial pain and is an essential component to general health and quality of life (WHO, n.d.). This case highlights the problem associated with dental and oral diseases. Dr. David Satcher, former Surgeon General of the United States, refers to these diseases as the "silent epidemic," a problem impacting Black men at a higher rate than any other group (Morehouse, 2012). In this scenario, although the quick solution of pulling all of his teeth was the most expedient way to go, it is definitely not optimal. Extra steps should have been taken to assist him, including having him meet with a social worker to explore other possibilities for accessing care and funding his dental care needs. Transportation possibilities could also have been considered to try to get him to a facility that could have assisted him.

Most people are less than thrilled to visit the dentist and are unaware of the potential ramifications of failing to do so. Oral health can be an indication of overall health quality, as gum disease can lead to, or be an indicator of, other serious health problems. Millions of people in the United States are without dental insurance, especially emerging majorities in low-income communities, who are not eligible for Medicaid. Economic barriers significantly impact the likelihood of seeking dental care. For those living in poverty and not eligible for Medicaid, dental care is not typically a priority; needs deemed more pressing, such as housing, food, and medical issues, must be met first. People in lower socioeconomic status scenarios will generally avoid visiting a dentist, particularly if they do not have insurance or have limited Medicaid coverage for dentistry, and opt for tooth extractions if their oral health situation becomes dire, as in this case. Even with insurance, there are usually additional fees, beyond insurance, which may make the process unaffordable. Thus, the inability to afford appropriate dental care is a major contributor to health disparities.

▶ Case Scenario 8: Testing and Health Disparities

A young Hispanic woman from Honduras, who has lived in the United States for most of her adult life, is proudly working, dating a successful physician assistant, and looking forward to a bright future. Her new boyfriend is only the second man with whom she has been intimate, and both relationships, to her knowledge, were/are completely monogamous. She visits the doctor for her annual checkup and is asked if she would like to undergo a full STD (sexually transmitted disease) panel as part of her bloodwork. Since she is sexually active, she agrees. To her shock and dismay, she is told that she is positive for HSV2—genital herpes. She panics and her life is disrupted in a state of hysteria as she wonders how this could have happened to her. Her new boyfriend, whom she has been dating for months, advises her to get a second test at a different lab. Because she is asymptomatic (as is he) and he indicates that he has been completely monogamous, he believes her test is a false positive. He discusses the flawed aspects of the test with her, including lack of specificity, cross-reactions, the various types of tests, and their high rates of false positives. She cries and explains to him that a few of her friends have taken this test and been given positive results and did not consider a second test, and their lives have been deeply impacted, psychologically and beyond, although they were all asymptomatic. She agrees to take another test, finding a different doctor who uses a different lab, as recommended by her boyfriend.

The new lab does not accept her insurance so she has to pay out of pocket for the test, which is costly for her, but she decides to do so anyway. Her second test result is negative, and after thorough review of her history and further exploration by her physician, a false positive for the first test is the conclusion. She is relieved but then wonders how often this scenario happens and how many people there are walking around, asymptomatic, who tested positive and did not get a second test. She recognizes that many of her friends and family living in the United States are unable to speak English, are poor, and have very little understanding of what their doctors explain to them.

Commentary

Health literacy is fundamental to self-advocacy. Often, people are unaware of the fact that Western medicine, like other types of medicine, is not flawless and that various kinds of tests are not standardized or specific and may lead to high rates of false-positive results. Furthermore, they have no idea what questions to ask and may not be able to afford a second opinion/test or consider that they need one. Unfavorable results may lead to psychological dismay, the need for costly medications, and unaffordable retests.

The psychological impact of such tests, without individuals understanding them, magnifies the problem, as explained by Krantz, Lowhagen, Ahlberg, and Nilstun (2004):

> One of the major problems with type-specific testing for genital herpes is false-positive results, particularly since the predictive value of the tests may be low given low prevalence. This may be the case even if the tests have high sensitivity and specificity. For example, in considering STD

clinics, diagnosis may occur that is absolutely wrong—10% or potentially 30–40% in lower risk populations. There is an approach to verify these tests, namely Western Blot for HSV2 but unfortunately, this is costly and often not available. When one is diagnosed with genital herpes, there is a psychological impact, particularly because it is an illness that is stigmatized. Therefore, when the diagnosis is not accurate, beyond the trauma caused for the individual there is a serious ethical problem.

Health literacy is a critical factor in terms of health disparities. Often, data, diagnosis, and ensuing remedies may lead to inaccuracies that further impact the health of communities, psychologically and beyond. In addition to access to care, health education and health literacy are imperative to ensure healthy minds and healthy bodies in emerging majority and low-income communities.

▶ Case Scenario 9: Children Need to See

A 6-year-old boy entering the first grade has been diagnosed with a severe vision problem, remedied by glasses. He is on Medicaid, as secured by his mother on his behalf. He lost his first pair of glasses. He is permitted to get a second pair, per Medicaid. Unfortunately, he dropped his second pair in the schoolyard and broke them. Medicaid provides only two pairs of glasses. His mother has no money to get him new glasses. He is doing very poorly in school because he cannot see without his glasses. His mother seeks help from many venues, but there is no solution. Her young son is now presenting with behavioral problems in the classroom, as he is unable to participate fully in schoolwork with his insufficient eyesight, and it is just halfway through the school year.

Commentary

Eyeglass frames and prescription lenses are extremely expensive, for both children and adults. A child's inability to see sufficiently, both in the classroom and while doing homework, presents a serious learning problem. Consequently, without glasses for those in need, learning will be limited and the overall outcome is the perpetuation of health illiteracy. Without health literacy, people are unable to resolve the health issues in their lives, which leads to health disparity. All obstacles leading to children's failure to learn in the K-12 system must be addressed. Children must be able to see in order to learn, and there must be provisions within the healthcare system to enable children to get or have their glasses replaced if their parents are unable to pay for them.

▶ Case Scenario 10: Why Must We Die So Young?

A teacher arrives at work at a predominantly White private school in his city. He notices tear-stained faces among teachers and students and is quickly pulled to the side by the school counselor and advised that one of their students committed suicide over the weekend. She was a Japanese seventh-grade student whom the teacher had taught 2 years prior. The teacher is deeply saddened, along with everyone else, as he wonders what could possibly cause a quiet and extremely bright student to kill herself. He finds himself weeping softly at the loss of such a young child with so much more life to experience.

Commentary

Evidence suggests that suicide is a frequent occurrence within the Japanese population for both adults and children, as explained by Lu (2015):

> Japan's overall suicide rate is roughly 60 percent higher than the global average, a 2014 World Health Organization report noted. In 2014 alone, 25,000 Japanese people took their own lives. Last year, suicide was the leading cause of death for Japanese children between the ages of 10 and 19. Among teens and young adults ages 10–24, there are roughly 4,600 suicide deaths in each year, and another 157,000 instances of hospitalization for self-inflicted injuries.

Some factors associated with the suicides include bullying, school pressures, and parental pressures, among other issues. For Japanese children, this unfortunate contribution to health disparities warrants observation of Japanese children to ensure that they are feeling safe, comfortable, and valued in their school and other spaces.

▶ Case Scenario 11: The Plumber

In 2016, A 63-year old, African American, homeless man, is sent from a community clinic with a prescription for medication and the advice from a physician to try to experience better nutrition as he is underweight and experiencing a severe cough. He also suggests that he visits an optometrist because his eyesight is weak, to see if he can at least attain glasses, if necessary, or determine if there is a greater problem. He does not have family, and has access to extremely limited funds, which he does not reveal to the physician. He appeared very clean and neat when he went to the doctor, as he visits local grocery stores and Walmart to wash up daily, and plays his guitar on the street for money and occasionally washes car windows for cars passing by. He doesn't beg as he wants to give some kind of service in order to earn his way. The physician is unaware that he is homeless.

The man is a convicted felon, who served time, twice, for low-level drug offenses, when he was a younger man, in the 1990s but was never able to sustain a job when he was released due to his felon status. Before prison, he was a plumber, and a good one at that, and always carried small quantities of marijuana, for personal use, and smoked it with some of his clients after providing plumbing services for them. Then he worked for a plumbing company. One of his clients turned him in to the police, unexpectedly, upon his arrival to complete plumbing work at their home. The customer was angry with him because he felt he had charged too much for plumbing services, on a prior visit, and he wanted marijuana to settle the matter. When the plumber did not provide the marijuana for him, on a subsequent visit for plumbing services, the customer set him up. The customer had notified the police that he believed that the plumber carried marijuana and the plumber was arrested with marijuana on his person, hence possession, when he arrived at the customer's house. He had experienced a similar possession conviction in the past, so this arrest was seriously problematic for him. Consequently, because of his felon status, he was not eligible for any of the societal safety nets (public housing, food stamps, etc.) and has lived quietly on the streets, after being released for ten years. No plumbing company will hire him, due to his felon status and he is unable to afford/acquire the necessary tools to work as a plumber on his own.

Upon leaving the clinic, he stops in a large pharmacy. He tries on some glasses and finds that with the higher-level readers, he can see better. He slips them into his pocket. He proceeds to the area for cough medicine and puts a bottle in his worn, jacket pocket, and thinks about using the small amount of money that he has to try and get fruit to eat along with the food he usually eats at the soup kitchen. As he heads out of the store, security pulls him over and asks him to empty his pockets. He explains that he just needed cough medicine and glasses and begs them not to call the police. They call the police anyway and he is arrested. Due to the three strikes law, he will spend the rest of his life in prison, based on the mandatory minimum. He is devastated as he realizes that he will most likely die behind prison walls. Although it was tough on the outside, at least he had his freedom.

Commentary

As of December 2018, laws have changed. If this man was arrested today, in 2019, perhaps life in prison would not be the outcome because the drug felony would have to be more serious than possession and would have to have happened within 15 years of the 2019 arrest. The law is entitled The First Step Act. This law is better, although it is indeed only a First Step, as ideally, the circumstances of this man's experience are such that at the age of 63, with no further convictions after his prior mistakes, perhaps community service would be a better approach to address his crime. Since the First Step Act is not retroactive, he will have no relief, based on this new law. It would seem that given his elderly status and his capability as a plumber, he would be in a position to offer plumbing instruction to young people and to be provided with glasses and the necessary medical care that he needs, rather then a sentence to spend his golden years in prison. Although he committed minor crimes of possession of low level drugs, out of necessity, and had a drug conviction previously, with no indication of committing the latter crime again, does he deserve life in prison? His serving in prison, for this minor infraction, will contribute to the statistics associated with mass incarceration of the elderly in the United States. What other approaches should be considered in examples like this? How does mass incarceration of elderly people contribute to health disparities?

▶ Case Scenario 12: The Suburban Gap

A 32-year-old, Black woman living in a beautiful suburb, with her husband and two children was delighted when she learned that she was pregnant with her third child. She and her husband were proud of their accomplishments as she worked as an

Executive at a health insurance company in her community and her husband was a science Professor at a local college. As the only Black executive at her firm, she often experienced or heard unfavorable remarks about her hair, Black people in general and other insults that she brushed off each day, but shared often with her husband. She was also concerned about the number of student loans that she and her husband had acquired while trying to achieve their educational goals and the daily burden of understanding how long it would take to pay them back. When she became pregnant again, she was concerned that perhaps she should discontinue working while pregnant, as it was so difficult to do so with two children, but she decided to press on to continue to help to pay bills for the family, although they lived rather comfortably. She was also concerned because she often worried about matters that were gravely impacting communities of color, namely the Black community, as she reviewed health statistics as part of her daily work and as she watched the news she would experience general anxiety. She continued to watch the news because she wanted to be informed but said to her husband "if I see another shooting of a Black child, I'm not sure if I'll be able to handle it." She tried not to think about what she read and heard too much, but she took many of these matters personally and felt it was her obligation to care. When it was time to deliver her baby, she was quite nervous because she had been experiencing hypertension throughout her pregnancy, which was carefully monitored by her doctor. She never missed a prenatal appointment and her husband was always by her side, for each visit. It was absolutely devastating to him and his family, that after she delivered their beautiful baby boy she suffered a stroke and died suddenly, just a few days after their baby was born. Her husband was shocked, when he began to read articles, subsequently, and learned that he was not alone in his grief, as many Black women, even if they are educated and have a higher socioeconomic status, die from maternal mortality. He was absolutely devastated as he thought of his loving wife and realized that he was not the sole parent of two small children and a newborn.

References

Crimmins, E., Hayward, M., & Seeman, T. (2004). Race/ethnicity, socioeconomic status, and health in National Research Council (U.S.) Panel on Race, Ethnicity, and Health in Later Life. In N. B. Anderson, R. A. Bulatao, & B. Cohen (Eds.). *Critical perspectives on racial and ethnic differences in health in late life.* Washington, DC: National Academies Press.

Emdin, C. (2016). *For White folks who teach in the hood and y'all too.* Boston, MA: Beacon Press.

Krantz, I., Lowhagen, G. B., Ahlberg, B. M., & Nilstun, T. (2004). Ethics of screening for asymptomatic herpes virus type 2 infection. *British Medical Journal, 329*(7466), 618–621.

Lu, S. (2015, September 22). The mystery behind Japan's high suicide rates among kids. *The Wilson Quarterly.* Retrieved from http://wilsonquarterly.com/stories/the-mystery-behind-japans-high-suicide-rates-among-kids/

Morehouse School of Medicine. (2012). Oral health, unmet needs, underserved populations, and new workforce models: An urgent dialogue. Retrieved from http://docplayer.net/8972006-Oral-health-unmet-needs-underserved-populations-and-new-workforce-models-an-urgent-dialogue.html

Nir, S. M. (2015, May 8). Perfect nails, poisoned workers. *The New York Times.* Retrieved from http://www.nytimes.com/2015/05/11/nyregion/nail-salon-workers-in-nyc-face-hazardous-chemicals.html?_r=0

Satcher, D. Quote available at https://www.brainyquote.com/quotes/david_satcher_405412

World Health Organization. (n.d.). Oral health. Retrieved from http://www.who.int/topics/oral_health/en/

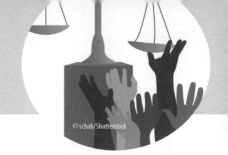
© schab/Shutterstock

CHAPTER 13

What Is Diversity and Who Defines It?

Our workforce and our entire economy are strongest when we embrace diversity to its fullest, and that means opening doors of opportunity to everyone and recognizing that the American Dream excludes no one.

—**Thomas Perez**

KEY TERMS

Alaska Native
Asian
Black/African American
cultural competence
diversity
Hispanic
Indian Health Service (IHS)

Indigenous population
nationality
Native American
Pacific Islander
predominantly white institution (PWI)
stereotypes

LEARNING OBJECTIVES

After reading this chapter, you should be able to do the following:

1. List the four racial groups in the United States.
2. Discuss the reason that Hispanics are an ethnic rather than a racial group per the Office of Management and Budget (OMB).
3. Define cultural competence.
4. Explain the difference between the terms *emerging majorities* and *minorities*.

▶ Introduction

On a National Public Radio (NPR) broadcast on May 26, 2015, an individual was being interviewed about the diversity that is beginning to take place in schools in American society. She was discussing Boston public schools and indicated that by 2025, the current students who are minorities will be majority minorities. Clearly she was utilizing the term that is used to describe congressional districts where the majority of the constituents are racial and ethnic minorities. It seems that the reality is that the term *majority* would be used to describe the larger group and the other group (Non-Hispanic Whites) would simply be referred to as the *minority* or *emerging majority*. However, what seems to be implied in this terminology is that although the minority students are the majority, they do not have the power associated with such numbers to hold the title of majority. Hence, the definitions are being determined beyond mere numbers and are based instead on how entities choose to define these terms. Such subjectivity is also the case for the term *diversity*. What does it mean and who defines it? This question will be pondered in more detail in this chapter, but as a start, Dr. David Satcher (2008) provides a critical perspective regarding diversity:

> There is a critical need for more diversity to focus on universal problems, to get providers in communities where they are needed, and to create a system that supports those needs. Diversity is important because it defines the parameters of opportunities to our children; it enriches the lives of future professionals; and because if we are going to achieve the goal of eliminating disparities in health, we'll need a diverse group of professionals to accomplish it. (p. 263)

Satcher further states that "diversity is an integral part of our environment. Diversity, or the lack of it, defines our environment" (2008, p. 1).

These statements make it clear that diversity matters in terms of public health and health professionals. Traditionally, the United States has been known for diversity based on an influx of individuals from all over the world. Often, the goal of immigrants is to seek greater opportunities beyond their homelands. This motivation explains the presence of practically all groups in the United States that are not **indigenous populations,** with the exception of African Americans, who were brought in as slaves by Europeans, in captivity, as chattel, to work the land. Native Americans are unique in that they are the only indigenous group to the United States, as they inhabited the land before any other group arrived and Europeans summarily took it from them. The resultant diversity in American society has made it necessary to understand the healthcare needs of various groups in an effort to provide optimal services. Understanding these needs involves recognizing the groups' distinctive health-seeking behaviors, attitudes, cultural nuances, and perceptions about health and beyond.

In an interview with Dr. Robert Fullilove, an interesting and perhaps controversial perspective is provided regarding the immigrant population in the United States. Dr. Fullilove, EdD, is the Associate Dean for Community and Minority Affairs, Professor of Clinical Sociomedical Sciences, and Co-director of the Cities Research Group at the Mailman School of Public Health, Columbia University. He has authored numerous articles in the area of minority health. From 1995 to 2001, he served on the Board of Health Promotion and Disease Prevention at the Institute of Medicine (IOM) at the National Academy of Sciences.[1]

Dr. Rose: In terms of health care in the United States, what are your thoughts regarding immigration?

Dr. Fullilove: Unless you're Native American, everybody here is either a direct immigrant or a second-, third-, or fourth-generation immigrant. I think that what that means is that it is impossible for Americans to claim some kind of unique, privileged status as if there are some of us who belong here and some of us who don't because we just got here. So, I think too much of what surrounds the current strategy on immigration reflects huge distortions about the impact that having a large immigrant population has on the structure of the labor force in the United States. American students do not go into mathematics and science, so 66 percent of all of our STEM jobs ranging from engineers to folks working in the area of scientific research—66 percent of that workforce comes from another country. If anything, were it not for our policy of training the brainpower of other nations so that we can meet our own economic and science base needs, if it were not for the brain drain, we would not have the privileged status that we occupy as the number one economic power in the world.

So, I think that in addition to there being a huge level of distortion around the role that immigration plays in American life, I also think that our inability to look at it in its totality so that we see what we do to promote our own interests and we also see what we do, or fail to do, which is to create the type of economic incentives that would make it possible for us to have a really rational policy with respect to immigration in this country. I think our failure to do that is something that hurts us enormously. I know that the one thing that will probably not change in the United States is this notion that if someone is ill, physicians, healthcare providers, clinics, and hospitals, if they have no other choice are going to be obligated to provide care. So the notion that somehow or other we can identify a scapegoat, call that scapegoat a bad guy and blame all our problems on the provision of health care on what's created because we have to care for their needs is once again a distortion of fact and not really an accurate way of understanding what's going on.

Dr. Rose: Do you think policies toward undocumented immigrants should be changed? Should their healthcare needs be covered?

Dr. Fullilove: At least in my mind, because the immigrants that we have on our shores probably do more to support the American economy than people imagine. We have a kind of obligational responsibility to make sure that their healthcare needs are covered. The fact that we are not able to have a national debate that is rational in scope and direction means that a lot of important issues are being ignored or swept under the table. And as a consequence, the health care of a large number of folk will suffer, as will the health care of just about all Americans, because we are unable to come up with the kind of policies that will ensure that we have appropriate health care for everyone.

Dr. Rose: How do you think that we can compare to other nations on this matter?

Dr. Fullilove: My belief is that, as I look at what's happening in Europe and in other parts of the world, the United States is not all that unique in the fact

---

1 Reproduced from https://www.mailman.columbia.edu/people/our-faculty/ref5

that, the economic inequalities that exist between the north and the south [in the United States] make it clear. People come to our shores trying to find a variety of opportunities, not the least of which would be the opportunity to gain access to health care. I think we have to accept that as a given and work both internationally as well as locally to make sure that access is as high a quality as possible. And that it doesn't create more problems than it solves, which is the case in all too many urban areas where there is an inability to treat critical conditions because people don't have access to health care. I think those are the types of problems that you have to worry about and also the problems that are ultimately going to bring us down if we don't do a better job of managing them.

Clearly, Dr. Fullilove is of the mind that the undocumented immigrant population is part of the diversity issue in the United States and that they deserve to have access to health care. However, there are differing definitions regarding diversity.

▶ **What Is Diversity and Who Defines It?**

It is important to focus on the most pertinent questions regarding diversity—namely, what is it and who defines it? The key factors, which help to define the term, begin with underrepresented groups in terms of race and ethnicity, who are the focus of this text. First, to be clear about the players involved in this discussion, the primary racial groups in the United States can be classified into four groups: White, **Black/African American**, **Asian** or **Pacific Islander**, and American Indian (**Native American**) or **Alaska Native**. **Hispanic** peoples are considered an ethnic group, as will be discussed in a moment. It is necessary to consider the specific groups because the term diversity, as applied institutionally, particularly in academic institutions, is defined very broadly. Universities, as an example, will often defer to international student enrollment and international faculty in indicating that their institution is racially and ethnically diverse. These factors do in fact lend to the diversity of institutions, but assessing diversity solely as an international matter precludes consideration of the very low representation of diverse individuals from the United States at many **predominantly White institutions**. For the purpose of this discourse, and this text in general, diversity refers to the racial and ethnic makeup of the workforce of a given healthcare organization or academic or any other type of institution. Generally, the term includes ethnic and racial backgrounds with the added emphasis of age, physical and cognitive abilities, family status, sexual orientation, socioeconomic status, religious and spiritual values, and geographic location (Betancourt, Green, & Carillo, 2002). However, the focus of this text is primarily racial and ethnic majority people as the emphasis is diversity as it relates to health disparities.

From that vantage point, the United States is a very diverse nation consisting of a predominant, or majority group, the White population, and emerging majority groups, which are Black/African American, Hispanic, Asian or Pacific Islander, and Native American or Alaska Native people. The White group is considered the current majority population based on their larger percentage of the total U.S. population, and the remaining groups are viewed as emerging majorities due to their smaller percentages and increasing numbers. It is important to reiterate that Whites,

Black/African Americans, Native Americans or Alaska Natives, and Asian or Pacific Islanders are racial groups, whereas Hispanics are an ethnic group. Race refers to "biological variation, including phenotypical differences in stature, skin color, hair color, facial shape, and other inherited characteristics that may or may not be mutually exclusive in each individual" (Perez & Luquis, 2014). Ethnicity refers to "a group or individual's conception of cultural identity, which includes a wide variety of learned behaviors that a human being uses in his or her natural and social environment to survive, which may result in cultural demarcation between and within societies" (Perez & Luquis, 2014). **TABLE 13·1** provides an overview of the various groups and the projected demographic changes in the United States.

Rubino, Esparza, and Chassiakos (2014) explain the effects of the racial and ethnic diversity in the United States as follows:

> People from diverse racial and ethnic backgrounds will make up the majority of the U.S. population by 2050 (Passel & Cohn, 2008). This increased racial and ethnic diversity will result in a more diverse workforce than in years past. Leaders of healthcare organizations will need to embrace this diversity and implement strategies that ensure that different cultural beliefs and attitudes are respected and valued by all members of the organization. (p. 58)

TABLE 13·1 The U.S. Population by Race and Ethnicity, and Projections

Race/Ethnicity	2010		2050	
White	246,630	79.5%	324,800	74.0%
Black	39,909	12.9%	56,944	13.0%
Native American	3,188	1.0%	5,462	1.2%
Asian/Pacific Islander	14,415	4.6%	34,399	7.8%
Native Hawaiian, Pacific Islander	592	0.2%	1,222	0.3%
Two or More Races	5,499	1.8%	16,183	3.7%
Hispanic	49,726	16.0%	132,792	30.2%
Totals	**359,959**		**571,802**	

Note: Percentage total is greater than 100% because some responders identify "Hispanic" as an ethnicity and identify an additional race designation.
Rubino, L. G., Esparza, S. J., & Chassiakos, Y. S. (2014). *New leadership for today's healthcare professions*. Burlington, MA: Jones & Bartlett Learning; Data from U.S. Census Bureau. (2008). National population projections. Retrieved from http://www.census.gov/population/projections/data/national/2008.html

▶ Hispanics/Latinos

Hispanic describes an ethnicity rather than a race, as one can be White Hispanic or Black Hispanic, as racial examples, where the terms *White* and *Black* serve as the racial identity and *Hispanic* as the ethnic identity. Hispanics can be further classified by **nationality**, which is an identity that can be defined by a person's place of legal birth or by a person's associational citizenship status governed by where an individual resides and works, which may defy national boundaries and sovereignty. People who identify their origin as Hispanic or Latino may be of any race, with commonality based on the language spoken—that is, Spanish. Although the terms Latino and Hispanic have been used interchangeably for decades, experts who have studied their meanings say the words trace the original bloodlines of Spanish speakers to different populations in opposite parts of the world. Hispanics derive from the mostly White Iberian Peninsula that includes Spain and Portugal. Latinos are descended from the Brown indigenous people of the Americas south of the United States and in the Caribbean, conquered by Spain centuries ago. Furthermore, the term Hispanic was given prominence during President Nixon's tenure more than 30 years ago through the Office of Management and Budget (OMB). It appeared not only on U.S. Census forms, but also on all other federal, state, and municipal applications for employment, general assistance, and school enrollment. Some sociodemographic characteristics of Hispanics and the percentage of racial and ethnic groups in Latin America are provided in **TABLES 13-2** and **13-3**.

TABLE 13-2 Sociodemographic Characteristics of Hispanics	
Characteristic	**Value**
Hispanic or Latino (2006)	47.5 million
In the 50 states	43.7 million
Commonwealth of Puerto Rico	3.8 million
Population not Hispanic or Latino	255.4 million
Total U.S. population (50 states) (2006)	299.1 million
Hispanic Subpopulations (2006)	
Mexican Americans	66.0%
Puerto Ricans	9.4%
Central Americans	7.8%
South Americans	5.2%

Hispanic Subpopulations (2006)		
Cuban Americans		4.0%
Other Hispanics		7.6%
Age	Hispanic Whites	Non-Hispanic Whites
Median age, Hispanics (2007)	27.4 Years	40.5 Years
≥65 years (2005)	6%	15%
Education: completed high school or more (2004)	58.4%	90%
Income; families with annual earnings ≥$35,000	50.9%	26%

U.S. Census Bureau. (2006). 2005 Puerto Rico survey (B03002-3-est). Washington, DC: Author; U.S. Census Bureau. (2004). The Hispanic population in the United States: March 2004. Retrieved from https://www.census.gov/population/socdemo/hispanic /ASEC2004/2004CPS_tab1.1a.html; U.S. Census Bureau. (2004). Current population reports: Educational attainment in the United States, detailed tables (PPL-169). Retrieved from http://www.census.gov/population/www/socdemo/education/cps2004.html; U.S. Census Bureau. (2007). Annual estimates of the population by sex, race, and Hispanic or Latino origin for the United States: July 1, 2006 (NC-EST 2006-04). Retrieved from https://www.census.gov/popest/data/national/asrh/2006/tables/NC-EST2006-03 .xls; U.S. Census Bureau. (2005). 65+ in the United States: 2005. Retrieved from http://www.census.gov/prod/2006pubs/p23-209 .pdf; U.S. Census Bureau. (2004). Current population survey, 2004 annual social and economic supplement. Retrieved from https:// www.census.gov/prod/techdoc/cps/cpsmar04.pdf

▶ Blacks/African Americans

Blacks/African Americans are now the second largest emerging majority group in America, after a long-held position as the largest, and they are also the largest racial emerging majority group. According to the Virginia Department of Health (n.d.), "the African American population is represented throughout the country, with the greatest concentrations in the Southeast and mid-Atlantic regions, especially Louisiana, Mississippi, Alabama, Georgia, South Carolina and Maryland." Black people have been referred to by many titles in America, including Colored, Negro, Black, Afro-American, and now African American, and other terms, not mentioned here, that are considered derogatory. These varying terms used to describe people of African descent in America were largely derived within political and historical contexts. Specifically, the term *colored* was used as a result of the following:

> The 1924 law restricting immigration might be the pivotal one here.... [It was] the first ever "comprehensive" immigration restriction law—with a "racial and national hierarchy that favored some immigrants over others." This immigration law treated "race" as obvious and visible as it split the world up into "colored" and "non-colored" races, and into European and non-European. (Rubin & Melnick, 2006, p. 8)

Racial/ Ethnic Group	Mestizo (%)	Mulatto (%)	Mixed (%)	Amerindian (%)	White (%)	Black (%)	Other (%)
Mexico	60			30	9		1
Cuba		51			37	11	1[a]
Columbia	58	14			20	4	
El Salvador	90			1	9		
Brazil	53.7	38.5				6.2	1.6
Peru	37			45	15		3[b]
Guatemala	59.4[c]			40.6[d]			

TABLE 13-3 Percentage of Racial and Ethnic Groups in Latin America

[a]Chinese
[b]Indigenous peoples (Mayans) including K´iche (9.1%), Mam (7.9%), Q´eqchi´ (6.3%), other Mayans (8.6%), and others (0.3%).
[c]Mestizo and European
[d]Blacks, Japanese, Chinese, and others
Central Intelligence Agency. (2009). *The world factbook.* Retrieved from https://www.cia.gov/library/publications/the-world -factbook/docs/profileguide.html

The term *Negro* has a different origination. One speculative perspective follows:

> Let us look back into history, then, and strive to discover the origin of this term "Negro." If you look at the unabridged edition of the *Oxford Dictionary*, you will be shown that the origin of the word "Negro," as far as is known in the English language, is in 1555. Nevertheless, that is not the beginning of the term because the English were not the first transgressors in this respect. The English adopted the word from the Spanish. The Spanish may have gotten it from the Portuguese; it isn't yet quite clear. (Moore, 1992, p. 35)

The term *Afro-American* was used to describe Blacks of African descent, and there are many theories regarding its origin, of which some are as follows, per Herbst (1997):

> Although sometimes said to date from the early 1850s, Flexner (1976) dates it to the 1830s and says it was used largely by Northerners or applied to free black people during the era of enslavement. Mencken (1962) cites a black leader, Dr. Kelley Miller, who in 1937 argued that *Afro-American* was coined in 1880 by T. Thomas Fortune, editor of *Age*. Miller also claimed that in the early twentieth century an English explorer of Africa, Sir Harry Johnston, shortened Afro-American to *Aframerican*,

suggested perhaps, as Mencken (1962) notes, by the coinage *Amerindian*; but Aframerican was never very popular. In any case, *Afro-American* was revived by the 1960s. (p. 4)

By the late 1980s, the term Afro-American was largely superseded by *African American*. However, *Afro-American* is still used by the Library of Congress for cataloguing purposes and is retained also in names of organizations or programs, such as Yale University's Afro-American Cultural Center.

Additionally, many still use the term *Black*. According to Spivey (2003), "Ninety Percent of all African Americans have their ancestral roots in the kingdoms of West Africa." (pg. 53) Consequently, the term African American is used to make a connection to this ancestral lineage. Some may prefer Black as a more unifying term, as they may identify themselves as persons from specific nations, such as Jamaican American and Trinidadian American. In these instances, African is not the lead term, although they are also of African descent. Others will solely use the nationality of their ancestry (i.e., the nation in which their parents were born or from which their family descends) to describe themselves, indicating that they are Jamaican or Haitian, for example, and leaving out the term *American* even if they were born in the United States.

▶ Native Americans

The notion of nationality as a key element of understanding culture applies to all of the groups mentioned previously. That said, Native Americans, who have been identified as indigenous to America, have a nationality that is unequivocally American. Other terms have been used to identify them, including Indian, but some are considered derogatory. Rubin and Melnick (2006) explain the erroneous nature of the term Indian in describing Native Americans:

> Writing in 1941, an Indian immigrant to the United States named Krishnalal Shridharani wrote, with tongue in cheek, about Columbus's "discovery" of America: "We Hindus take a pardonable pride in the fact that had it not been for us 'undiscovered' Indians, America would not have been the same America from 1492 on." (p. 139)

Shridharani is making light of the fact that Native Americans were given the title Indians because when Christopher Columbus arrived in the Americas during his exploratory voyages, he thought he was in India and incorrectly named the Native people "Indians." Hence, although the Office of Management and Budget (OMB) refers to this race of people as American Indians and Alaska Natives, it is important to note that they were native to American soil before Columbus arrived; therefore, the term Native American is somewhat more appropriate. This is not a definitive term, as the terms indigenous people and Indian are used, by some, as well as "tribal" names. Per Blackhorse (2015):

> This discussion varies in our ever-diverse culture. What I've learned is we can discuss this for hours on end but, when all is said and done, we call ourselves what we want because it is our choice. In fact, choice is something we did not have or were able to practice throughout the annals of U.S. history.

To that end, for the sake of discourse, the term Native American is used in this text, but the term should be used with understanding that there is controversy associated with it, and indigenous people should be asked what they prefer to be called.

The history of Native American people in the United States and the atrocities committed against them is complicated. Once Europeans set foot on American soil, the outcome for Native Americans was war, disease, hardship, and suffering. Ultimately, the U.S. government came up with laws, particularly related to the provision of health care for Native Americans and Alaska Natives. Hence, the **Indian Health Service (IHS)** was established and in 1955 was transferred to what was formally known as the Department of Health, Education, and Welfare, which is now the Department of Health and Human Services (Pfefferbaum, Strickland, Rhoades, & Pfefferbaum, 1996). The IHS provides health care through tribally contracted and operated health programs and service purchased from private providers (IHS, 2015). The result of this entity is significant improvement of the health of Native American and Alaska Native people. Nevertheless, their health status remains problematic.

There is no doubt that as an emerging majority population in the United States, Native Americans and Alaska Natives should have every opportunity to receive optimal health care to the same degree as their White counterparts and every other race/ethnicity. Although the relationship of this group with the United States has been challenging, the IHS has proven to be helpful. When the U.S. government decided to change its perception from the "termination" of Native Americans to "self-determination," as highlighted in the Indian Self-Determination Act of 1975, enabling transfer of programs under the Bureau of Indian Affairs, including the IHS, to tribal government (Pfefferbaum et al., 1996), there was the real opportunity to strive toward an improved health status. This is particularly true for Native American women, who, as in many other racial groups, are the primary caretakers of health in their families.

It should be noted that technically, Native American groups should not be equated with other ethnic minorities. The fact is that Native American tribes, by treaty rights, own their own lands and have other rights that are unique to the descendants of the real Natives of America. No other minority within the United States is in a similar legal position. Native peoples view themselves as separate nations within a nation. U.S. laws and treaties, officially endorsed by U.S. presidents and the Congress, confirm that status (Lanouette, 1990).

Despite steps in the right direction, such as establishment of the IHS, Native American and Alaska Native people suffer great health disparities, including alcoholism, obesity, diabetes, and heart disease. The leading causes of death among Native Americans are presented in **TABLE 13-4**. There are cultural nuances relative to the various Native American and Alaska Native groups, which often involve the need for healthcare providers to understand their traditional beliefs. The IHS helps to cross that barrier.

▶ Asian Americans and Pacific Islanders

Asian Americans are generally designated as people in the United States who arrived from Asia, namely from Vietnam, Indonesia, Japan, Korea, China, and other nations. Unlike with the Hispanic designation, language is not a factor in the Asian American designation. Culturally, there are significant differences among the Asian

Ranking	Cause of Death	No. of Deaths	Cause of Death	No. of Deaths
	2004		**1980**	
	All causes	13,124	All causes	6,923
1	Diseases of the heart	2,598	Diseases of the heart	1,494
2	Malignant neoplasms	2,392	Unintentional injuries	1,290
3	Unintentional injuries	1,520	Malignant neoplasms	770
4	Diabetes mellitus	746	Chronic liver disease and cirrhosis	410
5	Cerebrovascular disease	581	Cerebrovascular disease	322
6	Chronic lower respiratory diseases	486	Homicide	217
7	Suicide	404	Diabetes mellitus	210
8	Influenza and pneumonia	291	Certain conditions originating in the perinatal period	199
9	Nephritis, nephritic syndrome, and nephrosis	247	Suicide	181

TABLE 13-4 Leading Causes of Death Among Native Americans in 1980 and 2004

National Center for Health Statistics. (2006). *Health, United States, 2006. With Chartbook on Trends of the Health of Americans.* Hyattsville, MD: Author.

American groups. Asian Americans have distinct notoriety in the United States as the "model minority," given their tendency to assimilate into the mainstream.

Asian Americans are one of the fastest-growing racial categories in the United States (Reynolds, 2006). They are extremely diverse, coming from approximately

50 countries and speaking 100 different languages. Reeves and Bennet (2003) note the tendency of this emerging majority population to live in metropolitan areas:

> Ninety-five percent of all Asians and Pacific Islanders lived in metropolitan areas, a much greater proportion than of non-Hispanic Whites (78 percent). Of the two populations, Asians and Pacific Islanders were twice as likely to live in central cities located in metropolitan areas (41 percent compared with 21 percent). However, among those living in metropolitan areas but not in central cities, Asians and Pacific Islanders were only 3 percentage points below non-Hispanic Whites (54 percent and 57 percent, respectively). (p. 2)

▶ Emerging Majorities

Emerging majorities is a term used to describe an inevitable change taking place in American society based upon the prediction that by the years 2042–2050, in certain geographic areas in the United States, the majority populations will be Hispanic and Black people and other non-majority groups, and Whites will be the minority group. Therefore, understanding key aspects of Hispanic and Black people and other racial and ethnic groups is imperative in the provision of health care and public health services to diverse populations in the United States. In particular, the main racial and ethnic groups, as determined by the OMB (as described previously), are designated by category for federal statistics and administrative reporting (OMB, 1997). The categories determined by the OMB are delineated in **TABLE 13-5**. These categories are considered essential in the provision of health care in the United States, with specific attention focused on nationality and other aspects of individuals and their culture. Note, however, that the categories are under intense scrutiny and criticism, as some people feel that they do not accurately reflect the increasing diversity of the U.S. population.

It is essential that healthcare organizations learn to meet the needs of individuals served; otherwise, optimal, efficacious care may not be provided. There are consistent reports indicating racial and ethnic disparities in health. The IOM investigated such disparities in 2003 and provided concrete recommendations aimed at reducing them in a report titled *Unequal Treatment: Confronting Racial and Ethnic Disparities in Health Care* (Smedley, Stith, & Nelson, 2003). Some of the recommendations included increasing awareness of such disparities, integrating cross-cultural education into the training of healthcare professionals, using evidence-based guidelines to promote consistency and equity of care, and continuing research to assess disparities further and provide appropriate interventions. The IOM introduced a second report in 2005 titled *In the Nation's Compelling Interest: Ensuring Diversity in the Healthcare Workforce*, which focused on institutional and policy-level strategies aimed at increasing diversity within the healthcare workforce (IOM, 2004). Although the focus of this report was diversification of the fields of medicine, nursing, and psychology, diversification is necessary in all fields of health. Ensuring a diverse and culturally competent healthcare environment necessitates a top-down approach, beginning with the board of directors, administrators, and public health officials. Failure to recognize the need for diversity at these levels may preclude an understanding of the inherent needs of specific racial and ethnic groups. Insight from leaders that are representatives of ethnic and racial minority groups and who understand the need to

TABLE 13-5 Offices of Management and Budget—Racial and Ethnic Categories/Standards

Race	Description
American Indian or Alaska Native	A person having origins in any of the original peoples of North America, and who maintains cultural identification through tribal affiliations or community recognition.
Asian/Pacific Islander	A person having origins in any of the original peoples of the Far East, Southeast Asia, the Indian subcontinent, or the Pacific Islands. This area includes, for example, China, India, Japan, Korea, the Philippine Islands, and Samoa.
Black/African American	A person having origins in any of the Black racial groups of Africa.
White	Person having origins in any of the original peoples of Europe, North Africa,[a] or the Middle East.
Hispanic	A person of Mexican, Puerto Rican, Cuban, Central or South American, or other Spanish culture or origin, regardless of race.

[a]Note that there is great debate regarding North Africa, as it is located in Egypt, which is in Africa, and the people are largely Arab and African.
Office of Management and Budget (OMB). (1995). Standards for the classification of federal data on race and ethnicity. Retrieved from https://www.whitehouse.gov/omb/fedreg_race-ethnicity

diversify the workforce at every level in health care will prove to be extremely helpful in delivering efficacious health care for the individuals and populations served and would be a significant step toward reducing health disparities.

▶ Students and Diversity

The process of ensuring a racially and ethnically diverse workforce in the field of health must begin with educational institutions and students. The first step is to ensure that students who are representative of racial and ethnic emerging majority groups are admitted to programs that will train them to work in these fields. Additionally, healthcare administration and public health curriculums must include information about racial and ethnic health disparities, **cultural competence**, **diversity**, and the rapid change in demographics in the United States. Additionally, assessment must take place to identify any biases and **stereotypes** that students may hold, which may restrict their ability to develop and implement comprehensive and effective cultural competence plans in their respective work environments. (See Appendices II, III, and IV for cultural competence assessment tools.)

Health services administration and public health schools, departments, and programs must include research that focuses on health disparities, cultural competence, and diversity issues. Further, they must instill an understanding that failing to appreciate these dynamics will negatively impact the quality of care provided to patients and, ultimately, the fiscal bottom line of healthcare organizations and public health entities. There are educational institutions in America that remain predominantly White. This arguably needs to change if the needs of diverse populations are to be met and the health status gap is to be closed.

Diverse Healthcare Leadership

Optimal health care cannot be achieved without diversity and strong leadership within healthcare organizations. Assessment must take place over time to ensure that there is an understanding of demographic changes. The board of directors of healthcare organizations and academic institutions training healthcare professionals and staff should ideally be a representative microcosm of the communities served in the field. Consequently, boards should strive to choose leaders, namely the president/chief executive officer/administrator, of institutions who value diversity. Furthermore, human resources and education staff should be leaders in development of criteria for the hiring of diverse staff and training of employees at all levels to ensure an optimum level of cultural competence. Within healthcare organizations, it is not only processes that must be adapted to embrace racial and ethnic diversity, but also the people who serve as frontline staff. It cannot be expected that every individual within an organization will have insight into every racially and ethnically diverse group, because there are simply so many racial and ethnic groups. Hence, first and foremost, individuals in an organization should acknowledge that diverse patients/clients/customers will often have different values and customs based on their racial and ethnic backgrounds.

▶ Diversity as a Factor in the Doctor–Patient Relationship

The idea of physician bias was popularized in the IOM's 2003 report *Unequal Treatment: Confronting Racial and Ethnic Disparities in Health Care*. This report concluded that an important dynamic in race-related treatment difference was bias, prejudice, and discrimination within the doctor–patient relationship. It is also believed that the patient–doctor relationship has an important impact on disparities in medical care (Street, 2008). Although some research has supported the idea that race, ethnicity, and culture play a crucial role in the doctor–patient relationship, others have argued that socioeconomic status is also a critical factor (LaVeist, 2002).

Specifically, in terms of diversity, race and ethnicity have been cited as important cultural barriers in patient–doctor communication; yet cross-cultural factors have been relatively unexplored (LaVeist, 2002). Research has shown that racial and ethnic differences between doctor and patient influence not only physician communications but also decision making. However, these studies also show an enhancement of communication and decision making when the doctor and patient are of the same race or culture (LaVeist, 2002). This finding indicates that racial, ethnic, and cultural differences may be significant barriers to partnership and effective communication. A number of factors may account for this barrier in communication. One of these factors may be "unintentionally incorporated racial biases" (LaVeist, 2002), which is the idea that unconscious racial stereotypes may have been integrated into patients' symptoms and predictions of patients' behaviors and thus have become part of medical decision making. Hence, the notion of diverse providers to serve diverse populations makes sense.

The term *stereotype* was coined in 1978 during the onset of the modern industrial age. The image-setting process was called stereotyping, and over time, the word stereotype came to apply to the fixing of intellectual, as opposed to printed, images (Fuligni, 2007). Defining the term stereotype today, in terms of people, is complex. There are hundreds of possible definitions, even though they are all based on the idea that stereotypes are knowledge structures that serve as mental "pictures" of the group in question. With some exceptions, the general consensus is that stereotypes represent the traits viewed as characteristics of social groups or of individual members of those groups, particularly those characteristics that differentiate groups from each other (Wheeler, Jarvis, & Petty, 2001). In short, stereotypes are exaggerated beliefs or fixed ideas about a person, and the term is taught within the context of a particular example that expresses how this process can impact the provision of services to an individual. However, the tendency to oversimplify the definition has led to abandoning some of the presumed characteristics of stereotyping that were so critical to its early conceptualization as a result of inaccuracy, negativity, and over-generalization. Stereotypes are usually negative, inaccurate, and unfair; otherwise, they would simply be part of the broad study of human perception (Lee, Jussim, & McCauley, 1995). In terms of cultural competence, stereotypes matter because they influence judgment and behavior. Social categorization often occurs as a consequence of stereotyping, which usually transpires upon first meeting another person, without any real intention or awareness on the part of the person who is doing the categorizing (Nelson, 2009).

Another cause of barriers between patients and providers may be the lack of understanding of the patients' ethnic and cultural models or attributions of symptoms. This lack of understanding could lead to the patient being misdiagnosed. The final cause of barriers, suggested by LaVeist (2002), is that physicians and patients have different expectations of the visits, or physicians are unaware of patients' expectations of visits. Other factors that may contribute to communication barriers between doctors and patients are language barriers, low health literacy, and educational status.

Essentially, communication barriers between physicians and patients, no matter the cause, in terms of race, culture, and ethnicity, contribute to ongoing health disparities. When a doctor and patient are of the same race and culture, they are likely to have more in common than if they are of different races. Physicians and patients of the same race or ethnic group are more likely to share cultural beliefs, values, and experiences. These commonalities enable more effective communication because the individuals may be more comfortable with each other. Physicians have indicated that when their patients are from similar backgrounds, empathy is present automatically and that when treating patients that have different racial and cultural backgrounds from their own, there are fewer shared experiences (Chen, 2008).

▶ Treatment-Seeking Behaviors

Based on race, culture, and ethnicity, particular treatment-seeking behaviors exist that, on a generalized basis, need to be taken into consideration. As examples, the cultures of Mexican, Haitian, Native American, and Southern Black people and their definitions of health and illness will be explored. One should not view the perspectives offered here as representative of all members of these groups because that would lead to stereotyping. However, based on research pertaining to the groups, some commonalities have surfaced among people within the same groups (see **TABLE 13-6**).

Mexican people, in general, view health as a gift from God and a reward for good behavior. Health results from maintaining balance in the universe between "hot" and "cold" forces. Illness in an individual's body is considered a punishment

TABLE 13-6   Selected Behaviors/Perspectives of Various Groups That May Impact Treatment-Seeking Behaviors

Culture	Behaviors/Perspectives
Mexican People	■ Health is a gift from God and a reward for good behavior. ■ Health results from maintaining balance in the universe between "hot" and "cold" forces. Illness in an individual body is considered a punishment meted out for some wrong doing.
Haitian People	■ Health is a state of harmony with nature. Illness is a state of disharmony and is also caused by movement of blood, problems with gas, imbalance between "hot" and "cold" forces, and voodoo or a spell placed on a person. To maintain health, the spirit and body must be linked together by the soul. ■ Individuals may not feel comfortable discussing their spirit and soul with a medical practitioner for fear that their explanation may be misunderstood.
Native American People	■ Health is a state of total harmony with nature; human beings have an intimate relationship with nature. ■ Illness is considered a price paid for something that happened in the past or that will happen in the future. Illness may also be due to evil spirits.
Southern Black People	■ Individuals may feel that their illness is due to sin or evil. ■ Individuals may feel that an illness such as a cold is due to weather rather than a microbiologic factor (e.g., going out in cold weather will cause one to catch a cold).

Data from Giger, J. N., & Davidhizar, R. E. (1991). *Transcultural nursing: Assessment and intervention*. St. Louis, MO: Mosby Year Book.

meted out for some wrongdoing. Haitian people, on the other hand, view health as a state of harmony with nature and illness as a state of disharmony. To maintain health, the spirit and the body must be linked together by the soul. Illness is caused by movement of blood, problems with gas imbalance between "hot" and "cold" forces, and voodoo or a spell placed on a person. Additionally, although there are many different groups/tribes with different cultural norms, Native American people generally believe that health is a state of total harmony with nature and that human beings have an intimate relationship with nature. Illness is considered a price being paid for something that happened in the past or that will happen in the future. Some Native Americans believe that illness may also be due to evil spirits. Southern Black people may feel that their illness is due to sin or evil. They may also feel that their illnesses are a result of weather rather than microbiologic factors (Giger & Davidhizar, 1991); for example, they might believe that if one goes outside in cold weather, he or she will catch a cold as a result, rather than the cold being a result of a microbiologic (bacterial or viral) cause.

As a consequence of these beliefs, people from different cultures may have different treatment-seeking behaviors. Specifically, southern Black people may not seek care if they feel that their illnesses are due to sin or evil, and they may not want to reveal the supposed sin to healthcare practitioners. Haitians may not feel comfortable discussing their spirit and soul with a medical practitioner for fear that their explanation will be misunderstood. Hence, these examples illustrate how cultural perspectives may affect treatment-seeking behaviors within the context of cultural competence. Health service administrators and public health officials should ensure that all staff and providers are trained in the cultures of the specific groups served by their organization based on demographic data. This competence will build trust with patients.

Wrap-Up

Chapter Summary

The term diversity is often diluted by including too many categories in the definition. Hence, this chapter focused exclusively on racial and ethnic diversity, which is the focus of this text, along with health disparities. Demographics are rapidly changing in the United States, with the expectation that by 2050, emerging majorities will be the actual majority. This population includes immigrants to the United States. As pointed out in Dr. Fullilove's interview: "Unless you're Native American, everybody here is either a direct immigrant or a second-, third-, or fourth-generation immigrant."

Furthermore, in order to understand racial and ethnic diversity, detail is necessary about the four racial groups (White, Black/African American, American Indian or Alaska Native, and Asian or Pacific Islander) and the one ethnic group (Hispanic people), as provided in this chapter. The importance of diverse healthcare leadership, attention to diversity in the doctor–patient relationship, and racial and ethnic treatment-seeking behaviors are also covered.

Chapter Problems

1. Explain the meaning of diversity according to the former Surgeon General, Dr. David Satcher.
2. How is diversity defined in terms of emerging majorities?
3. List two key characteristics for each of the four racial groups and the one ethnic group in the United States.
4. Discuss the primary government organization that provides health care for the Native American population.
5. Why is attention to diversity important in the doctor–patient relationship?

References

Betancourt, J. R., Green, A. R., & Carillo, E. J. (2002). *Cultural competence in healthcare: Emerging frameworks and practical approaches.* New York, NY: The Commonwealth Fund.

Blackhorse, A. (2015, May 21). Blackhorse: Do you prefer "Native American" or "American Indian"? 6 prominent voices respond. *Indian Country.* Retrieved from http://indiancountrytoday medianetwork.com/2015/05/21/blackhorse-do-you-prefer-native-american-or -american-indian-6-prominent-voices-respond

Chen, P. (2008, November 14). Confronting the racial barriers between doctors and patients. *The New York Times.*

Fuligni, A. (2007). *Contesting stereotypes and creating identities: Social categories, social identities, and educational participation.* New York, NY: Russell Sage Foundation.

Giger, J. N., & Davidhizar, R. E. (1991). *Transcultural nursing: Assessment and intervention.* St. Louis, MO: Mosby Year Book.

Herbst, P. (1997). *The color of words: An encyclopedic dictionary of ethnic bias in the United States.* Boston, MA: Intercultural Press.

Indian Health Service: The Federal Health Program for American Indians and Alaska Natives. (2015). "Quick look". Retrieved from https://www.ihs.gov/newsroom/factsheets/quicklook/

Institute of Medicine. (2004). *In the nation's compelling interest: Ensuring diversity in the health-care workforce.* Washington, DC: Author.

Lanouette, J. (1990). Native American stereotypes (teacher's corner). *Anthropology Notes, 12*(3), 1. Retrieved from http://anthropology.si.edu/outreach/Indbibl/sterotyp.html

LaVeist, T. (2002). *Race, ethnicity, and health: A public health reader.* San Francisco, CA: Wiley and Sons.

Lee, Y., Jussim, L., & McCauley, C. (1995). *Stereotype accuracy.* Washington, DC: American Psychological Association.

Moore, R. B. (1992). *The name "negro": It's origin and evil use.* Baltimore, MD: Black Classic Press.

Nelson, T. (2009). *Handbook of prejudice, stereotyping, and discrimination.* New York, NY: Psychology Press.

Office of Management and Budget (OMB). (1997). Revisions to the standards for the classification of federal data on race and ethnicity. Federal Register Notice, October 30. Retrieved from https://www.whitehouse.gov/omb/fedreg_1997standards

Passel, J., & Cohn, D. (2008). *U.S. population projections: 2005–2050.* Washington, DC: Pew Research Center. Retrieved from www.pewhispanic.org/files/reports/85.pdf

Perez, M., & Luquis, R. (2014). *Cultural competence in health education and health promotion* (2nd ed.). San Francisco, CA: Jossey-Bass.

Perez, T. Quote available at https://www.brainyquote.com/quotes/tom_perez_643948

Pfefferbaum, B., Strickland, R., Rhoades, E. R., & Pfefferbaum, R. L. (1996). Learning how to heal: An analysis of the history, policy, and framework of Indian health care. *American Indian Law Review, 20*(2): 365–397.

Reeves, T., & Bennett, C. (2003). *The Asian and Pacific Islander population in the United States.* Washington, DC: U.S. Census Bureau.

Reynolds, D. (2006). Improving care and interactions with racially and ethnically diverse populations in health care organizations. *Journal of Healthcare Management, 49*(4), 243.

Rubin, R., & Melnick, J. (2006). *Immigration and American popular culture.* New York, NY: New York University Press.

Rubino, L., Esparza, S., & Chassiakos, Y. (2014). *New leadership for today's health care professions.* Burlington, MA: Jones & Bartlett Learning.

Satcher, D. (2008). The importance of diversity to public health. *Public Health Reports, 123*(3), 263.

Smedley, B. D., Stith, A. Y., & Nelson, A. R. (Eds.). (2003). *Unequal treatment: Confronting racial and ethnic disparities in health care.* Washington, DC: The National Academia Press.

Spivey, D. (2003). *Fire from the soul of the African-American struggle* (p. 53). Durham, NC: Carolina Academic Press.

Street, R. (2008). Understanding concordance in patient–physician relationships. *Annals of Family Medicine, 6*(3), 198–205.

Virginia Department of Health. (n.d.). African-American/Black population. Retrieved from http://www.vdh.virginia.gov/OMHHE/healthequity/minoritypopulations/africanamerican.htm

Wheeler, S. C., Jarvis, B. G., & Petty, R. E. (2001). The effects of stereotype activation on behavior: A review of possible racial stereotypes. *Journal of Experimental Social Psychology, 37,* 173–180.

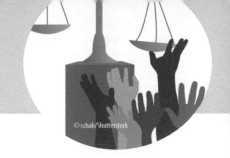

CHAPTER 14

Diversity in Health Care: Making It Happen and Sustaining It

Annie Daniel, PhD

Dominator culture has tried to keep us all afraid, to make us choose safety instead of risk, sameness instead of diversity. Moving through that fear, finding out what connects us, reveling in our differences; this is the process that brings us closer, that gives us a world of shared values, of meaningful community.

—bell hooks¹

KEY TERMS

diversity initiative
diversity plan
evidenced-based practice
pipeline

STEM
underrepresented student in medicine
 (URM)

LEARNING OBJECTIVES

After reading this chapter, you should be able to do the following:

1. Determine the key elements of an effective diversity program and the importance of planning.
2. Explain how an institution's positive climate and environment support racial and ethnic diversity and inclusion.

---

1 Reprinted with permission of Dr. bell hooks.

3. Identify the resources needed to support a highly effective diversity and inclusion plan.
4. Discuss the most effective methods to increasing diversity by comparing initiatives that drive institutionally-based programs, policies that suggest program implementation, policies within accreditation standards, or suggested resources to be used in diversity and inclusion activities by national organizations.

▶ Introduction

This chapter will discuss diversity in health care and effective programs that have been developed to sustain it. In recent years, it has become apparent that further work needs to be done to diversify the health professions. Although many methods have been integrated in professional schools to promote racial and ethnic diversity, much work needed is still needed. When the numbers of actual people of color are revealed, the health professions are not as diverse as the general population. A review of the literature and activities that most health education professional institutions have done to increase racial and ethnic diversity in the health professions reveals that pipeline programs are the most effective means of increasing diversity. **Pipeline** can be defined as a line of connected systems for identifying, developing, preparing, and producing an individual or group of individuals to enter a profession to fill organizational needs, which can be used to increase racial and ethnic diversity, starting at any level of education from K-12 to graduate levels.

In 2009, the U.S. Department of Health and Human Services, Health Resources and Services Administration, Bureau of Health Professions, and the U.S. Department of Health and Human Services, Office of Public Health and Science, Office of Minority Health, published a report of pipeline programs in the health professions. The report was an inventory of federal programs to improve racial and ethnic diversity titled *Pipeline Programs to Improve Racial and Ethnic Diversity in the Health Professions: An Inventory of Federal Programs, Assessment of Evaluation Approaches, and Critical Review of the Research Literature*. The findings of this report will be discussed later in the chapter.

Looking at models of success in the sciences, we can identify **evidence-based practices** that are working to increase diversity. In the report *Creating and Maintaining Excellence: The Model Institutions for Excellence Program*, Rodriguez, Kirshstein, and Hale (2005) identified seven core components in the Model Institutions for Excellence program that aimed to increase the presence of minorities in science, technology, engineering, and math **(STEM)**. These seven essential components were recruitment and transition initiatives, student support, undergraduate research, faculty development, curriculum development, physical infrastructure development, and STEM graduate school and employment initiatives. Although programs were different at each institution, Rodriguez et al. (2005) identified the common component at all institutions as student support, which included social, financial, and academic assistance.

In addition to Rodriguez and colleagues' report of 7 core components for programs to increase diversity, Thomas J. Durant, Jr. (2015), in his recently published book, identified 12 core components of a **diversity plan** (see Appendix IX). His model includes scholarships, mentorship, summer bridge, minority faculty and administrative representatives, recruitment, support groups, institutional linkages, multimedia advertising, direct visits (outreach), direct visits to the institution, referrals from alumni, and diversity environment. He stresses the importance of the environment and that it will be difficult to retain and recruit more students in an institutional setting that is not open to people racially and ethnically diverse from the majority group.

Both the work of Rodriguez et al. and Durant will be reviewed in this chapter to show the importance of including the core components in diversity planning and how developing a diversity plan with these components will yield greater success for increasing diversity.

▶ Current Standards for Diversity in Health Education Programs

A review of the current literature and research on the progress made to diversify the health professions, with its primary focus on African Americans, reveals that some progress has been made. Veterinary medicine and veterinary medical education, as an example, have never had the level of diversity of other healthcare professions. The U.S. Census projections illustrate that underrepresented minorities' composition will increase to become the majority population by the year 2042. Accordingly, the racial and ethnic minorities, when combined, will be the majority of the U.S. population (Day, 1996; Wang, 2002).

These population trends seem to be the driving force behind the current push to increase diversity in health care and healthcare education. Increasing diversity in these areas continues to be an issue with all of the healthcare professions, but it is more critical in veterinary medicine and veterinary medical education. At one point (during the academic year of 2003–2004), it was reported that of the 1,232 students enrolled in four different U.S. veterinary medicine schools, none were African American (Morse, 2008). The presence of underrepresented minorities has continually been below 10 percent in both veterinary medicine and veterinary medical education.

While other health professions have developed and implemented multiple programs and standards for increasing diversity, those with the least diversity have not consistently addressed the issue of diversifying their institutions. One very bold move by the Liaison Committee on Medical Education (LCME), the accreditation organization for medical education, was to change its standards for accrediting medical schools by including in Standard 3, Academic and Learning Environments, the following: "A medical education program occurs in professional, respectful, and intellectually stimulating academic and clinical environments that recognize the benefits of diversity and that promote students' attainment of the knowledge, skill, attitudinal, and behavioral competencies required of future physicians" (LCME, 2016). Furthermore, Standard 3.3 indicates that medical education programs must have diversity/pipeline programs and partnerships. This standard states the following:

> An institution that sponsors a medical education program has effective policies and practices in place, and engages in ongoing, systematic, and focused recruitment and retention activities, to achieve mission-appropriate diversity outcomes among its students, faculty, administrative staff, and

other members of its academic community. These activities include the development of programs and/or partnerships aimed at broadening diversity among qualified applicants for medical school admission and the evaluation of program and partnership outcomes. (LCME, 2016, p. 4)

With this move, we should look for increased diversity in medical education programs.

A more in-depth look into other health professions' standards for diversity in health education programs reveals that the accrediting group for medical education is the only one to make diversity a part of the standards for a program to receive accreditation.

▶ Meeting the Demands of a Changing Population

As reported, the U.S. Census projects by the year 2042 that racial minorities will be the majority of the U.S. population. The Pew Research Center reports that White Americans will go from making up 85 percent of the U.S. population to 43 percent, while Black and Hispanic Americans will reach 45 percent of the population by 2060. With these statistics in mind, the client base across all health professions, including veterinary medicine, is changing. The Association of American Veterinary Medical Colleges and the American Veterinary Medicine Association realize that such compositional changes in the general population require an increased strategic effort to recruit, educate, and graduate a diverse veterinary workforce that will be positioned to meet the myriad of health care, biomedical, and agricultural research and food sourcing and safety needs of the future. However, unlike medical education accreditors, veterinary medicine is known as the least diverse of all healthcare professions and does not address the issue as seriously and boldly as does the LCME and other accreditors of healthcare educational programs.

▶ Increasing Racial Diversity in Health Professions

In the fall of 2003, the *Journal of Blacks in Higher Education* published an article declaring the veterinary profession as the most "segregated field in graduate education" ("Holy Cow!" 1996). Nearly a decade later, an article in *The Atlantic* broadened the dubious distinction by labeling the profession as the "Whitest" profession in America (Thompson, 2013).

The absence of racial and ethnic diversity in the veterinary profession is often easily dismissed given the very narrow view of the profession as inheritors of the legacy of James Herriot, the gentle pet doctor; such characterizations of the profession, while noble and somewhat true, ignore the numerous societal roles of veterinarians as biomedical scientists and integral protectors of the public health, among others. The relative absence of diversity in the veterinary profession has significant implications, much like those seen in human medicine. Talented applicants of color may be excluded from opportunities to enter the profession (Chubin & Mohamed, 2009; Greenhill, 2009; "Holy Cow!" 1996). Additionally, the academic environment may be suboptimal (Greenhill, 2009; Greenhill & Carmichael, 2014), and underrepresented racial and ethnic communities are more likely to be underserved by the profession (Lowrie, 2009; Strayhorn, 2009). Lastly, the homogeneity of the profession limits its long-term social impact on clinical practice, research, and human and animal health (Lowrie, 2009; Strayhorn, 2009).

The *Journal of Blacks in Higher Education*'s 2003 article triggered the creation of a national **diversity initiative** by the Association of American Veterinary Medical Colleges focused on increasing the representation of underrepresented students and faculty. At the time, the percentage of racially and ethnically underrepresented students (*all* racial/ethnic groups excluding White/Caucasian) had never exceeded 10 percent; in fact in 2003, the total number of minority students at veterinary schools in the United States was only 877, and 140 of those students attended Tuskegee University. (See Appendix XIV.)

As in veterinary medicine, most racial and ethnic minorities in the United States are also severely underrepresented across various health professions, including medicine, dentistry (Grumbach & Mendoza, 2008), and nursing (Bednarz, Schim, & Doorenbos, 2010). Compelling evidence shows that the lack of diversity in the workforce effectively limits access to quality health care by minority and poor communities (Institutional Committee, 2004; Sullivan Commission, 2004). The result is a myriad of health disparities, which not only negatively impact the health outcomes for underserved populations, but also serve to economically stunt these communities (LaVeist, Gaskin, & Richard, 2011). Increases in racial, ethnic, gender, and sexual diversity in health care have all been advocated as one approach to increasing access to healthcare services, reducing health disparities, and increasing positive health outcomes. It has been documented that health disparities in humans who own pets are transferred to their ability to satisfy the health needs of pets and animals (LaVeist, Gaskin, & Richard, 2011).

The healthcare workforce can be changed only through the health education system. The application by and admittance, of a more diverse population, to health professions education programs are essential to changing the racial and ethnic composition. A curriculum designed to help students achieve cultural competence prepares them for working in a more diverse environment and has the long-term effect of addressing health disparities. These efforts are strengthened by data showing that increases in racial and ethnic diversity in the classroom are tied to eventual increases in the delivery of culturally competent care (Pacquiao, 2007).

▶ Determining Evidence-Based Practices for Increasing Diversity in Healthcare Education and Healthcare Professions

A review of literature and interviews with healthcare educators identified 12 common themes or elements that have been proven to increase diversity. In some cases, the institution may not have all 12 elements in its diversity plan, but are including three or more of the elements results in a successful plan to increase people of color in a healthcare education program. Research has also shown that these practices work for increasing the number of faculty of color as well.

However, diversity efforts may fail due to the absence of recruitment plans, retention, plans, mentoring models, and resources; a lack of involvement (isolation); and, finally, the element that tends to damage any diversity progress, the environment. An institution may have excellent plans, models, and resources in place, but if the people in the institution create a negative environment and are not open to receive and interact with people of color, these people will not remain in the institution, and diversity and inclusion will not be successful. An institution's diversity climate may cause faculty of color to face diversity pressures, isolation, and racism. In addition, faculty of color may have a lack of mentoring and support for advancement. Rodríguez, Campbell, Fogarty, and Williams (2014) advise that to sustain minority faculty, it is important to have a mentoring program and faculty development programs established.

▶ Medical Education National Diversity and Inclusion Initiatives

As previously discussed, medical education has taken the boldest position in promoting diversity and inclusion within the schools accredited by the LCME. This accrediting body has set a standard for other healthcare education programs. In addition to these standards, the support for diversity in medical colleges is bolstered through one of the most robust diversity and inclusion programs of all of the healthcare professions, that of the Association of American Medical Colleges (AAMC). The AAMC has very carefully and strategically planned many initiatives to purposefully increase diversity and inclusion, especially for people of color. This organization has invested resources in human capital, organizational capacity building, and public health initiatives—initiatives known as the AAMC Diversity Portfolios. (See Appendix X.)

To determine if medical schools are prepared to implement the LCME's robust standards of developing pipeline programs and/or partnerships that will lead to increased diversity and inclusion, this author contacted Dr. Gaarmel Funches at the University of Mississippi Medical Center (UMMC). UMMC has, including medical education, 28 health care-related degree programs offered through the Schools of Dentistry, Graduate Studies in the Health Sciences, Health Related Professions, Medicine, and Nursing. Dr. Funches joined the UMMC in July 2000 and serves as the Director of Community Education and Outreach. She is responsible for initiatives involving recruitment, outreach, pipeline, and enrichment programming, and she provides support to the university medical center students as well as the community. She has a three-phase focus of prepping and recruiting qualified students to attend UMMC and retaining them once enrolled.

According to Dr. Funches (in an interview conducted in 2016), the University of Mississippi School of Medicine was established on the Oxford, Mississippi, campus in 1903 as a 2-year program. Students completed their 3rd and 4th years of study at various other American medical schools. A School of Nursing was added in 1948. The Mississippi Legislature passed legislation in the early 1950s to construct the

UMMC, including a 4-year School of Medicine, a teaching hospital, and the School of Nursing. The faculty, facilities, and students at Oxford were transferred to the Jackson, Mississippi, campus, which opened in 1955.

DR. DANIEL: Please tell me a little bit about your programs. How did it get started?

DR. FUNCHES: It was established over 30 years ago, in an effort to increase the number of underserved, underrepresented students pursuing health careers. Pipeline programs were established to expose area middle school, high school, and college students to health careers through multidimensional outreach efforts such as health career exploration, health science readiness, and simulated rigor using a science-based college preparatory curriculum.

DR. DANIEL: What is the mission and vision of your program?

DR. FUNCHES: The Office of Health Careers Opportunity (OHCO), formally the Division of Multicultural Affairs, supports the Medical Center's efforts to train a diverse healthcare workforce for the state of Mississippi. The OHCO's overarching mission is to foster an environment that recognizes the benefits of diversity and inclusiveness through academic preparation, instruction, community outreach, and professional development. It also seeks to disseminate valuable resources and research on cultural competence, quality, and equity in health care to the UMMC community.

The vision of our programs is to:

■ Increase enrollment and retention of underrepresented, underserved students in all UMMC programs, including medicine, dentistry, nursing, pharmacy, graduate education, and health-related professions;

■ Provide programming designed to ensure academic progression and timely graduation;

■ Provide support services, including academic counseling, mentoring, etc., in efforts to support the academic and professional growth of students;

■ Provide a health careers pipeline to support efforts to maintain a competitive and diverse applicant pool;

■ Foster a sense of community among students through support of student organizations; and

■ Support and implement institutional initiatives that promote an inclusive and diverse UMMC community.

DR. DANIEL: When did it get started?

DR. FUNCHES: The program actually started in 1971 in the Office of Minority Student Affairs here on UMMC's campus.

DR. DANIEL: What are the statistics for students participating in the programs?

DR. FUNCHES: One hundred percent of our medical students (147) are Mississippi residents. Thirty percent (44) of the current medical students participated in the pre-matriculation program last summer. Fifteen of our 16 (93%) African American students participated in the pre-matriculation program last year, which accounts for (34%) of the 44 slots taken by medical students.

One hundred percent of our dental students (35) are Mississippi residents. Seventeen percent (6) of the current dental students participated in our pre-matriculation program last year. One hundred percent (4) of our African American students participated in the pre-matriculation program last year, which accounts for (67%) of the 6 slots taken by dental students.

DR. DANIEL: What are the demographics of current students at UMMC?

DR. FUNCHES: There are 147 current medical students, and 16 (11%) are African American. There are 35 current dental students, and 4 (11%) are African American.

DR. DANIEL: What are the statistics of students that were in the pre-enrollment programs?

DR. FUNCHES: In the past 10 years, we have had a 100 percent passing rate of pre-enrollment students in the first year of medical and dental courses that we offer during the summer, which are biochemistry and gross anatomy, and in the last 5 years histology.

DR. DANIEL: How many of the pipeline students applied and were admitted to your programs?

DR. FUNCHES: One hundred percent of our students that participated in any of our programs are given priority over others to participate on the next level to continue our "pipeline." This is providing they continue to have the qualifications as stipulated for each program.

DR. DANIEL: How do you promote your program to recruit students from diverse backgrounds?

DR. FUNCHES: We visit all of our state schools twice a year. Our admission departments for both the school of medicine and dentistry encourage the incoming students to participate upon their acceptance, and they send us a referral list.

DR. DANIEL: Describe your process for students' selection.

DR. FUNCHES: We have students who participated in earlier programs apply to our programs upon being accepted to medical and dental school here at UMMC. The students are given information about our pre-matriculation program during revisit day as well as recruitment visits to the schools and the information on our website. Of the accepted students who are accepted from HBCUs [historically Black colleges and universities], small schools or programs that did not offer biochemistry, gross anatomy, and histology as undergraduates, the School of Medicine and School of Dentistry send our office a referral list. The program is not mandatory for the students to participate in. We reach out to students on the referral list first and from there we reach out to the students that actually apply to the program if slots are available.

DR. DANIEL: What are your criteria for entrance?

DR. FUNCHES: Being accepted to our school of medicine and dentistry here at UMMC.

DR. DANIEL: Tell me about the application process for applying to the schools.

DR. FUNCHES: In the last 3 years we have implemented an electronic application for all of our programs. Before then it was paper and pencil. The application process opens up in December of each year and the deadline date for application is April 1 each year.

DR. DANIEL: Do you partner with HBCUs?

DR. FUNCHES: We partner with Alcorn State University, Jackson State University, and Tougaloo College.

DR. DANIEL: How do you select faculty and mentors for students?

DR. FUNCHES: Our students have peer mentors with whom they are paired before starting their academic year. The peer mentors are responsible for ensuring that all students become acclimated to campus in the best way possible.

DR. DANIEL: What are the areas of impact of the different programs? Any particular curriculum content?

DR. FUNCHES: Our areas of potential impact for our students include biochemistry, gross anatomy, and histology. These are areas that for the longest had a negative impact upon incoming students that was evident by their grades.

DR. DANIEL: What are the evidence-based practices that you have integrated in the program?

DR. FUNCHES: Practical application of lecture and labs and having the students to perform the skills taught by way of hands-on application or testing. Our academic enrichment and outreach programs begin at the elementary school level, extending to pre-professional levels. Annually, approximately 170 students are exposed to appropriate age and grade level academics in science, mathematics, critical thinking, and computer application and technology. Students are nurtured through practical experiences on practice examinations such as ACT, MCAT, and DAT exams. Coordinated outreach efforts have created sustainable and long term partnerships with public school districts, colleges and universities, associations, and other educational organizations. As a result of our long-term commitment in increasing the number of **underrepresented students in medicine or URM** (as defined by the American Association of Medical Colleges), we have recently extended our programming efforts by launching our STEP program [Science, Training Enrichment Program] as a satellite program in two off-campus locations. In 2016, our goal is to have served nearly 600 students from across the state.

DR. DANIEL: What practical lessons were learned from implementing the programs?

DR. FUNCHES: We learn to get feedback from our students in order to make the programs better. In December of each year, we hold focus groups with the students who participated in the summer program and ask them how we can make the program better for them to be more successful. Five years ago, the students wanted us to add histology to the summer program because they thought it would be beneficial. So, as of 5 years ago, the students have three summer classes instead of two.

DR. DANIEL: What would you do differently?

DR. FUNCHES: Nothing at the current time because we have programs that reach students from elementary school to preentry into medical and dental school.

DR. DANIEL: The literature identifies about 12 evidence-based practices a successful diversity and inclusion program should include. Please tell me how you have incorporated these into your different programs.

DR. FUNCHES: We include all of the practices in our diversity and inclusion programs. We have scholarships, mentorship, summer bridge, minority faculty/administrative representatives, support groups, institutional linkages, multimedia advertising, direct visits, direct visits to school, referrals from alumni, and a positive environment for diversity.

DR. DANIEL: Do you have any closing thoughts about your programs and school that you would like to share or final thoughts for those developing a pipeline program for racial and ethnic diversity?

DR. FUNCHES: Do not get discouraged about your numbers as far as minorities are concerned because students still need to have an interest in health care and be given the right guidance during undergraduate years.

DR. DANIEL: Thank you so much, Dr. Funches, for sharing your knowledge and experience.

Wrap-Up

Chapter Summary

This chapter addressed major initiatives by healthcare professions' education programs and reviewed core elements of highly effective diversity and inclusion programs. The evidence-based practices that work implement 3 or more of 12 core components identified by Durant (2015) for programs to increase diversity. Durant (2015) identified these components in his recently published book that chronicled his and others' efforts to desegregate the university at which he worked as professor of sociology for 36 years (1973–2009). The group of faculty, staff, and students developed a plan of evidence-based practices in 1983 to recruit African American graduate students. Today, these practices are still implemented across the campus in various departments, with much success. To review, the model incorporates scholarships, mentorship, summer bridge, minority faculty and administrative representatives, recruitment, support groups, institutional linkages, multimedia advertising, direct visits (outreach), direct visits to the institution, referrals from alumni, and diversity environment. Durant (2015) stresses the importance of having a positive environment and climate for diversity and inclusion because it will be difficult to recruit and retain more students of color in an institution that is not open to people from racially and ethnically diverse backgrounds—that is, people who are not from the majority group.

Chapter Problems

1. Using the following list, identify the current practices in medical education, nursing education, dental education, and veterinary education aimed at meeting the 12 core components outlined by Durant, and list an example of the practice that is in place:

Evidence-Based Practices That Work

1. *Scholarships*
   a. Medical education
   b. Nursing education
   c. Dental education
   d. Veterinary education

2. *Mentorship*
   a. Medical education
   b. Nursing education
   c. Dental education
   d. Veterinary education

3. *Summer Bridge*
   a. Medical education
   b. Nursing education
   c. Dental education
   d. Veterinary education

4. *Minority Faculty/Administrative Representative*
   a. Medical education
   b. Nursing education
   c. Dental education
   d. Veterinary education

5. *Recruitment*
   a. Medical education
   b. Nursing education
   c. Dental education
   d. Veterinary education

6. *Support Groups*
   a. Medical education
   b. Nursing education
   c. Dental education
   d. Veterinary education

7. *Institutional Linkages*
   a. Medical education
   b. Nursing education
   c. Dental education
   d. Veterinary education

8. *Multimedia Advertising*
   a. Medical education
   b. Nursing education
   c. Dental education
   d. Veterinary education

9. *Direct Visits (Outreach to K-12 and Undergraduate Education)*
   a. Medical education
   b. Nursing education
   c. Dental education
   d. Veterinary education

10. *Directs Visits to the Institution*
    a. Medical education
    b. Nursing education
    c. Dental education
    d. Veterinary education

11. *Referrals From Alumni*
    a. Medical education
    b. Nursing education
    c. Dental education
    d. Veterinary education

12. *Diversity Environment*
    a. Medical education
    b. Nursing education
    c. Dental education
    d. Veterinary education

2. Using the information you collected for Question 1, show the effectiveness of the initiatives by reviewing the diversity data for medical education, nursing education, dental education, and veterinary education:

Healthcare Education Profession	Diversity Data of Enrollees Prior to Implementing the Initiatives (People of Color)	Diversity Data of Enrollees After Implementing the Initiatives (People of Color)
Medical education		
Nursing education		
Dental education		
Veterinary education		

3. Review the initiatives and the data discussed in the chapter. What can you conclude about the effectiveness of having a systematic, strategic plan to increase diversity and inclusion in healthcare education, at a national or local level, as discussed in the UMMC interview?

4. This chapter has discussed the diversity initiative of medical education and the move to require a diversity plan as a criterion for accreditation. Research the other healthcare education programs and summarize their diversity requirements for accreditation, if such requirements are in place.

5. After reviewing the data for diversity, the initiatives, and policies, which do you believe is most effective at increasing diversity, initiatives that drive institutionally based programs, policies that suggest program implementation, policies within accreditation standards, or suggested resources to be used in diversity and inclusion activities by national organizations?

References

Bednarz, H., Schim, S., & Doorenbos, A. (2010). Cultural diversity in nursing education: Perils, pitfalls, and pearls. *The Journal of Nursing Education, 49*(5), 253–260.

Chubin, D. E., & Mohamed, S. (2009). Increasing minorities in veterinary medicine: National trends in science degrees, local programs, and strategies. *Journal of Veterinary Medical Education, 36*(4), 363–369.

Day, J. C. (1996). *Population projections of the United States by age, sex, race and Hispanic origin: 1995 to 2050.* U.S. Census Bureau, Current Population Reports, Series P25-1120. Washington, DC: Government Printing Office.

Durant, T. J. (2015). *A view from the inside: Thirty-six years of desegregation.* Baton Rouge, LA: Durant Publishing Company.

Greenhill, L. M. (2009). DiVersity matters: A review of the diversity initiative of the Association of American Veterinary Medical Colleges. *Journal of Veterinary Medical Education, 36*(4), 359–362.

Greenhill, L. M., & Carmichael, K. P. (2014). Survey of college climates at all 28 U.S. colleges and schools of veterinary medicine: Preliminary findings. *Journal of Veterinary Medical Education, 41*(2), 111–121.

Grumbach, K., & Mendoza, R. (2008). Disparities in human resources: Addressing the lack of diversity in the health professions. *Health Affairs (Millwood), 27*(2), 413–422.

Holy Cow! The Near-Total Racial Segregation in Veterinary Higher Education. (1996). *The Journal of Blacks in Higher Education, Autumn*(13), 46–48.

Institutional Committee. (2004). *In the nation's compelling interest: Ensuring diversity in the health care workforce.* Washington, DC: The National Academies Press.

LaVeist, T. A., Gaskin, D., & Richard, P. (2011). Estimating the economic burden of racial health inequalities in the United States. *International Journal of Health Services, 41*(2), 231–238.

Liaison Committee on Medical Education (LCME). (2016). *Functions and structure of a medical school: Standards for accreditation of medical education programs leading to the MD degree.* Retrieved from https://med.virginia.edu/ume-curriculum/wp-content/uploads/sites/216/2016/07/2017-18_Functions-and-Structure_2016-03-24.pdf

Lowrie, P. M. (2009). Tying art and science to reality for recruiting minorities to veterinary medicine. *Journal of Veterinary Medical Education, 36*(4), 382–387.

Morse, E. M. (2008). *Minority student perceptions of the veterinary profession: Factors influencing choices of health (MA dissertation).* Cleveland State University, Cleveland, OH.

Pacquiao, D. (2007). The relationship between cultural competence education and increasing diversity in nursing schools and practice settings. *Journal of Transcultural Nursing, 18*(1), 28S–37S.

Rodríguez, J. E., Campbell, K. M., Fogarty, J. P., & Williams, R. L. (2014). Underrepresented minority faculty in academic medicine: A systematic review of URM faculty development. *Family Medicine, 46*(2), 100–104.

Rodriguez, C., Kirshstein, R., & Hale, M. (2005). *Creating and maintaining excellence: The Model Institutions for Excellence Program.* Washington, DC: American Institutes of Research.

Strayhorn, T. L. (2009). The absence of African-American men in higher education and veterinary medicine. *Journal of Veterinary Medical Education, 36*(4), 351–358.

Sullivan Commission. (2004). *Missing persons: Minorities in the health professions.* Washington, DC: Author.

Thompson, D. (2013, November 6). The 33 Whitest jobs in America. *The Atlantic.* Retrieved from http://www.theatlantic.com/business/archive/2013/11/the-33-whitest-jobs-in-america/281180/

Wang, C. (2002). *Evaluation of Census Bureau's 1995–2025 state population projections.* U.S. Census Bureau. Current Population Reports. Working Paper Series No. 67. Washington, DC: Government Printing Office.

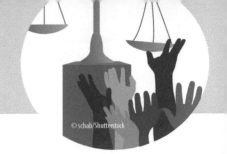
© schab/Shutterstock

CHAPTER 15

Cultural Competence Versus Diversity: Why Cultural Competence Also Matters

Cultural competence requires that organizations have a defined set of values and principles, and demonstrate behaviors, attitudes, policies, and structures that enable them to work effectively cross-culturally.

— **National Center for Cultural Competence**

KEY TERMS

cultural filtration
cultural nuances
linguistic competence

nationality
refugee

LEARNING OBJECTIVES

After reading this chapter, you should be able to do the following:

1. Define cultural competence.
2. Define diversity.
3. Differentiate between cultural competence and diversity.
4. Understand rapid demographic changes in the United States.

5. Explain the terms race, culture, and ethnicity.
6. Discuss cultural nuances and their relevance to particular racial/ethnic groups.
7. Explore cultural competence as a developmental process.
8. Describe linguistic competence within the context of cultural competence.

▶ Introduction

There is a distinct difference between the concepts of cultural competence and diversity, although the terms are often used interchangeably. This chapter will explore those differences by reviewing the terms and discussing strategies to increase cultural competence and diversity as separate but interrelated entities. It is essential to explore current and projected demographics pertaining to the majority and emerging majority groups in the United States. Through this exploration, a basis is established for the fact that cultural competence is an imperative for health service administrators and public health practitioners to ensure optimal services to all people as they interact with, and seek, services from those individuals who serve in these fields.

▶ Demographic Changes

There are currently significant demographic changes taking place in the United States that are having a direct impact on health care. Traditionally, the United States has always been known for diversity based upon an influx of individuals from all over the world. **TABLE 15-1** provides recent details regarding foreign-born residents.

Kosoko-Lasaki, Cook, and O'Brien (2009) provide statistics in regard to specific groups of undocumented immigrants:

TABLE 15-1 Foreign-Born Residents, 2000	
Statistic	**Value**
Total U.S. population, 2000	281,421,906
Foreign-born population, 2000	31,107,889
Percentage of residents who were foreign born, 2000	11
Percentage of foreign-born population who arrived 1900–2000	43
Percentage of Foreign-Born Population in 2000 From Top Five Countries of Origin	
Mexico	30
China	5

Statistic	Value
Philippines	4
India	3
Vietnam	3
Percentage of Foreign-Born Population in 2000 by Region	
Latin America	52
Asia	26
Europe	16
Africa	3
North America	3
English Proficiency	
Percentage of the total U.S. population ages 5 or older with limited English proficiency	8
Percentage of foreign-born population ages 5 or older with limited English proficiency	51

U.S. Department of Homeland Security, U.S. Citizenship and Immigrant Services, Office of Citizenship. (2004). Helping immigrants become new Americans: Communities discuss the issues. Retrieved from http://www.uscis.gov/files/article/focusgroup.pdf. Also see U.S. Census Bureau at http://quickfacts.census.gov

> In the 1900s an estimated 350,000 undocumented immigrants entered the United Sates in 2004, 81% were from Latin America, 9% from China, 6% from Europe and Canada, and 4% from Africa and other countries. Children under 18 years of age (1.7 million) accounted for 17% of the undocumented population in 2004. (p. 255)

Diversity in American society has made it necessary to understand the healthcare needs of various groups in an effort to provide optimal services and to understand health-seeking behaviors, attitudes, cultural nuances, and perceptions about health. This discussion begins with an exploration of cultural competence, its meaning, and why it is imperative as an undertaking for healthcare organizations and public health.

Additionally, the **refugee** population must be taken into consideration. Kosoko-Lasaki et al. (2009) explain this group as follows:

> According to the United Nations, a refugee is a person who, "owing to a well founded fear of being persecuted for reasons of race, religion, **nationality**,

membership in a particular social group, or political opinions outside the country of his nationality, and is unable to or owing to such fear, is unwilling to avail himself of the protection of that country." More than 2 million refugees were admitted to the United States between 1975 and 2000. (p. 255)

TABLE 15-2 provides insight in terms of the number of refugees in the United States. The numbers presented have changed dramatically in recent years, as there has been an influx of refugees into the United States, and at the time of this writing, current data are unavailable as to the number of refugees in the United States. They are mainly from Syria and other nations that have experienced war in recent years. Often, the goal of immigrants is to seek greater opportunities beyond their homelands. As mentioned elsewhere in this text, this motivation for immigrating is true for practically all groups found in the United States that are not indigenous populations, with the exception of African Americans, who were brought, in captivity as slaves, by Europeans as chattel to work the land.

TABLE 15-2 Statistics on Refugees in the United States

Area	Period	Number
Africa	1980–2000	Total >85,000; >30,000 Ethiopian; 25,000 Somali; the remainder Sudanese, Liberian, Zairian, Rwandan, Ugandan, and Angolan
Southeast Asia	1975–2000	Total >1.4 million; ~900,000 Vietnamese; the remainder Laotian, Cambodian, and Burmese
Near East, South Asia	1980–2000	Total 112,500; ~47,000 Iranian; ~31,200 Iraqi; ~28,000 Afghan
New Independent States and the Baltic	1989–2000	Total >378,000
Former Soviet Union	1989–2000	Total 546,516
Yugoslavia	1992–2000	Total ~107,000
Latin America	1975–2000	Total 79,634

Data from U.S. Department of State, Bureau of Population. (2000). Refugees admissions and resettlement. Retrieved from http://www.state.gov/www/global/prm/admissions_resettle.html#fact; Kemp, C., & Rasbridge, L. (2004). *Refugee and immigrant health: A handbook for health professionals*. Cambridge, UK: Cambridge University Press.

▶ Cultural Competence

In recent years, cultural competence has become a significant concept in health. In some settings, it generates controversy because of concerns regarding its necessity and cost-effectiveness. To many, it is a misunderstood concept that does not seem to have relevance to health care. Thus, it is important to spend some time exploring the definition of cultural competence. The overriding definition of cultural competence, as there are many, is provided by the Office of Minority Health (OMH) of the U.S. Department of Health and Human Services (DHHS), which states, "Cultural and linguistic competence is a set of congruent behaviors, attitudes, and policies that come together in a system, agency, or among professionals that enables effective work in cross-cultural situations" (DHHS, 2005).

Rubino, Esparza, and Chassiakos (2014) explain cultural competence as follows:

> Cultural competence was initially viewed as a way to eliminate cultural and language barriers between providers and patients with limited English proficiency (LEP). By 2005, efforts to enhance cross-cultural health delivery had broadened beyond the acknowledgement and addressing of language differences to include an understanding of how patients from different cultures viewed health and illness. Researchers studied various cultural traditions and perspectives to develop tools for enhancing communication in clinical encounters between healthcare providers and their patients.

Ultimately, the CLAS (Culturally and Linguistically Appropriate Services) standards were developed by the U.S. Office of Minority Health to provide guidance relative to cultural and linguistic competence. (See Appendix I for more on the CLAS standards.)

▶ Cultural Proficiency

Cultural proficiency takes the process of cultural competence a step further as the focus is on cultural expertise, ensuring assessment and training efforts, and reviewing policies and procedures that ensure the inclusion of culturally competent language. At this level, the active pursuit of resource development is maintained with advocacy with and on behalf of populations that reflect the various cultures served by health organizations to ensure maximum efficacy in meeting their needs (Cross et al., 1989). Cultural proficiency is considered the highest level of the overall concept of cultural competence.

▶ Linguistic Competence

Linguistic competence involves understanding the fact that many people in the United States do not speak English or have limited English proficiency and seek health care in environments where their predominant language is not spoken; hence, there is a need for linguistic competence in the provision of health care and public health to ensure effective communication. Unfortunately, many individuals who do not speak English do not receive optimal care because of language barriers.

Per Goode and Jones (2004), the definition of linguistic competence, according to the National Center for Cultural Competence at Georgetown University, is as follows:

> The capacity of an organization and its personnel to communicate effectively, and convey information in a manner that is easily understood by diverse audiences including persons of limited English proficiency, those who have low literacy skills or are not literate, and individuals with disabilities.

Often, healthcare organizations will use interpreters to assist with language barriers. Kosoko-Lasaki et al. (2009) describe medical interpreting as follows:

> Medical interpreting is a specialty in high demand as healthcare systems strive to improve language access. Healthcare systems from mega hospitals to neighborhood clinics develop language access plans to comply with governmental regulations, attain facility certification, increase patient certification and improve public health. Plans include how and where to find language services including volunteers, bilingual staff, independent contractor interpreters and telephonic language bureaus. (p. 106)

The use of family members (particularly children) as interpreters can be a precarious situation because it is inappropriate (due to confidentiality or reversal of parent–child relationships, which is problematic in some cultures). It is also inappropriate to use nonclinical and bilingual staff because medical terminology may be misinterpreted by nonclinical staff, and bilingual staff may confuse dialects/terms that are unique to a given culture. For example, regarding the latter, a word in Spanish spoken by a person from Costa Rica may not have the same meaning as the same word in Spanish spoken by a person from Puerto Rico. Therefore, to strive toward accuracy, it is appropriate to use only trained interpreters (either in person or by telephone). The use of untrained interpreters may also cause other problems beyond incorrect interpretation of words and concepts, including the wrong use of health-related terminology, the inclusion of personal perspectives in the interpretation process, and violation of confidentiality. The trained interpreter is aware of all of the possible errors mentioned and is better prepared to avoid them. The goal is to avoid **cultural filtration**, which is when cultural beliefs or ideas are either included or removed from the interpretation process by the interpreter. The considerations discussed here for spoken language apply also to written communication.

Another definition of linguistic competence is the ability to communicate effectively and accurately with individuals whose primary language is not English. Understanding of culture and respect for differences will allow healthcare managers to make more appropriate planning and intervention decisions. Patient satisfaction is reliant upon an organization's ability to communicate and understand the cultural factors that affect health behavior (Betancourt, Green, Carrillo, & Park, 2005). It is also important to take linguistic factors into consideration because language barriers can adversely affect the delivery of healthcare services in communities. Patients/clients/customers who are not proficient in English will often enter a healthcare facility or receive public health information and have no idea how to proceed because they cannot understand what is said to them, read the signage, or understand written materials provided to them. This experience can cause fear, apprehension, and miscommunication and impact treatment-seeking behaviors, compliance regarding instructions provided to them, treatment follow-up, and adherence to medication requirements. For example, in many states in the United States, disaster preparedness is critical. Public health organizations will often provide information on how to prepare for a disaster. If the literature, public service announcements, and other materials are in English only, individuals who are monolingual—speaking only Creole or Spanish, for example—will be without insight if a disaster impacts their Haitian or Spanish-speaking (e.g., Cuban, Dominican, Costa Rican) communities.

Cultural competence is a developmental process that takes place over time. It requires an understanding of key social determinants, namely socioeconomic status and its impact on health disparities from a racial and ethnic vantage point. Furthermore, treatment-seeking behaviors, based on diversity and cultural nuances specific to cultural and ethnic groups, must be understood. Linguistic competence is also a critical factor because language can serve as a barrier and impact treatment-seeking behaviors, leading to health disparities. Such language barriers may also impact expectations of care for individuals seeking optimal health care. Linguistic competence is a key component of cultural competence because language is also a part of culture, and it is the responsibility of the health service organization and public health practitioners to meet the needs of their customers on every level.

▶ Culture

Depending upon one's culture, there are nuances that may be significant to health-seeking behaviors, attitudes, diet, whom individuals prefer to receive care from, whether or not individuals will return for care, and so on. Culture is an integrated pattern of learned beliefs and behaviors that can be shared among groups. It includes thoughts, styles of communicating, ways of interacting, views on roles and relationships, values, practices, and customs (Donini-Lenhoff & Hendrick, 2000; Robins, Fantone, Hermann, Alexander, & Zweifler, 1998). Culture also includes a number of additional influences and factors, such as socioeconomic status, physical and mental ability, sexual orientation, and occupation (Betancourt, Green, & Carrillo, 2002).

It is essential that health care and public health organizations learn to meet the needs of individuals served; otherwise, optimal, efficacious care may not be provided. There are consistent reports indicating that there are racial and ethnic disparities in health. The Institute of Medicine (IOM) investigated such disparities in 2003 and provided concrete recommendations aimed at reducing them in a report titled *Unequal Treatment: Confronting Racial and Ethnic Disparities in Health Care* (Smedley, Stith, & Nelson, 2003). Some of the recommendations included increasing awareness of such disparities, integrating cross-cultural education into the training of healthcare professionals, use of evidence-based guidelines to promote consistency and equity of care, and continued research to assess disparities further and to provide appropriate interventions.

▶ Cultural Nuances

A key aspect of cultural competence is recognizing **cultural nuances**, which are the subtle differences between particular cultures. Subtleties of individual cultures define a people's view of themselves and the perception of the world around them.

By understanding these nuances, better interaction can be achieved in terms of culture and communication. For example, a cultural nuance specific to the Japanese population is the removal of one's shoes upon entering a home. This is a very strict requirement among many Japanese people, requiring the use of provided slippers prior to walking on the floors of their homes. Nonadherence to this requirement is considered rude, inappropriate, and unhygienic.

As another example, in certain sects of the Muslim community, women are mostly covered and can reveal only certain body parts, usually their faces (in some instances, limited to their eyes, hands, and feet), when in public in an effort to maintain modesty, respect, and privacy for the women per their religious scripture, the Koran. Consequently, when a Muslim woman is cared for by a male physician, it is often required that a female relative be present for any examination of the patient. The best approach is for the woman to be seen by a female practitioner to avoid violation of the modesty requirement (Hollins, 2006). This cultural nuance requires sensitivity, understanding, and adherence to the requirement in order to maintain female Muslim patients/clients/customers and ensure respect and dignity for their culture.

As a final example, people from Spain find stretching and yawning to be very bad manners and in poor taste. They are also very casual about keeping appointments (Graff, 2001). Keeping these nuances in mind is important so as not to insult them by yawning or stretching in their presence or being overly upset if they miss an appointment, but rather explaining the impact of their doing so in terms of scheduling. Awareness of cultural nuances over a broad base of cultures, races, and ethnicities will optimize the provision of services for individuals.

▶ Fiscal Accountability and Cultural Competence

Without cultural competence, the fiscal bottom line of healthcare organizations may be impacted because cultural groups may decide not to use facilities that do not service them appropriately, and hence the facilities lose market share. This is particularly true as diversity continues to expand in the United States and varying racial and ethnic groups grow larger in their respective communities and beyond. Although there is a great deal of altruism involved in cultural competence and diversity within healthcare organizations, there is also a bottom-line aspect to moving in this direction. Healthcare administrators and public health officials are interested in optimal financial and strategic performance. Therefore, the need for cultural competence and diversity in healthcare organizations should be reflected in their directive strategies, which include the mission, vision, and values statements; policies; and strategic plans of these organizations. The benefits for health service administrators and their organizations, and public health entities where appropriate, will include profitability based upon maintaining and growing current and future market share, enhancing the reputation of health care and public health organizations with ethnic and racial minorities, developing a sustainable competitive advantage over organizations that are not proceeding with cultural competence and diversity efforts, improved customer service, motivation of staff as they experience better relationships with the individuals they serve, and ultimately enhanced productivity. Conceivably, these efforts would lead to earnings growth, acceptable return on investments (because there is an expense factor associated with cultural competence and diversity initiatives), and cost reduction over time.

▶ Cultural Competence as a Developmental Process

In addition to optimizing the provision of services, cultural competence is a developmental process that evolves over an extended period of time, for both individuals and organizations, at various levels of awareness, knowledge, and skills along the cultural competence continuum (Cross, Bazron, Dennis, & Isaacs, 1989). Assessment of staff, providers, and the executive team is an important aspect of development to first determine people's attitudes toward cultural competence. In an effort to assess the level of cultural competence, from an attitudinal vantage point, a cultural competence tool was developed by the author of this text. Three distinct surveys were developed based on questions that are particularly relevant to healthcare organizations. (See Appendices II through IV for the three survey tools.) The surveys were designed to assess boards of directors, executive teams, and managers; providers; and staff. The response categories are based on a Likert-type format of Strongly Agree, Agree, Strongly Disagree, Disagree, and N/A, enabling numeric scoring of each response category, of which there are seven content areas: (1) concern for others, (2) self-awareness, (3) patient/customer/client contact, (4) cultural sensitivity, (5) workshops/training, (6) knowledge, and (7) communication and language.

In an effort to establish reliability and validity, a study was conducted involving four stages. The first step was to review and evaluate the survey tool. The next step was survey data collection followed by data entry. The last step was statistical analysis. Several techniques were used to measure reliability and validity. The techniques used to test reliability were test–retest, alternate/parallel forms, and Cronbach's alpha estimate (internal consistency). For validity, content-related strategy and construct-related strategy were used. All survey tools passed the rigorous statistical tests for reliability and validity. In terms of reliability, based on parallel form, the average estimates for reliability were 0.81 for the executive survey; 0.72 for the board of directors survey; 0.71 for the providers survey; and 0.77 for the staff survey. The Cronbach's alpha estimates were all within the acceptable range of >0.7 for all survey instruments. Furthermore, all surveys demonstrated good content, construct, and item-discriminant validity.

▶ The Importance of Reliable and Valid Assessment Tools

Surveys are important tools to gather data, but without established reliability and validity, the results from them have little or no meaning. Gaining insight regarding the level of cultural competence of health professionals through a survey tool is useful in identifying the areas of weakness that must be targeted in training efforts to improve attitudes about important cultural competence constructs. Tailoring the surveys to specifically address categories/types of health professionals ensures that queries are specific to the correct intended respondents. Often, by merely responding to items on an attitudinal survey, respondents gain insight as they explore questions that they may not have considered previously in terms of cultural competence. A number of factors may influence attitudes over time, including education, socioeconomic status, personality traits, and beyond, so it is important to reassess on an ongoing and consistent basis to ensure that attitudes that may remain, or that have become unfavorable, are addressed through training and workshops, specifically geared to address areas of concern.

▶ Cultural Competence Plan

The development and implementation of a robust cultural competence plan by health service organizations and public health entities must be a key strategy for success. (See Appendix VII for key components.) The aim of such a plan should be to change from a one-size-fits-all system to one that is responsive to diverse populations. This change requires diversity among board members, staff, and providers, enhanced data collection capacities, effective interpretation and translation services, and cultural competence education. Cultural competence and diversity are inextricably intertwined. These efforts require that organizations recognize and address their needs through both internal and external assessment processes. These processes should include consideration of the factors that currently define the delivery of health care in the United States, along with the compelling need for cultural competence to be incorporated into organizational policy.

Additionally, some reasons that cultural competence is necessary include the changing demographics of the population; the need to eliminate disparities in the health status of people of diverse racial, ethnic, and cultural backgrounds; the need to improve the quality of services and health outcomes; compliance with legislative, regulatory, and accreditation mandates; strategies to gain market share; and strategies to decrease potential liability and/or malpractice claims (Cohen & Goode, 1999). Lack of awareness of differences, such as the cultural nuances described earlier (and additional insight in terms of health-seeking behaviors, expectations of care by specific racial/ethnic groups, cultural values and beliefs, and so on), and failure to provide translation and interpretation services may result in a lack of understanding and, subsequently, breaches of professional standards of care or the presumption of negligence.

Wrap-Up

Chapter Summary

A paradigm shift is needed to accomplish the comprehensive process of incorporating cultural competence as a key component in the healthcare field. This requires an investment of time, people, money, and information. Each organization needs to diversify its workforce at every level based on race, nationality, ethnicity, and other key factors to ensure that it reflects the community served throughout its hierarchy. Linguistic competence is imperative to ensure that no matter the language spoken by individuals, they will be served optimally within healthcare organizations and within the context of public health efforts. As stated by Betancourt et al. (2002),

> "In the end the ultimate goal is a healthcare system and workforce that can deliver the highest quality of care to every patient, regardless of race, ethnicity, cultural background, or English proficiency" (p. 2).

A number of factors must be taken into consideration when trying to understand cultural nuances and barriers to cultural understanding. It is very difficult for health service administrators and public health practitioners to ensure optimal services without considering the needs of various racial and ethnic groups and making sure providers and staff have an understanding of cultural nuances, cultural beliefs and values, and treatment-seeking behaviors and their relevance. Diversity in healthcare leadership and the workforce provides a better basis for moving in the direction of understanding because it sets the tone for overcoming barriers to care among racial and ethnic minorities. Diversification alone, however, is insufficient. Making sure specific skills pertaining to cultural and linguistic competence are provided at every level of health service and public health organizations is paramount, with the goal being to offer top-notch services leading to the elimination of racial and ethnic health disparities.

Chapter Problems

1. A Haitian woman arrives at a healthcare facility in pain and in need of desperate care. She tries to explain that a spell has been placed on her and she needs an immediate remedy. She is monolingual, speaking only Creole. What steps should be taken at the healthcare facility to handle her situation?
2. *Cultural competence* and *diversity* are two distinct but interrelated terms. Explain the difference between the two.
3. At a monthly board meeting, a board member expresses that the health center that he serves is in the United States and that the predominant language spoken in the United States is English. Therefore, he sees no need for linguistic competence to be an aspect of concern for the organization because patients who seek care need to learn to speak English. What might the CEO say to the board member when she emphasizes the need for a fundraiser to acquire funds to implement costly translation and interpretation services throughout the healthcare facility, necessitating board participation?
4. Public health workers are assigned to conduct research in a metropolitan community to determine potential reasons for obesity, diabetes, and other issues. The researchers are advised by their supervisor in a preparation meeting that although the community members are solely people who are Haitian or African American, there is no need to present the research findings on the two groups distinctively because all of the community members are Black and hence their cultural and social characteristics,

including diets and exercise habits, will be the same. Explain the problem(s), if any, with this directive.

5.   A children's hospital in the United States has a contract to serve families from a small Arab-speaking nation who will fly in their children for specialty care when needed. The marketing director of the hospital advises his staff to develop a brochure in English for the incoming patients. One of the staff members objects, suggesting that the patients will not understand the brochure because they do not speak English. The marketing director responds, "If a patient wants to receive care here and read our informational materials, they better learn English and fast." Is there a problem with this director's perspective regarding the patients to be served, and does he need cultural competence or linguistic competence training? If so, describe possible approaches.

References

Betancourt, J. R., Green, A. R., & Carrillo, E. J. (2002). *Cultural competence in health care: Emerging frameworks and practical approaches.* New York, NY: The Commonwealth Fund.

Betancourt, J., Green, A., Carrillo, M., & Park, E. (2005). Cultural competence and health care disparities: Key perspectives and trends. *Health Affairs, 24*(2), 502–505.

Cohen, E., & Goode, T. D., (1999), revised by Goode, T. D., & Dunne, C. (2003). *Policy brief 1: Rational for cultural competence in primary care.* Washington, DC: National Center for Cultural Competence, Georgetown Center for Child and Human Development.

Cross, T., Bazron, B., Dennis, K., & Isaacs, M. (1989). *Towards a culturally competent system of care* (Vol. 1). Washington, DC: Georgetown University Child Development Center, CASSP Technical Assistance Center.

Donini-Lenhoff, F. G., & Hendrick, H. L. (2000). Increasing awareness and implementation of cultural competence principles in health professions education. *Journal of Allied Health, 29*(4), 241–245.

Goode, T., & Jones, W. (2004). *Definition of linguistic competence, National Center for Cultural Competence.* Washington, DC: National Center for Cultural Competence, Georgetown University Center for Child and Human Development.

Graff, M. L. (2001). *Culture shock! A guide to customs and etiquette: Spain.* Portland, OR: Graphic Arts Center Publishing Company.

Hollins, S. (2006). *Religions, culture and healthcare: A practical handbook for use in health care environments.* Oxford, UK: Radcliffe Publishing.

Kosoko-Lasaki, S., Cook, C., & O'Brien, R. (2009). *Cultural proficiency in addressing health disparities.* Sudbury, MA: Jones and Bartlett Publishers.

National Center for Cultural Competence. Quote available at https://nccc.georgetown.edu /culturalbroker/8_Definitions/index.html

Robins, L. S., Fantone, J., Hermann, J., Alexander, G., & Zweifler, A. (1998). Improving cultural awareness and sensitivity training in medical school. *Academic Medicine, 73*(10 Suppl), S31–S34.

Rubino, L., Esparza, S., & Chassiakos, Y. (2014). *New leadership for today's health care professionals.* Burlington, MA: Jones and Bartlett Learning.

Smedley, B. D., Stith, A. Y., & Nelson, A. R. (Eds.). (2003). *Unequal treatment: Confronting racial and ethnic disparities in health care.* Washington, DC: The National Academies Press.

U.S. Department of Health and Human Services. (2005). What is cultural competency? Retrieved from http://minorityhealth.hhs.gov/omh/browse.aspx?lvl=1&lvlid=6

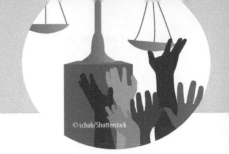
© schab/Shutterstock

CHAPTER 16

Case Studies and Diversity

People of different religions and cultures live side by side in almost every part of the world, and most of us have overlapping identities which unite us with very different groups. We can love what we are, without hating what—and who—we are not. We can thrive in our own tradition, even as we learn from others, and come to respect their teachings.

—**Kofi Annan**, Former Secretary-General of the United Nations

LEARNING OBJECTIVES

At the end of this chapter, you should be able to do the following:

1. Discuss scenarios in which lack of diversity impacts the overall delivery of services in the healthcare field.
2. Explain specific steps that would be useful in diversifying healthcare organizations.
3. List healthcare fields in which there is a significant lack of diversity and provide insights as to why.
4. Identify at least three distinct solutions for at least three different scenarios presented in the various cases.

▶ Introduction

The purpose of this chapter is to review eight case studies relevant to diversity in the United States as it relates to health care and education in healthcare fields. There are reasons for lack of diversity that often remain unexplored, and often solutions to the problems are not sought. Examples of such scenarios are indicated with commentary toward solutions. Tolerance and linguistic competence are also discussed in relation to diversity matters. Although case studies are not provided for every issue associated with diversity, the following eight examples will serve as a guide to help individuals approach similar situations in their own life experiences.

▶ Case Scenario 1: Veterinary Medicine

An African American man living in a low socioeconomic community in the city of Baton Rouge, Louisiana, has two mixed-breed dogs and one cat that he acquired from a shelter. He has lost his job, and with it his healthcare insurance. Now living on unemployment and dealing with his ongoing severe rheumatoid arthritis, he is having difficulty caring for his beloved pets. One of his dogs has a problem in which he seems to have to urinate, but when trying to do so, very little urine emerges. The man does not know what to do so he takes his animal to a private veterinarian near his home.

As he sits and waits, he notes that all of the magazines primarily show White people and their pets and that there are paintings on the walls with White people in various stages of activity with their pets, including cats, dogs, horses, etc. The veterinarian, his assistants, and everyone else at the facility are White except for the receptionist at the front desk. After explaining the dog's symptoms, the veterinarian advises the man that X-rays and bloodwork will have to be done and ultimately medication or beyond will be needed, depending on the outcome. The man has no money to proceed, so he is advised to go to the veterinary hospital at the nearby university where maybe they can help him. He does but with great trepidation, as he is told by the Black woman working at the receptionist desk, "There are no Black people at that veterinary hospital either. I doubt they will help you and yours." He clutches his dog and heads there with worry and concern.

Commentary

A healthcare profession that is rarely included in discussions of health care is veterinary medicine. Veterinarians spend 4 years in professional school, becoming educated in the same subjects as medical doctors as well as public health concerns. Health disparities exist in their field in that there is a correlation between animal health and the socioeconomic status of pet owners. Basically, when people are unable to ensure their own health care due to lack of insurance or accessibility, it can be expected that the animals in their possession as pets will have the same experience. In fact, recent research has shown that if humans experience premature deaths in poor neighborhoods, so will their animals.

In a study conducted by Dr. Gary Patronek, VMD, PhD, of the Animal Rescue League of Boston and also a veterinary epidemiologist, a definite link was established between the socioeconomic status of human pet owners and their health and the health of their pets. Essentially, "The same kinds of things that lead to poor health outcomes in people are leading to poor health outcomes in animals" (Zimlich, 2010).

Additionally, veterinary medicine is the Whitest profession in the United States (Davis, n.d.). The numbers of Black people, and people of color in general, in the profession are dismally low, as is the case with many predominantly White institutions.

Furthermore, according to the August 2014 Bureau of Labor Statistics Report, "Labor Force Characteristics by Race and Ethnicity," 97.3 percent of veterinarians in the labor force in 2013 were White. The man in this case scenario has reason to be concerned. In the first location, there was no visual affirmation of him in the waiting room area. There was nothing to indicate in the images that surrounded him that he was welcome there, hence a seemingly culturally incompetent environment. The receptionist was clearly indicating to him that race matters in terms of the provision of services to his animal. Perhaps the customer should go to the veterinary teaching hospital for care, but his trepidation is due to his concern that he will have the same experience at the next facility. Veterinary schools and the profession at large need to diversify so that people will feel comfortable and affirmed in these facilities, eliminating the health disparity of pets of low socioeconomic people of color, as animals need their owners to serve as their healthcare seekers.

▶ Case Scenario 2: Tolerance

A Chinese American professor, Dr. Wang, starts a new position as a faculty member at a predominantly White university in a public health program and attends the university orientation for all new employees. Within the context of orientation, a representative of the human resources department announces, with pride, that they have a tolerance program as part of their diversity initiatives. Dr. Wang is concerned about the term, ponders it, and then raises her hand to ask the following questions: How is that term, tolerance, appropriate within the context of this institution? While tolerance refers to acceptance, it's usually within the mindset of accepting something that one really disagrees with. Is a parent merely to tolerate his/her children? Should a husband/wife tolerate his/her spouse? What about parents? Should they be tolerated? What about classmates in school? Should they tolerate each other? How about faculty? What if a teacher says to students, at any stage of their education, that in this classroom, I am going to tolerate your presence? The answer to some of these questions may be yes, but is that optimal?

Commentary

In a 2010 article, John Achrazoglou considers the implications of the term *tolerance*:

> Diversity needs to go beyond tolerance. Tolerance is a first step. It is much better than conflict. But tolerance is a somewhat negative word, according to the former lieutenant governor of British Columbia. To "tolerate" and to be "tolerated" involves an unequal relationship. Tolerance implies that the tolerator has the power to not tolerate.

Emerging majorities are members of American society and deserve to be in any place and any space that any other person occupies in the workforce, even if the numbers are low. Often, emerging majority people find themselves as part of a very small group or the only person from their race/ethnicity in an organization of predominantly White Non-Hispanic people. Emerging majority people do not want to be merely tolerated at such organizations that choose to move forward with diversity initiatives and hiring practices that are inclusive. Diversity is an effort of inclusiveness, to ensure that the workforce is not homogeneous. Homogeneity is not reflective of the American population as a whole. Hence, when an organization decides to ensure that diversity happens, it should not be within the context of tolerating people of color, but of valuing and appreciating individuals that will add to a vibrant milieu.

If an organization chooses to have a tolerance program, the term must be clearly defined from a positive vantage point. Recor (n.d.) offers an excellent definition of tolerance:

> Tolerance is respect, acceptance and appreciation of the rich diversity of our world's cultures, our forms of expression and ways of being human. It is fostered by knowledge, openness, communication, and freedom of thought, conscience and belief. Tolerance is harmony in difference.

But the question is, in reality, are organizations, on the whole, with tolerance programs defining the term this way? Tolerance, if not properly defined, is limiting and demeaning. It is not a start in the right direction. Valuing and appreciating is a better place to begin.

▶ Case Scenario 3: Visual Affirmation

Nurses and staff treated a volunteer at a pediatric hospital, whose child suffered from cancer and survived, beautifully. This is why she became a volunteer. It was a public hospital, so she decided to give back by decorating a wing of the hospital with art reflective of the varied cultural backgrounds of the patients. Although she is White, she realized that the hospital needed to visually affirm the patients and their families, largely emerging majorities, who spent much of their time there as their children were treated. The hospital president supported this endeavor, monetarily and administratively, which led to a wonderful, supportive, diversified atmosphere for the children and their families, allowing the volunteer to feel positive that she was giving back and making a difference.

Commentary

Diversity is not merely about the employees at a given organization but also the environment in which patients/customers are served. In healthcare facilities in which the majority of the patients are emerging majorities, the environment should reflect this diversity. Hallways and waiting rooms should have artwork or images that positively reflect the people being served. There should be magazines/materials available that are reflective of the people being served. If the majority of the patients/customers being served are Haitian people, for example, then images should be of Haitian people, with magazines and other information in both English and Creole. Visual affirmation is a concept that is easy; it works and it is the right thing to do. Knowing the demographics of patients and creating spaces for them where they feel welcome, comfortable, affirmed, and appreciated enhance the environment of care.

▶ Case Scenario 4: Linguistic Diversity

An elderly Cuban woman has been in a car accident in Miami, Florida. Subsequently, her doctor recommends that she visit a physical therapist so she can gradually work on her mobility again. Her physical therapist is English speaking and is not Hispanic. The family members (her adult son and daughter) request a Spanish-speaking therapist because their mother is unable to speak any English, having never found the need to learn English while living in Miami. The administrator at the physical therapy facility declines the request, indicating that the simple solution would be to have one of the staff members or one of her children who speaks Spanish present whenever the physical therapist is with her. The staff person selected is not a physical therapist, and she is Puerto Rican rather than Cuban. At their first session, the daughter and the staff person get into a conflict in which only Spanish is spoken. The physical therapist does not understand their conversation and becomes anxious and frustrated. He is watching the clock because he has another client on his schedule and does not want to be late. Ultimately, the discussion between the staff person and the patient's daughter ends and the staff person interprets the conversation to the physical therapist, but by then he is able to work with his patient for only about 10 minutes. The patient is very emotional during the remainder of the session, and very little is accomplished.

Commentary

In this situation, a number of steps could have been taken. First, the administrator should have considered the hiring of a Spanish-speaking physical therapist, preferably a Cuban person, given that many individuals seeking care at the facility are Cuban. If a Cuban therapist was not available, a trained, Spanish-speaking interpreter should have been sought, either in person or, if not available, via a language line to ensure understanding of cultural nuances within the communication process based on nationality. The health administrator should have been concerned regarding whether the diversity of his staff met the needs of the clients at the facility. The suggestion of the patient's daughter or a nonclinical staff member being at every one of the client's sessions seemed to be a violation of her privacy and posed a limit to her care.

▶ Case Scenario 5: The Student Loan Crisis and Its Impact

A young Black, first-generation college student, who always had an interest in serving low-income communities, given her own background, is eager to attend medical school after attending college and completing the medical track. She applies to medical school and is accepted to several. She needs additional funding, namely a graduate PLUS loan, to complete her financial aid needs. The PLUS loan is a federal student loan that is specifically geared toward graduate students. It requires a credit check. She was not timely with recent credit card payments because she used them to buy books for college and ran out of funds to make her monthly payments. She is denied the PLUS loan and sadly decides she is unable to attend medical school and fulfill her dream to serve in the community to help close the health disparity.

Commentary

Given that the current federal debt for student loans is above $1 trillion with substantial default rates, new ideas, besides student loans, are needed to assist young people in their endeavors to attend school for medical and healthcare professions and graduate schools. This student should have immediately explored other options, such as scholarships, and approached the universities to find out if they could help her in any way. If a solution were in place, the financial burden of attending graduate/professional school would not serve as an obstacle. Additionally, high tuition at most graduate schools precludes attendance for potential students. The barrier must be lifted, particularly to assist emerging majority students, who have the greatest financial need.

▶ Case Scenario 6: Cultural Competence Matters

Jenny is a White nurse practitioner at a large community hospital in Los Angeles. She was educated at one of the best nursing programs in a large urban city, and she prides herself on being fair and equal to all of her patients. She turned down many jobs at private hospitals because they did not have a diverse clientele. One day Jenny is assisting a Hispanic patient who speaks with a heavy accent. As she completes the intake process with him, she becomes a little frustrated and asks the patient to speak more slowly and clearly because she does not understand Mexican very well. The patient becomes visibly upset and short with his answers. When the session ends, the patient leaves the room, angrily speaking to himself in Spanish. He was highly offended by her use of the term Mexican, as he is from Guatemala, and that she confused nationality with language. Jenny does not understand why the patient was angry and from that point on avoids working with Hispanic patients, as she had experienced a similar situation on several occasions previously.

Commentary

The nurse in this case would have benefited greatly from cultural and linguistic competence courses as part of her training or as a requirement at the facility where she is working. Although she is eager to work with a diverse clientele, she is not prepared to do so. She makes a tremendous mistake by referring to the Spanish language as Mexican and assuming that because the patient is speaking Spanish he is Mexican, which shows a very weak skill set in terms of understanding the nationality aspect of Hispanic people. People who speak Spanish may be from many different Latin American or Central American countries or from Spain. Also, the nurse should have immediately sought out the interpreter at the facility (if available) or used a language line to assist her in communicating with the patient. Cultural competence is a skill set that, unfortunately, many health practitioners are lacking.

▶ Case Scenario 7: Cultural Connections

A hospital opens a new walk-in healthcare facility in a predominantly Jamaican community in South Florida. The administrator in charge of the facility anticipates that they will be serving a significant number of patients from Jamaica and has an opening to recruit several health professionals. He contacts the human resources department and asks them to take this into consideration while hiring. The human resources department decides that because they already hired two African American health professionals, Jamaican health professionals are not necessary.

Commentary

In this case, the human resources department is not recognizing that there are differences between Jamaican and African American people. Although Black Jamaican people are of African descent, as African Americans are, culturally, the two groups are different. They do not eat the same foods, as an example, and so dietary habits would have to be taken into consideration along with health behaviors. Although non-Jamaican people can serve the Jamaican patients optimally, having people who relate to the culture and fully understand it would go a long way. The human resources staff could clearly benefit from cultural competence training, with specific focus on Jamaican culture and beyond.

▶ Case Scenario 8: Mental Health

A young Black college student experiences serious health issues, one after another. She complains of lower back pain, pain in her legs, lethargy, and other symptoms. She visits a doctor for various tests, only to be told that there are no identifiable causes for her illnesses. Her mother, with whom she was very close, recently died unexpectedly of a heart attack. She is advised by a doctor to visit a therapist at the mental health center at her school to deal with her grief. Her father advises her that it would be ridiculous to do so. After considerable suffering with no relief, she locates a Black female psychologist at the center who was recommended by a classmate who meets with her regularly. They work through the grief associated with the sudden loss of her mother. Over time, her physical symptoms gradually dissipate. Her father observes her gradual healing and also decides to see a therapist. He is unable to find a Black male psychologist and refuses to see anyone else, deciding that he alone will handle his grief related to the loss of his beloved wife of 35 years. Within 2 years of her death, he also dies of a heart attack. His daughter is saddened but not surprised, as she had heard her father weeping in his room on many nights, grieving for her mother, when she visited him during school breaks. He had refused to discuss his grief with her, or anyone else, and merely endured his pain and sadness.

Commentary

Black men are particularly hesitant to seek mental health care, as pointed out by Dr. David Satcher, former U.S. Surgeon General. In a keynote speech for a Black fraternity event titled "Brother, You're On My Mind: Changing the National Dialogue Regarding Mental Health Among African-American Men," he stated the following in regard to the mental health needs of African American men: "We are less likely to seek care because of the stigma associated with mental illness in our community. [But] you shouldn't be embarrassed about having a mental disorder" (*Florida Times-Union* Editorial, 2015).

In response to Dr. Satcher's claim that "if you don't have mental health, you don't have good health at all," the *Florida Times-Union* (2015) stated the following:

> It's a fact that African-American men have been traditionally slow to accept, a crippling hesitancy that causes many black males to silently suffer from mental illness rather than seek care that could effectively treat them. And it is an issue that continues to put huge numbers of Americans

at risk, especially black men. It's estimated that at least 1.3 million African-American men will develop depression during their lifetimes.

Furthermore, research has supported the idea that race, ethnicity, and culture play an important role in the doctor–patient relationship. Racial and ethnic differences between doctor and patient influence physician communications, but these cross-cultural factors remain relatively unexplored. In fact, those studies that have been done show that communication is enhanced when the patient and physician are of the same race or culture (LaVeist, 2002). Perhaps in this case, if a Black male psychologist/psychiatrist had been identified, the father could have worked through his grief under less duress and suffering, possibly extending his life and avoiding his fatal heart attack, as it may have been related to his prolonged, unaddressed grief.

References

Achrazoglou, J. (2010, November 9). Perspectives: How diversity goes beyond tolerance. Retrieved from http://diverseeducation.com/article/14369

Davis, K. (n.d.). Diversity, inclusion, and veterinary medicine: At the least, we are changing. Insight Into Diversity. Retrieved from http://www.insightintodiversity.com/diversity-inclusion-and -veterinary-medicine-at-the-least-we-are-changing/

Florida Times-Union Editorial. (2015, July 16). African-American men must be engaged on mental illness. Retrieved from http://jacksonville.com/opinion/editorials/2015-07-16/story/african -american-men-must-be-engaged-mental-illness

JAVMA (2015). Grant aims to give minorities a boost in whitest profession. Retrieved from https:// www.avma.org/News/JAVMANews/Pages/150901t.aspx

LaVeist, T. (2002). *Race, ethnicity, and health: A public health reader.* San Francisco, CA: John Wiley and Sons.

Recor, A. (n.d.). Teaching tolerance. Learning to Give. Retrieved from http://www.learningtogive .org/resources/teaching-tolerance

United Nations. (2001, December 10). *"We can love what we are, without hating what – and who – we are not", Secretary General says in Nobel Lecture* [press release]. Retrieved from https://www .un.org/press/en/2001/sgsm8071.doc.htm

Zimlich, R. (2010, April 1). Cat health linked to social status, health of owners, study suggests. *DVM360 Magazine,* Retrieved from http://veterinarynews.dvm360.com/cat-health-linked -social-status-health-owners-study-suggests

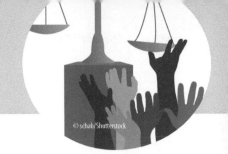
© schab/Shutterstock

CHAPTER 17

Closing the Health Status Gap: A Spiritual Approach Toward Resolution

Yolanda Richard, MDiv

They sang with all the strength that was in them, and clapped their hands for joy. There had never been a time when John had not sat watching the saints rejoice with terror in his heart, and wonder. Their singing caused him to believe in the presence of the Lord; indeed, it was no longer a question of belief, because they made that presence real. He did not feel it himself, the joy they felt, yet he could not doubt that it was, for them, the very bread of life—could not doubt it, that is, until it was too late to doubt.

—**James Baldwin**

KEY TERMS

Black Sacred Cosmos
Black spirituality
freedom

religion
spirituality

LEARNING OBJECTIVES

After reading this chapter, you should be able to do the following:

1. Understand the importance of religion and spirituality in the lives of racial and ethnic groups, with an emphasis on African American/Black people.

2. Offer alternative definitions and theoretical frameworks for engaging discussion on the role of spirituality in attempts to survey wellness.
3. Consider causes for cultural mistrust of the medical infrastructure.
4. Engage in greater discussion on the need for a broader national identity that includes ethnically and racially marginalized groups.

▶ Introduction

Belief is not simply what one recites at the moment of questioning. Belief is the composition of seemingly insignificant moments that expose the deep thoughts that drive one's engagement with self and others. Belief is the internal matter that accompanies the individual as they both define and navigate the terrain of life. Belief is that undiscovered criterion that lays the foundation for the inconspicuous work of meaning making. In *Go Tell It on the Mountain*, James Baldwin unveils the unique process of conversion within the African American religious tradition. John, the protagonist, sees God in the ecstatic shouts, songs, and praise of the Black and beaten faces around him. Now their faces, their worship, and their God was in him and it was too late to doubt it. In this revelatory experience, John sees, for the first time, spirituality as a viable resource for the whole of life, the bread of life itself.

Religion and spirituality have always held a central place in the narrative of Black existence in the United States. In the face of severe racism and government-mandated psychological and physical abuse, African American spirituality has operated as a barrier to the external insanity of the nation. It ought to be considerably challenging to discuss Black health without also discussing Black spirituality and its impact on the lives of African Americans. In this chapter, the intersection between Black spirituality and the health disparity crisis between Blacks and Whites will be explored. It is no secret that race, ethnicity, and socioeconomic status are determinant factors in shaping health outcomes.

Health disparity negatively impacts various groups in the United States, including, but not limited to, poor Whites, the newly immigrated, Native Americans, Non-White Hispanics, and African Americans. Though health disparity impacts various groups in the United States, the gap is widest between Black and White people. This reality is not a new phenomenon; it has held true since the beginnings of the nation. This relationship between White and Black people has also shaped the racial discourse of the United States in such a way that other racial and ethnic minority groups must also confront the consequences of this history. For this reason, this chapter will focus through the lens of the African American religious experience and widen into a discussion about health disparity generally. The goal of this chapter is to highlight the importance of **religion** and spirituality to African Americans, offer new definitions and theoretical frameworks for engaging discussion on the role of African American spirituality in attempts to evaluate Black wellness, explore the benefits and challenges of understanding religion and spirituality as a source of resolution for the health disparity crisis, and, finally, explore an expanded national identity as a conceptual response to disparity.

▶ Black Spirituality and the De-Christianization of America

In 2007 and 2014 the Pew Research Center administered virtually identical national surveys to a national sample to capture changes in America's religious landscape over the course of 7 years. This comparative study has been quite significant since the U.S government does not collect statistics on religious composition of the U.S. public. The 2014 results revealed that there are more Christians in the United States than anywhere else in the world. Seven in 10 Americans identify with some branch of Christianity. The jewel of the study was data showing that overall Christian affiliation in the United States is at a surprising decline. The percentage of American adults who identify with some branch of Christianity has declined by 8 percent, from 78.4 percent in 2007 to 70.6 percent in 2014. Adults who identify as being unaffiliated with any religion has increased by 6 percent, from 16.1 percent in 2007 to 22.8 percent in 2014. Overall, American Christians have declined somewhere between 2.8 and 7.8 million. In spite of the national decline of Christian affiliation, the Pew study reports that historically Black Protestants have remained stable, at nearly 16 million adults. African American Protestants have declined only 0.2 percent, from 15.9 percent in 2007 to 15.7 percent in 2014 (Pew Research Center, 2015).

The significance of Black religious stability is highlighted when juxtaposed to the Pew Research report on the religious portrait of African Americans published in 2009. The conclusions of this report were derived from data presented in the 2007 U.S. Religious Landscape Survey. According to this survey, African Americans are the most Protestant ethnic group in the country. African Americans (78%) far exceed Protestant affiliation compared to Whites (53%), Asians (27%), Latinos (23%), and the overall U.S. population (51%). The survey also showed that Blacks are the least likely group to be unaffiliated with any religion. White respondents ranked highest at 24 percent, compared to 20 percent of Hispanics and 18 percent of Blacks (Pew Research Center, 2009).

The results make clear that African Americans are the most religiously affiliated group among the U.S. population. Bolstering this claim, the study shows that 87 percent of African Americans belong to a religious group, while 83 percent report being affiliated with a specific religion. Beyond religious affiliation, the study shows that religion and involvement in religious life constitute a significant aspect of African American life. Eight in 10 African Americans say religion is very important to their lives, compared to 56 percent of the U.S. population. Even among African Americans who identify as being unaffiliated with any particular religion, spirituality is a significant aspect of their lives. According to the study, 45 percent of unaffiliated African Americans say that religion is very important in their lives. A higher percentage (72%) of unaffiliated African Americans reported that religion plays at least a somewhat important role in their lives (Pew Research Center, 2009).

African American involvement in religious life is also telling. When asked about prayer and attendance at religious services, 76 percent of African Americans say they pray daily, and more than half report attending religious services at least once a week (Pew Research Center, 2009). When asked about the existence of God, 88 percent report being absolutely certain God exists. Interestingly, unaffiliated

African Americans' response to these same categories mirrors the percentages of mainline Protestants and Catholics (Pew Research Center, 2009). Among unaffiliated African Americans, 48 percent pray at least daily compared to 53 percent of mainline Protestants. Similar to mainline Protestants (73%) and Catholics (72%), 70 percent of unaffiliated African Americans believe God exists with absolute certainty (Pew Research Center, 2009). Only 1 percent of African Americans describe themselves as atheists or agnostic (Pew Research Center, 2009).

▶ The Role of Spirituality in the Lives of African Americans and Wellness

It is essential to acknowledge the critical role of spirituality in the lives African Americans. An assessment of Black wellness without any consideration to spirituality ignores the significant ways in which this group has chosen to lift up religion as central to the Black ethos. The results make clear that religion, particularly Christianity, is not simply important but present in the everyday lives of African Americans through engagement with the historically Black church and daily prayer, among other factors.

Furthermore, the results highlight that **Black spirituality** is not only significant but also distinct from the greater population. The stability of religious affiliation is telling of the uniqueness of Black culture and life in the United States. It points to the need for definitions, theoretical frameworks, and models of wellness that do not simply seek to model the normativity of White culture but that generate meaning from a locus point of Black life. (The locus point of Black life and that of the greater populace are not to be seen as mutually exclusive or separate. In this instance, the locus point of Black life refers to a point of cultural saturation along a spectrum of Black embodiment, engagement, and connection with surrounding human expression). Spirituality has always carried potential for shaping behavior, influencing lifestyle, and defining the parameters for one's understanding of self, others, and the world. Black spirituality deals deeply with the inner workings of Black people and thus plays a major role in influencing the health outcomes of African Americans. To be explored later in this chapter is the notion that Black spirituality is not simply the profession of basic Christian tenets, but is a divinely inspired reframing of Christianity that affirms Black existence in the world. Many scholars have taken on the task of evaluating the role of religion and spirituality in the health outcomes of African Americans. In the process, one must determine a definitional framework that will shape how the data are understood in light of the demographic sample. Definitions of religion and spirituality play a major role in framing the discussion of the relationship between Black religious practice and health. Therefore, before delving into a discussion on resolutions, a conversation about definitions is at hand.

▶ Religion Versus Spirituality

Religion and *spirituality* are terms that are often used interchangeably, though they describe different aspects of one's relationship to faith. Religion is an infrastructure of belief surrounding a collective understanding of the divine identity. This infrastructure contains a series of theological premises, the conclusions of which determine the boundaries that make the religion distinct from other claims to divine revelation. These theological claims concerning the divine identity manifest into a set of subclaims about the human identity. Understandings of the human identity and the divine identity are not mutually exclusive; in fact, one informs the other knowingly and unknowingly. From an understanding of the divine and self emanates a set of practices and expectations that mediate an individual and collective relationship to the divine being.

In a sense, this religious infrastructure is helpful. Over time the structure will shortcut centuries of theological developments and debates within the tradition into a series of norms, expectations of membership, catechistic orientations, and periodic chastisement to make one aware of the behavioral boundaries of belonging. Also, devotees will discover language and ritual nuance, the utilization of which further integrates them into the institutional identity. These prepackaged theological bright lines are quite attractive to new converts and members because they ease the process of religious assimilation and create an in-house measurement to gauge religious performance. They are also helpful in providing alternative sources of allegiance. Belonging on the basis of belief subverts the requirements of cultural belonging on the basis of resources the devotee lacks. For marginalized groups, religion provides a sense of belonging to a higher moral order that trumps the social mores of the day. Finally, religion assumes the operationalization of divine engagement and spiritual growth. A common by-product associated with the religious structure is a tendency toward rigidity and the formation of dogma. Such outcomes bolster the pursuit of clearer institutional identity but simultaneously strain one's pursuit of a fluid, organic spirituality.

Spirituality evokes a different relationship to the divine that is not intrinsically associated with the expectations of the religious structure. Spirituality is marked by a comfort with the mysterious quality of the divine and the mysterious quality of the self. This engagement located in the space of mystery operates within a theological assumption of private intimacy with God that generates creative, innovative, and individualized theology. Many turn to spirituality in an attempt to break from the religious institution; however, such a task is quite difficult. Often, this spirituality finds itself bound by the expectations of the religious structure. In other words, how can one completely part from what may be his or her only reference point to divine engagement? The tools one acquires to engage the divine (e.g., prayer, songs of worship, folklore, reading of religious texts, meditation, contemplative practices, retreat to the divine temple) will influence the person's spirituality or at the very least remain as contours to his or her spirituality. In this way, religion and spirituality are bound to overlap. Spirituality makes possible the ability to transcend the religious structure, but the structure will often inform how one understands that transcendence. For example, one can transcend to a higher awareness of the finitude of life via deep reflection on a religious text that acts as a convenient springboard to the place of transcendence. In this sense, some find the contours of the institution as a comforting guide toward their development and connection with the divine. Others find these contours restricting and seek to balance the assumed truths of the structure with suspicion and the development of unique terms for their divine engagement.

Definitions are essential to set a base understanding of key concepts and determine the scope of discussion. Over the years, researchers have gone back and forth concerning definitions and potential distinctions between the terms religion and spirituality. Definitions have been provided above to weigh in on the matter and to mark the point beyond which we will explore deeper, nuanced, and complex definitions that match the movement of the African American religious experience. Additionally, general definitions are important to provide a context by which alternative definitions are highlighted.

▶ Spirituality, Religion, and Mental Health

In her 1998 dissertation, *The Relationship Among Spirituality, Religion, and Mental Health for African Americans*, Gwendolyn L. Jones provides a slew of definitions of spirituality and religion. Spirituality is described as "a quality deep within all human beings," and "its expression through the individual is one's spiritual perspective" (Jones, 1998, p. 13). Religion is understood as "an integrated set of beliefs, rituals, and institutions through which persons give expression about that which is holy or held in highest esteem in their lives" (Jones, 1998, p. 13). Jones hypothesizes that these two terms are distinct concepts in the lives of African Americans. Ultimately, her study shows that spirituality is a much better predictor for mental health than is religion, suggesting that African Americans understand these two terms as separate and distinct (Jones, 1998). She argues that the lack of definitional autonomy between the terms is due to the difficulty health professionals find in operationalizing these seemingly immeasurable concepts. Also, she finds that mental health practitioners simply lack knowledge about religion and spirituality. Jones argues that research on health outcomes of African Americans should consider not only an individual's relationship to the infrastructure of the church, but also one's perception of self in relation to others (Jones, 1998).

A recent 2010 report on the impact of the two terms showed different results. In the article "Importance of Religion and Spirituality in the Lives of African Americans, Caribbean Blacks and Non-Hispanic Whites," Robert J. Taylor and Linda M. Chatters evaluated the importance of religion and spirituality in the lives of African Americans. They cited religion as a three-fold concept: "(1) a multidimensional construct encompassing public and private behaviors, attitudes and beliefs, (2) organizing around a structured system of tenets, practices, and ritual and (3) characterized as community-focused, formal, and behaviorally oriented" (Taylor & Chatters, 2010, p. 281). Spirituality is defined as "a higher-order endeavor with individual quest that facilitates both greater personal expression and enhanced personal benefits and outcomes, a viewpoint that is particularly ardent among those who are estranged from organized religion" (Taylor & Chatters, 2010, p. 282). The report of Taylor and Chatters is based on the National Survey of American Life: Coping With Stress in the 21st Century survey administered by the Program for Research on Black Americans at the University of Michigan. This survey is one of only a few national probability samples that explore the connection between religion and spirituality (Taylor & Chatters, 2010). The survey sample was composed of 6,082 face-to-face interviews from 3,570 African Americans, 891 Non-Hispanic Whites, and 1,621 Blacks of Caribbean descent. Respondents were asked two questions: "How important is religion in your life?" and "How important is spirituality in your life?" The study found that African Americans are more likely to report that religion and spirituality are very important to their daily lives, at 93 percent. When the results of African Americans and Caribbean Blacks are viewed together, results show that both groups were likely to report that spirituality and religion are very important to them (90%). Taylor and Chatters argue that the results are indicative of two things. First, studies that simply concern themselves with institutional engagement with religion (i.e., church attendance and membership) miss the mark at displaying the full range of one's relationship to faith. Second, the results indicate that the larger Black community does not perceive any particular distinction between the two terms religion and spirituality to describe the importance of faith in their lives (Taylor & Chatters, 2010).

Both studies confirm that a sole focus on African American involvement to the religious institution does not fully capture what African Americans mean when they report that religion and spirituality are important to them. The two studies differ in that Jones reports that spirituality is a better indication of African American religious expression, while Taylor and Chatters contend that recent data reveal that African Americans do not see these two constructs as mutually exclusive and actually find both valuable for their religious expression. It is clear that African Americans engage the terms spirituality and religion when asked to relate them to their religious experience. What is not clear is how effectively these terms capture the religious structure of African Americans. Taylor and Chatters (2010) confess the following:

> The present study in conjunction with previous research on self-rated religiosity and self-rated spirituality provide an in-depth and complementary understanding of these constructs and demonstrate the need for continued exploration of the meaning of religion and spirituality, both across and within racial/ethnic groups. (p. 288)

Taylor and Chatters aptly posit that the next step in properly evaluating the self-rated engagement with religiosity and spirituality in the lives of African Americans and other racial and ethnic groups is exploring the meaning of these terms across and within racial and ethnic communities. This effort would assume that a definition of religion and spirituality when interfaced with African Americans must also consider these terms from a locus point of Black life and across racial and ethnic groups.

▶ The Black Religious Cosmos and Its Impact on Health

In *The Black Church in the African American Experience*, C. Eric Lincoln and Lawrence H. Mamiya provide a descriptive and historical overview alongside statistical data on the current state of the Black church. Their study is the latest major empirical study of Black churches in the United States since Benjamin E. Mays and Joseph W. Nicholson's study in 1924, published in their book *The Negro's Church*. Lincoln and Mamiya interviewed a national sample of pastors from seven historically Black denominations serving in 2,150 urban and rural churches. The study occurred over the span of 8 years, from 1978 to 1986. They provide sociology of the Black church and contribute much-needed theoretical assumptions for engaging the study of the African American religious tradition. They assume a religious dimension spanning over the entirety of Black life they call "the Black Sacred Cosmos."

Like other scholars, Lincoln and Mamiya provide a base definition of religion as a starting point of discussion on the Black religious tradition. They site David Émile Durkheim's 1965 claim in his book *Elementary Forms of Religious Life* that religion is "a social phenomenon, a shared group experience that has shaped and influenced the culture as screens of human communication and interpretation" (Lincoln & Mamiya, 1990, p. 2). Lincoln and Mamiya, however, push beyond this definition and do the work suggested by Taylor and Chatters. They present the concept of the **Black Sacred Cosmos** as a theoretical framework for understanding the religious composition of African Americans. For Lincoln and Mamiya, The Black Sacred Cosmos is "the religious worldview of African Americans... related to their African Heritage, which envisaged the whole universe as sacred, and to their conversion to Christianity during slavery and its aftermath" (Lincoln & Mamiya, 1990, p. 2). This definition moves beyond base definitions and is tailor-made for a deeper understanding of the African American religious tradition.

The Black Sacred Cosmos provides the framework many researchers lack when trying to evaluate the impact of religious tradition on Black health. Lincoln and Mamiya suggest that scholars have consistently struggled to see African American history, culture, and religion as being distinctly generated from the locus point of Black life. It is only in recent years that scholars have recognized Black cultural creations without assuming Eurocentric origin or the mimicking of mainstream culture. Lincoln and Mamiya make clear that Black culture is a culture valid in itself and generative of itself against external pressures. Assumed lack of innovation on the part of African Americans, Lincoln and Mamiya argue, points to the common practice of not granting African Americans the same presuppositions as other "hyphenated Americans" (Lincoln & Mamiya, 1990, p. 3), the presupposition that prior to contact with North America they had viable cohesive, and valid cultures through which they developed new creative American identities (Lincoln & Mamiya, 1990). Such an acknowledgement is crucial when one considers the enormity of research on the connection between spirituality and health of African Americans that lack a definitional framework specific to the religious cosmos in which African Americans operate. In other words, to simply ask questions of religious involvement or whether religion and spirituality are important not only misses the full picture of the impact of religion on the lives of African Americans but also reinforces the idea that the Black religious infrastructure is not unique, independently developed, and distinct from mainstream conceptions of religion and spirituality. It is important for scholars not to dismiss the creative and generative quality of the Black religious infrastructure. To do so is to dismiss a reservoir of unexplored and untapped resolutions to Black health that derive from the locus point of Black life. Lincoln and Mamiya teach us how to appropriately match conceptual framework with demographic sample.

Lincoln and Mamiya's theoretical assumption of the Black Sacred Cosmos also allows them to redefine terms typically associated with definitions of religion. For example, they define culture as "the sum of the options for creative survival" (Lincoln & Mamiya, 1990, p. 3). This definition, when situated within the locus of Black life, takes unique shape. When centered on the heritage of African Americans, survival is the designated end to the pursuit of cultural production. Lincoln and Mamiya's redefinition of terms through the lens of Black life is indicative of the definitional potential of the use of Black-centered paradigms when surveying African

American communities. This is not to say that all Black people will articulate their religious experience specifically as "the Black Sacred Cosmos" or even articulate that survival is at the center of culture. Such theoretical assumptions are meant to posit the unarticulated, lived experience of African Americans and frame research in such a way that one's results and discussion of data are appropriately understood in light of the arch of Black religious heritage and history. The Black Sacred Cosmos is marked by the African religious tradition of having a central sacred object. For African Americans, the Christian God revealed in Jesus Christ is the central sacred object of the Black Sacred Cosmos (Lincoln & Mamiya, 1990).

Though African Americans have operated within the religious structure of White Christians, African Americans are generative in where they choose to place emphasis in the vast tapestry of Christian theology. For example, the imagery of God as a liberating force that avenges on behalf of his children is a powerful emphasis made by African Americans. The idea of being children of God directly confronts Constitutional definitions of Blacks as being three-quarters of a person. Even today, several Black churches still place emphasis on this kind of divine imagery. The suffering and humiliation of Jesus is also a point of emphasis that resonates with this community (Lincoln & Mamiya, 1990).

A central concept in the Black Sacred Cosmos is the concept of **freedom**. For Lincoln and Mamiya, freedom is "the absence of any restraint which might compromise one's responsibility to God" (Lincoln & Mamiya, 1990, p. 4). Freedom through the lens of the Black Sacred Cosmos presupposes a call to total allegiance to God alone and free reign over one's life to do as God requires. To not be free would then complicate one's assurance of salvation. If one belongs to an earthly master, how can he or she also belong to God? Freedom through the lens of Eurocentric normativity has always highlighted an American pursuit toward individualism. The pursuit of freedom to follow one's destiny has always been at the center of American identity. For African Americans, though, the collective nature of slavery and the preeminent identification as Black above all else generated an understanding among African Americans that freedom is a communal pursuit (Lincoln & Mamiya, 1990).

Also at the center of the Black Sacred Cosmos is the concept of individual conversion. Though the idea of being "born again" was a theology widely propagated during the first and second religious awakenings in the United States, African Americans engaged this theological concept differently than did their White counterparts. Though White Christians also emphasized personal conversion, African Americans encountered conversion with a marked element of ecstatic expression. From its inception, the ecstatic nature of the Black church has remained its most marked distinction and unique quality among other American churches (Lincoln & Mamiya, 1990).

For Lincoln and Mamiya, religion "raises the core values of that culture to ultimate levels and legitimates them" (Lincoln & Mamiya, 1990, p. 7). At the center of the Black Sacred Cosmos are the values of "freedom, justice, equality, an African Heritage, and racial parity at all levels of human intercourse" (Lincoln & Mamiya, 1990, p. 7). Within the cosmos, these values are legitimated (Lincoln & Mamiya, 1990) and may inform how individuals evaluate their life and determine their level of satisfaction.

Lincoln and Mamiya's work is an optimal example of how one ought to engage definitions and theoretical models for research on the African American religious tradition. It is also significant for its acknowledgement of the role of religion in the formation of Black culture and points to our initial claim that any resolution for health disparity for African Americans must be rooted in the locus point of Black life, which naturally assumes a deep engagement with the African American religious tradition and the reclaiming of that tradition as American.

In *Black Spirituality and Black Consciousness* (1999), Carlyle Fielding Stewart provides a definition of African American spirituality that is similar to the definition offered by other scholars:

> Spirituality is… a process by which people interpret, disclose, formulate, adapt, and innovate reality and their understanding of God within a specific context or culture. It signifies a style or mode of existence, an ethos and mythos that creates its own praxis and culture, and compels identification and resolution of human problems through divine intervention. These processes involve adaptation and transformation of internal, as well as external conditions. (p. 1)

Stewart, however, goes beyond this definition and describes what spirituality means from the perspective of African Americans: "To be spiritual from an African-American perspective, is to live wholly from the divine soul center of human existence. This center is the core of the universe and the quintessential impetus driving the quest for human fulfillment" (1999, p. 2). For Stewart, this definition connotes possession of a "soul force" that allows the individual to transcend the realities of human existence. This soul force "divinely mediates, informs, and transforms a human being's capacity to create, center, adapt, and transcend the realities of human existence" (Stewart, 1999, p. 2). From this soul force derives a "cultural soul" where Black existence resides. This cultural soul force is where African Americans discover, analyze, celebrate, valuate, corroborate, and transform the meaning of Black life in society.

Soul force can be understood through a dual praxis: creative soul force and resistant soul force. Creative soul force refers to the elements of spirituality that enable African Americans to creatively confront and manage their current reality through the generative construction of Black culture. Resistant soul force is the ability to creatively transcend the barriers and constraints that seek to "enforce the complete domestication to those values, processes, behaviors, and beliefs that reinforce human devaluation and oppression" (Stewart, 1999, p. 2). Simply put, creative soul force is the spirit of creativity to transform and bend reality to support one's existence in the world. Resistant soul force is the part of Black spirituality that resists all attempts to domesticate and annihilate the creative mechanisms of survival of the Black spirit. Culture soul is thus the "archive of values, beliefs, behaviors, practices, and passions that empower and confer value on African-American life" (Stewart, 1999, p. 3).

The concept of creative and resistant soul forces derives from Black people's unique view of themselves as spiritual beings who are yoked with the divine in such a way that freedom, liberation, and positive change are consistently birthed from the connection. African American spirituality is particularly essential to acknowledge because it is the "ultimate reference point for black existence" (Stewart, 1999, p. 3). Since Christianity's introduction to North American Black captives, God and the spirit of the divine became the guarantee that survival was inevitable and freedom imminent.

This definition of spirituality marries well with the concept of the Black religious cosmos, as it is rooted in the belief that freedom is at the center of the Black religious tradition. These two definitions will carry through the rest of this chapter as we consider additional ways of understanding Black spirituality and its impact on the health disparity crisis.

▶ A Spiritual Approach Toward Resolution of Health Disparities: A Personal Case Study

I had a dream that God gave me medicine.

—**Seul Dieu Richard** (father of this chapter's author)

When my father repeated these words, I paused in wonder and in terror. As a person of faith, I didn't disregard the idea entirely. I myself have had dreams, so vivid and mysterious that it could be, for me, nothing less than the presence of the divine revealing itself to me. But this religious declaration seemed to be lodged in a different category entirely. Did he believe that his connection with God somehow made him immune to sickness and death? Was the medicine of God better than the medicine of science? Was he simply avoiding yet another doctor's visit? Was this a classic example of how religion gets in the way of health care?

My father's perspective is quite unsettling for many of us. Immediately, the mind travels to the many consequences of a lack of preventive care. A desire to somehow show him the power of modern medicine and draw him to an enlightened modern socio-perspective subsequently follows. Often, this enlightened modern socio-perspective requires a deconstruction of the divine identity, a psycho-emotional detachment from the divine presence, and a tempering of one's level of dependence on the amorphous acts of the divine. It is believed then that the image of the divine, assumedly crowding the rational judgment of the devotee, will be displaced to make room for the clear choice of modern medicine.

We must move away from cheap evaluations that overestimate religiosity as the Achilles' heel of African Americans and other affected communities as it relates to health disparity. To do so is not simply to appease affected groups to make them feel "welcomed"; rather, to highlight an assumed mutual exclusivity between religion and science is to avoid the real issues of health disparity altogether. There is a mountain of sociopolitical, socioeconomic, racial, gender, and sexuality-based factors that keep affected groups sick, tired, and poor. Plainly, at the center of health disparity is not a question of one's ability to believe in the efficacy of modern medicine (the long-held biased focus of Western European concern), but one's ability to trust institutions of health that seem to work in tandem with the socioeconomic and sociopolitical forces that have historically pursued, in overt and latent fashions, the domestication and annihilation of non-normative life in the United States. Sadly, the health system has proven over and over again, particularly in the lives of African Americans, to be antithetical to the existence of non-normative life.

In her essay "The Underutilization of Health Services in the Black Community: An Examination of Causes and Effects," Daphne Chandler discusses the roots of the Black community's cultural mistrust toward the generally White medical infrastructure. She sees cultural mistrust as being "characterized by a lack of trust in Whites, suspicion of their motives, uncertainty about the sequence of events, a sense of individual powerlessness, and a belief that caution is necessary to avoid trouble" (Chandler, 2010, p. 926). Another source of mistrust is connected to the fear of being misdiagnosed and overdiagnosed. Chandler states, "Blacks are disproportionately misdiagnosed and over-diagnosed for such mental disorders as schizophrenia, due to such factors as counselor incompetence, an outcome of little or no knowledge of the Black culture, and racial or cultural bias" (2010, p. 926). Mistrust is deepened when one considers the history of surgical and disease experimentation on Black bodies and access to these bodies through the medical and prison infrastructure. Unsurprisingly, when interacting with the medical infrastructure, Blacks generally have low expectations for the quality of care they will experience, even while being treated by a Black doctor. Ultimately, Chandler posits that this mistrust is rooted in the institutional legacy of racism in the United States (2010, p. 296).

When the conversation centers on trust, the weight of responsibility bares heavily on normative locations of power to restore, retain, and maintain healthy relationships with affected communities. It is imperative that these relationships are mutually committed to fostering a kind of trust that conveys the utmost commitment to affirming the flourishing and survival of people affected by health disparity. Furthermore, centering the conversation on trust reveals that religion and science are not at odds with one another. When imagined comparative evaluations on the efficacy of God versus the efficacy of modern medicine are marginalized, suddenly centuries of historical anecdotes that progressively fostered general mistrust of wellness efforts for marginalized groups materialize. Under such circumstances, normative efforts to engage wellness of non-normative people simply do not carry the same credence as institutions centered on the survival and flourishing of that group (i.e., religion and spirituality). Perhaps there is a reality where religiosity and science will not contend or reach for intellectual authority, but will collaborate in assuring the survival and flourishing of non-normative life. As we have seen, to disregard the role of spirituality is to disregard the cultural psychology of several groups to whom spirituality defines culture and identity. These groups include, but are not limited to, African Americans and Native Americans. These groups have historically suffered greatly as a result of health disparity. Thus, it is essential to defend the role of spirituality from swift attempts to supplant it entirely with Eurocentric demands to maintain a mutually exclusive dependence on the efficacy of modern medicine.

How is spirituality a viable lens, though, for envisioning the resolution to health disparity? I begin this exploration by returning to my father's words: "I had a dream that God gave me medicine." What was he saying? And why is it important? In true theological fashion, I have interpreted his statement while considering what I know about the historical context of his life and faith. His beliefs may be expressed in these words:

> I believe in the benevolence of God so deeply that this God can heal me in my sleep of any unknown and known diseases. My connection to the divine does not make me immune to sickness and death, but it says to me everyday that I, like anyone else, deserve to live. I believe this so deeply that I do not fear life or death, but am comforted to know that I will be comforted in my departure. If sickness were to take me, I would prefer it

be the will of God and not the wielding of strange and unknown men. In this I am utterly satisfied.

After much coaxing and theological gymnastics, I have still not been able to get my father to the doctor's office. The last I asked, he said, "They might give me medicine that could end up killing me if it doesn't work with my body." In this comment I sensed not only a fear of being mishandled or misdiagnosed, but a deeper awareness that his body would not be seen as valuable enough for extraordinarily excellent and accurate care. He was challenging the competence of the medical system in engaging his Black body. He is not a famous Black man, nor does he have many riches. In the walls of a big hospital and local clinic, he is not the beloved Pastor Richard of the local storefront church. He is not immediately known, as I know him, as father, counselor, and friend. He is another patient whose death could be easily explained away by medical jargon, without any fear of national press or criticism among colleagues. The fear of being inconsequential in the hands of strange men is real and should not be taken lightly. But God—God, for him, is the only assurance of his survival and existence in this world. Who am I to say that in this day and age he has no right to depend on the divine? One cannot expect those who suffer from health disparity to trust a system that defines them as inconsequential. It is imperative that health frame itself within the various cultural loci of affected groups, which often implies a locus of spirituality. Looking through the lens of Black life reveals spirituality as an integral mode of survival in light of micro-aggression and the external hostility of the nation. In this sense, while we wait for the nation to appropriately respond to health disparity, to create an atmosphere of trust, we will let faith do its work.

▶ The Connection Between Spirituality and Religiosity, Health Outcomes, and Solutions/Resolutions

Several years of research have concluded that there is, in fact, a connection between religiosity and health outcome. Generally, those who are deeply religious often avoid high-risk behavior, exhibit higher levels of life satisfaction, possess social networks and tools useful to cope with stress and recover from depression from stressful life events, and heal at a much faster rate than do their non-religious counterparts. They also exhibit stronger immune systems, have better cardiovascular health, and fare well as they age and encounter end of life (Koenig, 1999).

Generally, religion and spirituality aid in building resilience, a high level of life satisfaction, and much-needed peace in moments of severe stress and life difficulty that often circumvent risk of disease and sickness. In the face of the effects of health disparity, religion and spirituality provide an internal shield to protect one's internal system of approval and sense of happiness. The more negative the external environment, the deeper the dependence on the internal shield.

Chandler sees this internal protective mechanism as useful but also as a potential hindrance to wellness. She understands the effects of spirituality as creating a "pseudo-harmony" within the self that makes the stress caused by disparity bearable and manageable. Though she sees this as a positive trait of religion, she also sees the potential danger, stating the following:

> In light of the detrimental health and socioeconomic milieu plaguing the Black community, it is very likely that the adverse effects of internal pseudo-harmony would result in increased health disparity. Consider the effects of accepting repression and oppression as God's plan, or as manageable only with God's help, turning a blind eye to the racist institutions and the need for activism. (Chandler, 2010, p. 925)

From this thought, she proposes, "Spirituality can act as a positive or a negative coping strategy depending on one's degree of reliance" (Chandler, 2010). She provides an example cited by Fowler and Hill (2004), who found that deeply religious Black women in abusive relationships tend to stay with their partners to uphold religious values of marriage, forgiveness, and steadfast waiting on God to restore the marriage. Chandler concludes that spirituality is not the answer to disparity, but a way of dealing with the stress caused by disparity. She argues that resolution would require a dismantling of the repressive and oppressive forces that are at the root of disparity (Chandler, 2010). It is for this reason that this chapter is subtitled "A Spiritual Approach *Toward* Resolution."

Chandler is right. There can be theological assumptions that emanate out of one's understanding of the divine identity that keep the individual in high-risk unhealthy situations. One's spirituality may be an effective solution to the stress of the situation but is not a solution to the root cause of disparity. The potential of pseudo-harmony does not mean that religion ought to be discarded, but that it is part of a whole approach to address the main issue of disparity. Chandler's critique draws us back to a need to understand spirituality from a perspective of cultural singularity. Spirituality is not a stagnant affair. It is ever evolving as we encounter new and old ideas within our culture. Through the lens of the Black Sacred Cosmos, for example, the value of freedom is viewed in highest esteem, and survival the end of any attempt of cultural production. One's spirituality, when confronted with moments of oppression, can take the shape of the oppression itself, while simultaneously presenting abundant theological resources for liberation. Such resources will go unnoticed if the religious infrastructure has not been liberated. Chandler's critique is not a wholesale dismissal of spirituality but truly a critique on the impact of dogmatic religious infrastructure that would rather maintain theological claims over the liberation of its people from oppressive forces. Clearly this thinking is not descriptive of all religious encounters, but it is essential to note as a call to religious clergy and spiritual sojourners to actively evaluate the impact of theological claims, affirming claims that liberate, rejecting claims that bind, and creating claims needed to affirm the lives of those we have utterly overlooked.

Furthermore, health disparity points to a greater issue of national identity. Spirituality is not simply understating who God is but also who we are. Definitional frameworks that consider religion and spirituality across racial/ethnic groups are, as we've seen, quite necessary. Taylor and Chatters's request for such definitions ought not be considered as a type of ritualistic checks and balances for academic study. In fact, their request speaks to a greater need for a type of emphasis on cultural singularity that ushers an integration and expansion of the national American identity. In other words, a spiritual approach provokes discourse on identity in such a way that a conversation about national inclusion in inventible. The hyphen sometimes sandwiched between the terms *African* and *American* is pregnant with the unfinished work of claiming American identity. In the *Souls of Black Folks*, first published in 1903, W. E. B. DuBois wrote the following:

> Freedom, too, the long-sought, we still seek,—the freedom of life and limb, the freedom to work and think, the freedom to love and aspire. Work, culture, liberty,—all these we need, not singly but together, not successively but together, each growing and aiding each, and all striving toward that vaster ideal that swims before the negro people, the ideal of human brotherhood, gained through the unifying ideal of Race; the ideal of fostering and developing the traits and talents of the Negro, not in opposition to or contempt for other races, but rather in large conformity to the greater ideals of the American Republic, in order that some day on American soil two world-races may give each to each those characteristics both so sadly lack. (2005, p. 15)

A conceptual emphasis on an integrated national identity speaks directly to the concept of disparity. It short-circuits attempts at making culture the distinctive factor that determines and simplifies methods of care. Establishing cultural singularity is important, but it runs the risk of conceptual reinforcement of racialized binaries that either propagates disengagement by the dominant culture or reaches for parentalist control and judgment of non-normative ways of existing. In other words, when an emphasis on cultural difference is taken too far, cultural difference becomes the scapegoat through which the dominant culture evades responsibility for health disparity. Under such circumstances, narrowing the health disparity gap becomes the task of the non-normative communities and White sympathizers instead of, more appropriately, the responsibility of the national community. Conceptual frameworks for the study of the impact of religion and spirituality on the health outcomes of African Americans, for example, must claim the uniqueness of the African American religious tradition, while maintaining a rightful understanding of the broader history of the American religious tradition.

Wrap-Up

Chapter Summary

This chapter enabled the discovery of the significant role and importance of religion and spirituality in the lives of African Americans. It provided the potential for alternative considerations for framing discussions on the impact of religion and spirituality to health outcomes of marginalized groups, through engaging the Black Sacred Cosmos and Black spirituality as definitions that move beyond general and imprecise attempts at matching conceptual frameworks to a demographic sample. Finally, the chapter explored a spiritual approach toward resolving the health disparity crisis. Though research shows that there are major health benefits to religiosity, religion and spirituality are not, per se, the resolution to health disparity but are factors that must be present in any attempt at a resolution, particularly for non-normative ethnic and racial groups who identify deeply with a spirituality as unique to their identity. Approaches to the healthcare disparity crisis must call upon the concepts of religion and spirituality to (1) provoke a deeper definitional framework for discussion that appropriately matches the demographic sample, (2) engage the importance of a psycho-emotional safety net to skillfully manage sickness-inducing stresses caused by disparity, (3) identify misguided attempts at obscuring the central causes of health disparity by a disregard of the importance of spirituality, and (4) engage a discussion on the need for an expanded national identity that embraces the cultural singularity of non-normative groups, particularly those impacted by disparity. A call for an expanded national identity speaks directly to the concept of disparity without reinforcing cultural binaries that re-legitimate segregation-based treatment.

One's unique understanding of the divine, the self, and others is at the center of spirituality. It resides at the core of one's being. To know this core, to see this core, and to affirm its existence is the coeffort of the nation and its Gods. Hand in hand, both must incite belonging and affirm life and wellness.

Chapter Problems

1.   Explain the notion of a Black Sacred Cosmos as a conceptual framework and its relevance to health disparities.
2.   Is spirituality a concept that should be considered in terms of reducing/ resolving health disparities? Explain why or why not.
3.   Explain how spirituality may be unique to some individuals.
4.   What is the difference between religiosity and spirituality?
5.   What racial and ethnic groups are negatively impacted by health disparity in the United States?

References

Chandler, D. (2010, May). The underutilization of health services in the Black community: An examination of causes and effects. *Journal of Black Studies, 40*(5), 915–931.

Dubois, W. E. B. (2005). *The souls of Black folks*. New York, NY: Simon & Schuster.

Jones, G. L. (1998, May). *The relationship among spirituality, religion, and mental health for African Americans* (Doctoral dissertation, University of New Orleans).

Koenig, H. G. (1999). *The healing power of faith: Science explores medicine's last frontier*. New York, NY: Simon & Schuster.

Lincoln, C. E., & Mamiya, L. H. (1990). *The Black church in the African American experience*. Durham, NC: Duke University Press.

Pew Research Center. (2009, January 30). A religious portrait of African Americans. Retrieved from http://www.pewforum.org/2009/01/30/a-religious-portrait-of-african-americans/

Pew Research Center. (2015, May 12). America's changing religious landscape. Retrieved from http://www.pewforum.org/2015/05/12/americas-changing-religious-landscape/

Stewart, C. F. (1999). *Black spirituality and Black consciousness: Soul force, culture, and freedom in the African-American experience*. Trenton, NJ: Africa World Press.

Taylor, R. J., & Chatters, L. M. (2010). Importance of religion and spirituality in the lives of African Americans, Caribbean Blacks and Non-Hispanic Whites. *The Journal of Negro Education, 79*(3), 280–294.

Appendix I

The National Standards for Culturally and Linguistically Appropriate Services in Health and Health Care (The National CLAS Standards)

In *Essentials of Health, Culture, and Diversity*, Edberg (2012) describes the CLAS Standards as follows:

> These standards... have become the key document used to guide cultural competence efforts in the United States.... They are organized by theme: standards 1–3 address culturally competent care; 4–7 refer to language access services; and 8–14 refer to organizational supports for cultural competence. (p. 160)

Edberg (2012) describes the first seven clinical/service-oriented standards as follows:

- **Standard 1:** Healthcare organizations should ensure that patients/consumers receive from all staff members effective, understandable, and respectful care that is provided in a manner compatible with their cultural health beliefs and practices and preferred language.
- **Standard 2:** Healthcare organizations should implement strategies to recruit, retain, and promote, at all levels of the organization, a diverse staff and leadership that are representative of the demographic characteristics of the service area.
- **Standard 3:** Healthcare organizations should ensure that staff at all levels and across all disciplines receive ongoing education and training in culturally and linguistically appropriate service delivery.
- **Standard 4:** Healthcare organizations must offer and provide language assistance services, including bilingual staff and interpreter services, at no cost to each patient/consumer with limited English proficiency at all points of contact, in a timely manner, during all hours of operation.
- **Standard 5:** Healthcare organizations must provide to patients/consumers, in their preferred language, both verbal offers and written notices informing them of their right to receive language assistance services.

- **Standard 6:** Healthcare organizations must assure the competence of language assistance provided to limited English proficient patients/consumers by interpreters and bilingual staff. Family and friends should not be used to provide interpretation services (except on request by the patient/consumer).
- **Standard 7:** Healthcare organizations must make available easily understood patient-related materials and post signage in the languages of the commonly encountered groups and/or groups represented in the service area.

Edberg (2012) describes the organization-oriented standards as follows:

- **Standard 8:** Healthcare organizations should develop, implement, and promote a written strategic plan that outlines clear goals, policies, operational plans, and management accountability/oversight mechanisms to provide culturally and linguistically appropriate services.
- **Standard 9:** Healthcare organizations should conduct initial and ongoing organizational self-assessments of CLAS-related activities and are encouraged to integrate cultural and linguistic competence-related measures into their internal audits, performance improvement programs, patient satisfaction assessments, and outcomes-based evaluations.
- **Standard 10:** Healthcare organizations should ensure that data on the individual patient's/consumer's race, ethnicity, and spoken and written language are collected in health records, integrated into the organization's management information systems, and periodically updated.
- **Standard 11:** Healthcare organizations should maintain a current demographic, cultural, and epidemiological profile of the community as well as a needs assessment to accurately plan for, and implement, services that respond to the cultural and linguistic characteristics of the service area.
- **Standard 12:** Healthcare organizations should develop participatory, collaborative partnerships with communities and utilize a variety of formal and informal mechanisms to facilitate community and patient/consumer involvement in designing and implementing CLAS-related activities.
- **Standard 13:** Healthcare organizations should ensure that conflict and grievance resolution processes are culturally and linguistically sensitive and capable of identifying, preventing, and resolving cross-cultural conflicts or complaints by patients/consumers.
- **Standard 14:** Healthcare organizations are encouraged to regularly make available to the public information about their progress and successful innovations in implementing the CLAS standards and to provide public notice in their communities about the availability of this information.

These standards were initially derived from an analysis of current practices and policies on cultural competence and shaped by the experiences and expertise of healthcare organizations, policy makers, and consumers and were developed over a 3-year period based upon input from a number of sources, as sponsored by the U.S. Department of Health and Human Services, Office of Minority Health (Rose, 2013).

References

M. Edberg (2012). *Essentials of health, culture, and diversity.* Burlington, MA: Jones & Bartlett Learning.

P. Rose (2013). *Cultural competency for the health professional* (pp. 171–172). Burlington, MA: Jones & Bartlett Learning.

Appendix II

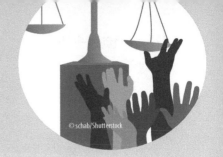

Cultural Competence Assessment Survey

▶ Executive Team and Management

Site: _____

Date: _____

Please place a check mark ✓ next to the selection that best represents your thoughts.

1. I display pictures, posters, and other materials that reflect the cultures and ethnic backgrounds of patients/clients/customers served by my site.

   ☐ Strongly Agree   ☐ Disagree
   ☐ Agree   ☐ N/A
   ☐ Strongly Disagree

2. I speak up when someone is humiliating another person or acting inappropriately.

   ☐ Strongly Agree   ☐ Disagree
   ☐ Agree   ☐ N/A
   ☐ Strongly Disagree

3. I avoid using language that reinforces negative stereotypes.

   ☐ Strongly Agree   ☐ Disagree
   ☐ Agree   ☐ N/A
   ☐ Strongly Disagree

4. I ensure that magazines, brochures, and other printed materials in reception areas reflect the different cultures of patients/clients/customers served by my site.

   ☐ Strongly Agree   ☐ Disagree
   ☐ Agree   ☐ N/A
   ☐ Strongly Disagree

5. When using videos, films, or other media resources for health education, treatment, or other interventions, I ensure that they reflect the culture of the patients/clients/customers served by my site.

   ☐ Strongly Agree   ☐ Disagree
   ☐ Agree   ☐ N/A
   ☐ Strongly Disagree

6.   I assist my new staff members, including people of various cultures, ages, and sizes, to feel welcome and accepted.

☐ **Strongly Agree**   ☐ **Disagree**
☐ **Agree**   ☐ **N/A**
☐ **Strongly Disagree**

7.   I disregard physical characteristics when interacting with others and when making decisions about competence and ability.

☐ **Strongly Agree**   ☐ **Disagree**
☐ **Agree**   ☐ **N/A**
☐ **Strongly Disagree**

8.   I am culturally competent.

☐ **Strongly Agree**   ☐ **Disagree**
☐ **Agree**   ☐ **N/A**
☐ **Strongly Disagree**

9.   I know the definition of cultural competence.

☐ **Strongly Agree**   ☐ **Disagree**
☐ **Agree**   ☐ **N/A**
☐ **Strongly Disagree**

10. I know the definition of cultural proficiency.

☐ **Strongly Agree**   ☐ **Disagree**
☐ **Agree**   ☐ **N/A**
☐ **Strongly Disagree**

11. I am culturally proficient.

☐ **Strongly Agree**   ☐ **Disagree**
☐ **Agree**   ☐ **N/A**
☐ **Strongly Disagree**

12. I intervene in an appropriate manner when I observe my staff or clients/patients/customers engaging in behaviors that exhibit cultural insensitivity or prejudice.

☐ **Strongly Agree**   ☐ **Disagree**
☐ **Agree**   ☐ **N/A**
☐ **Strongly Disagree**

13. Cultural proficiency training sessions/workshops will be helpful to my staff in their overall work performance.

☐ **Strongly Agree**   ☐ **Disagree**
☐ **Agree**   ☐ **N/A**
☐ **Strongly Disagree**

14. My work responsibilities include direct patient/client/customer contact.

☐ **Strongly Agree**   ☐ **Disagree**
☐ **Agree**   ☐ **N/A**
☐ **Strongly Disagree**

15. I have difficulty communicating with patients/clients/customers who cannot speak English.

☐ Strongly Agree   ☐ Disagree
☐ Agree   ☐ N/A
☐ Strongly Disagree

16. All patients/clients/customers who visit my work site for service should know how to speak English if they want help.

☐ Strongly Agree   ☐ Disagree
☐ Agree   ☐ N/A
☐ Strongly Disagree

17. Translation and signage should be available for patients/clients/customers with limited English proficiency (LEP).

☐ Strongly Agree   ☐ Disagree
☐ Agree   ☐ N/A
☐ Strongly Disagree

18. Ongoing training and education for executives, management, and staff is necessary to promote culturally and linguistically competent/proficient service delivery.

☐ Strongly Agree   ☐ Disagree
☐ Agree   ☐ N/A
☐ Strongly Disagree

19. I am interested in attending cultural competency/proficiency workshops/training sessions.

☐ Strongly Agree   ☐ Disagree
☐ Agree   ☐ N/A
☐ Strongly Disagree

20. I use bilingual staff or trained volunteers to serve as interpreters during assessment, meetings, or events for clients/patients/customers who would require this level of assistance.

☐ Strongly Agree   ☐ Disagree
☐ Agree   ☐ N/A
☐ Strongly Disagree

Thank You

Appendix III

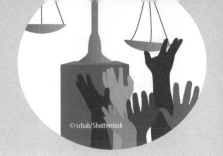

Cultural Competence Assessment Survey

▶ Staff

Site: _____

Date: _____

Please place a check mark ✓ next to the selection that best represents your thoughts.

1. I avoid imposing values that may conflict, or be inconsistent, with those of cultures or ethnic groups other than my own.

   ☐ Strongly Agree   ☐ Disagree
   ☐ Agree   ☐ N/A
   ☐ Strongly Disagree

2. I speak up when someone is humiliating another person or acting inappropriately.

   ☐ Strongly Agree   ☐ Disagree
   ☐ Agree   ☐ N/A
   ☐ Strongly Disagree

3. I avoid using language that reinforces negative stereotypes.

   ☐ Strongly Agree   ☐ Disagree
   ☐ Agree   ☐ N/A
   ☐ Strongly Disagree

4. I get to know people from different groups and cultures as individuals.

   ☐ Strongly Agree   ☐ Disagree
   ☐ Agree   ☐ N/A
   ☐ Strongly Disagree

5. I accept and reinforce the fact that not everyone has to act or look a certain way to be successful or valuable.

   ☐ Strongly Agree   ☐ Disagree
   ☐ Agree   ☐ N/A
   ☐ Strongly Disagree

6.   I assist new people at the site where I work, including people of various cultures, ages, and sizes, to feel welcome and accepted.

☐ **Strongly Agree**   ☐ **Disagree**
☐ **Agree**   ☐ **N/A**
☐ **Strongly Disagree**

7.   I disregard physical characteristics when interacting with others and when making decisions about competence and ability.

☐ **Strongly Agree**   ☐ **Disagree**
☐ **Agree**   ☐ **N/A**
☐ **Strongly Disagree**

8.   I am culturally competent.

☐ **Strongly Agree**   ☐ **Disagree**
☐ **Agree**   ☐ **N/A**
☐ **Strongly Disagree**

9.   I know the definition of cultural competence.

☐ **Strongly Agree**   ☐ **Disagree**
☐ **Agree**   ☐ **N/A**
☐ **Strongly Disagree**

10.   I know the definition of cultural proficiency.

☐ **Strongly Agree**   ☐ **Disagree**
☐ **Agree**   ☐ **N/A**
☐ **Strongly Disagree**

11.   I am culturally proficient.

☐ **Strongly Agree**   ☐ **Disagree**
☐ **Agree**   ☐ **N/A**
☐ **Strongly Disagree**

12.   I intervene, in an appropriate manner, when I observe other staff or clients/patients/customers within my worksite engaging in behaviors that exhibit cultural insensitivity or prejudice.

☐ **Strongly Agree**   ☐ **Disagree**
☐ **Agree**   ☐ **N/A**
☐ **Strongly Disagree**

13.   Cultural proficiency training sessions/workshops will be helpful to me in my overall work performance.

☐ **Strongly Agree**   ☐ **Disagree**
☐ **Agree**   ☐ **N/A**
☐ **Strongly Disagree**

14.   My work responsibilities include direct patient/client/customer contact.

☐ **Strongly Agree**   ☐ **Disagree**
☐ **Agree**   ☐ **N/A**
☐ **Strongly Disagree**

15.   I have difficulty communicating with patients/clients/customers who cannot speak English.

☐ **Strongly Agree**   ☐ **Disagree**
☐ **Agree**   ☐ **N/A**
☐ **Strongly Disagree**

16.   All patients/clients/customers who visit my worksite for service should know how to speak English if they want help.

☐ **Strongly Agree**   ☐ **Disagree**
☐ **Agree**   ☐ **N/A**
☐ **Strongly Disagree**

17.   Translation and signage should be available for patients/clients/customers with limited English proficiency (LEP).

☐ **Strongly Agree**   ☐ **Disagree**
☐ **Agree**   ☐ **N/A**
☐ **Strongly Disagree**

18.   Ongoing training and education for staff to promote cultural and linguistically competent/proficient service delivery is important.

☐ **Strongly Agree**   ☐ **Disagree**
☐ **Agree**   ☐ **N/A**
☐ **Strongly Disagree**

19.   I am interested in attending cultural competency/proficiency workshops/training sessions.

☐ **Strongly Agree**   ☐ **Disagree**
☐ **Agree**   ☐ **N/A**
☐ **Strongly Disagree**

20.   I recognize and challenge the biases that support my own thinking.

☐ **Strongly Agree**   ☐ **Disagree**
☐ **Agree**   ☐ **N/A**
☐ **Strongly Disagree**

Thank You

Appendix IV

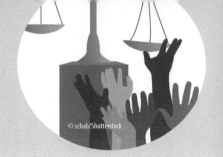

Cultural Competence Assessment Survey

▶ Health Professionals

Site: _____

Date: _____

Please place a check mark ✓ next to the selection that best represents your thoughts.

1. I display pictures, posters, and other materials that reflect the cultures and ethnic backgrounds of patients served by my site.

   ☐ Strongly Agree   ☐ Disagree
   | | Agree   ☐ N/A
   ☐ Strongly Disagree

2. I make extra efforts to educate myself about the various cultures of my patients.

   ☐ Strongly Agree   ☐ Disagree
   ☐ Agree   ☐ N/A
   ☐ Strongly Disagree

3. I avoid using language that reinforces negative stereotypes.

   ☐ Strongly Agree   ☐ Disagree
   ☐ Agree   ☐ N/A
   ☐ Strongly Disagree

4. I ensure that magazines, brochures, and other printed materials in reception areas reflect the different cultures of patients served by my site.

   ☐ Strongly Agree   ☐ Disagree
   ☐ Agree   ☐ N/A
   ☐ Strongly Disagree

5. When using videos, films, or other media resources for health education, treatment, or other interventions, I ensure that they reflect the cultures of the patients served by my site.

   ☐ Strongly Agree   ☐ Disagree
   ☐ Agree   ☐ N/A
   ☐ Strongly Disagree

6. I attempt to determine any family colloquialisms used by patients that may impact an assessment, treatment, or other intervention.

☐ **Strongly Agree**   ☐ **Disagree**
☐ **Agree**   ☐ **N/A**
☐ **Strongly Disagree**

7. I accept that religion, and other beliefs, may influence how families respond to illness, disease, and death.

☐ **Strongly Agree**   ☐ **Disagree**
☐ **Agree**   ☐ **N/A**
☐ **Strongly Disagree**

8. I am culturally competent.

☐ **Strongly Agree**   ☐ **Disagree**
☐ **Agree**   ☐ **N/A**
☐ **Strongly Disagree**

9. I know the definition of cultural competence.

☐ **Strongly Agree**   ☐ **Disagree**
☐ **Agree**   ☐ **N/A**
☐ **Strongly Disagree**

10. I know the definition of cultural proficiency.

☐ **Strongly Agree**   ☐ **Disagree**
☐ **Agree**   ☐ **N/A**
☐ **Strongly Disagree**

11. I am culturally proficient.

☐ **Strongly Agree**   ☐ **Disagree**
☐ **Agree**   ☐ **N/A**
☐ **Strongly Disagree**

12. I use bilingual staff or trained volunteers to serve as interpreters during assessment of patients who require this level of assistance.

☐ **Strongly Agree**   ☐ **Disagree**
☐ **Agree**   ☐ **N/A**
☐ **Strongly Disagree**

13. Cultural proficiency training sessions/workshops will be helpful to me in the provision of health care.

☐ **Strongly Agree**   ☐ **Disagree**
☐ **Agree**   ☐ **N/A**
☐ **Strongly Disagree**

14. When possible, I ensure that all communiqués to patients are written in their language of origin.

☐ **Strongly Agree**   ☐ **Disagree**
☐ **Agree**   ☐ **N/A**
☐ **Strongly Disagree**

15. I have difficulty communicating with patients who cannot speak English.

☐ **Strongly Agree**   ☐ **Disagree**
☐ **Agree**   ☐ **N/A**
☐ **Strongly Disagree**

16. All patients who need care should know how to speak English if they want help.

☐ **Strongly Agree**   ☐ **Disagree**
☐ **Agree**   ☐ **N/A**
☐ **Strongly Disagree**

17. Translation and signage should be available for patients with limited English proficiency (LEP).

☐ **Strongly Agree**   ☐ **Disagree**
☐ **Agree**   ☐ **N/A**
☐ **Strongly Disagree**

18. Ongoing training and education for health providers is necessary to promote culturally and linguistically competent/proficient service delivery, which is important.

☐ **Strongly Agree**   ☐ **Disagree**
☐ **Agree**   ☐ **N/A**
☐ **Strongly Disagree**

19. I am interested in attending cultural competency/proficiency workshops/training sessions.

☐ **Strongly Agree**   ☐ **Disagree**
☐ **Agree**   ☐ **N/A**
☐ **Strongly Disagree**

20. I recognize that the meaning or value of medical treatment and health education may vary greatly among cultures.

☐ **Strongly Agree**   ☐ **Disagree**
☐ **Agree**   ☐ **N/A**
☐ **Strongly Disagree**

Thank You

Appendix V

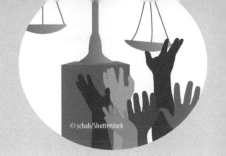

Sample Components of a Diversity Plan

Although diversity is a broad term, inclusive of many types of individuals and groups that warrant emphasis, the focus of this brief sample plan is racial and ethnic diversity, as is the case for this text throughout, with the understanding that the information provided may be applicable and revised to suit the needs of groups beyond the scope of this text. The goal of this sample plan is to provide guidelines and key insight into potentially useful objectives, methods, and action steps relating to the process, and to identify the leaders who may be involved with implementation. This table is intended only to serve as a guide as to components that should be considered. These cursory suggestions are provided in a simple format, as the process should not be complicated but rather easily doable.

Objective	Methods	Action Steps	Leaders
Develop/revise the institutional mission statement to include an emphasis/focus on diversity.	■ Review existing mission statements that have accomplished this. ■ Define the term "diversity" so that it is clear to all members of the organization. ■ The mission and vision statements should be displayed throughout the organization and on the security badges worn by all members of the organization, the organization's web page, and all ingoing and outgoing communications per letterhead or below email signatures.	■ Have a strategic mission statement development/revision meeting with the president and CEO and his cabinet and key staff. ■ Get approval of the board of directors/trustees for the new/revised mission statement.	■ President and CEO ■ Cabinet of the president and CEO ■ Key staff (administrative and nonadministrative) ■ Faculty, administrators, and staff at academic institutions
Create a fully staffed (racially and ethnically diversified) Diversity and Cultural and Linguistic Competence Office with the sole responsibility of racially and ethnically diversifying the organization and handling multicultural affairs.	■ Ensure cultural and linguistic competence training for the board of directors, administrators, faculty, and staff. ■ Maintain and manage a comprehensive budget for all diversity, cultural, and linguistic competence efforts (exclusive of fundraising). ■ Seek ongoing continuing education and developmental training for all diversity and cultural and linguistic staff. ■ Offer educational conferences at the institution to ensure that all members of the organization are provided with timely information about racially, ethnically diverse, cultural and linguistic competence issues.	■ Hire staff for the office that are reflective of the diversity goals of the organization, in terms of administration and staff. ■ Develop a full calendar of events for diversity and cultural competence initiatives (conferences, guest speakers, training sessions workshops, etc.) to be distributed to all members of the organization encouraging and requiring (where appropriate) attendance.	■ Diversity and Cultural and Linguistic Competence Office's vice president and all office staff ■ Chief financial officer ■ President and CEO ■ Board of Directors ■ Human Resources

Create marketing materials that are reflective of a commitment to serve diverse populations and (visual affirmation).	■ Collect data specific to the definition of diversity for the organization so that efforts are true to the mission of the organization in terms of diversity. ■ Analyze the sociodemographic characteristics and data of clients/customers/patients/students served. ■ Determine the predominant racial/ethnic groups served by the organization.	■ Provide ongoing assessment, evaluation, and review of the efficacy of the office to ensure that all efforts are being met while simultaneously developing and implementing solutions where gaps may exist. ■ Budget for, and develop, marketing materials (paper and technological) that are reflective of the populations served based on culturally relevant images and linguistic requirements.	■ President and CEO ■ Marketing and relevant administrative staff ■ Chief financial officer and staff ■ Practitioners, faculty, and other staff who have direct interactions with clients/customers/students ■ Technological staff ■ Human resources ■ Diversity and Cultural and Linguistic Competence Office

(continues)

Objective	Methods	Action Steps	Leaders
Recruit a workforce (of clinical and nonclinical staff, administrators, faculty, and beyond) whose demographic makeup is reflective of the population served.	■ Train and advise all staff who will be involved with diversity recruitment on how and where to do so.	■ Develop long-term and short-term recruitment efforts. ■ Develop a multicultural recruitment advisory committee (consisting of members of the recruitment target population). ■ Ensure that all job descriptions include the organization's diversity recruitment aims.	■ Diversity and Cultural and Linguistic Competence Office ■ Human resources ■ Supervisors, managers, directors, and department chairs ■ Marketing department
Organize diversity-related activities that enable cross-cultural learning at all levels of the organization in an atmosphere of positive lighthearted activities.	■ Example: Encourage staff to submit recipes for the development of a company- or institutional-wide cookbook. ■ Have select staff, clinicians, students, faculty present a lecture, in an ongoing seminar series about their culture, language, and family lineage to ensure cross-cultural understanding of diverse cultures.	■ Develop and publish the company- or institution-wide cookbook for all staff to enjoy and experience and for the opportunity to learn about diversity. ■ Prioritize the lecture series as an important and significant aspect of the organization, offering time release and some type of accolades for participation and attendance.	■ Diversity and Cultural and Linguistic Competence Office ■ Human Resources ■ All members of the organization/staff

Appendix VI

Cultural Competence Plan

Company Analysis

Brief organizational history with cultural competence emphasis.

Community Analysis

- Local demographics
- Patient/client/customer demographics
- Executive and management demographics
- Board of directors demographics
- Provider/health professional demographics
- Staff demographics

Cultural Competence Assessment

- Board and executive team
- Health professionals/providers
- Staff

Facility Assessment (Visual Affirmation and Bi-/Multilingual Signage)

- Waiting areas
- High-traffic areas
- Treatment protocols
- Staff-accessible areas
- Reading materials and written information
- Website review
- Review of procedures and protocols, mission and vision statements

Strategic Cultural Competence Marketing Plan and Development

Strategic Approach

- Expected cultural competence goals and outcomes
- Achieving diversity
- Cultural competence champions (committee)
- Internet cultural marketing and training

Community Partnering

- Community leaders
- Key organizations
- Supporting affiliates/stakeholders

Cultural Competence Project Timeline

- Key elements
- Key points and dates
- Checkpoints

Post-Project Assessment/Evaluation

- Goal measurement
- Continued cultural competence assessment (ongoing)

Appendix VII

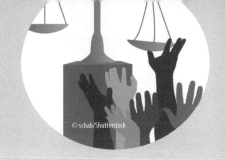

Abbreviations

Glossary

AAMC	Association of American Medical Colleges
ACA	Affordable Care Act (short for Patient Protection and Affordable Care Act)
ACLU	American Civil Liberties Union
AFDC	Aid to Families with Dependent Children
AHRQ	Agency for Healthcare Research and Quality
AACTE	American Association of College Teachers
AGS	American Geriatrics Society
ACLU	American Civil Liberties Union
AVMA	American Veterinary Medical Association
CAASP	Child and Adolescent Service System Program
CBO	Congressional Budget Office
CDC	Centers for Disease Control and Prevention
CEO	chief executive officer
CFO	chief financial officer
CHC	community health center
CIA	Central Intelligence Agency
CLAS	Culturally and Linguistically Appropriate Services
DHHS	Department of Health and Human Services
ELLs	English Language Learners
FPL	federal poverty level
FQHC	federally qualified health center
HBCUs	historically Black colleges and universities
HCOP	Health Careers Opportunity Program
HRSA	Health Resources and Services Administration
IHS	Indian Health Service
IMR	infant mortality rate
IOM	Institute of Medicine (now known as the National Academy of Medicine)
LBW	low birth weight
LEP	limited English proficiency
MSAW	migrant and seasonal agricultural worker
MSFW	migrant seasonal farmworker

NAACP	National Association for the Advancement of Colored People
NAWS	National Agricultural Workers Survey
NCFES	National Association for Education Statistics
NCACTE	National Council for the Accreditation of Teacher Education
NHDR	*National Healthcare Disparities Report*
NHQR	*National Healthcare Quality Report*
NIH	National Institutes of Health
NIMHD	National Institute on Minority Health and Health Disparities
OMB	Office of Management and Budget
OMH	Office of Minority Health
PPACA	Patient Protection and Affordable Care Act
PSSA	Pennsylvania System of School Assessment
SCF	Survey of Consumer Finances
SDOH	social determinant of health
SIDS	sudden infant death syndrome
SES	socioeconomic status
STEM	science, technology, engineering, and math
TANF	Temporary Assistance for Needy Families
URM	underrepresented in medicine
USDA	U.S. Department of Agriculture
USDOE	U.S. Department of Education
WHO	World Health Organization

Appendix VIII

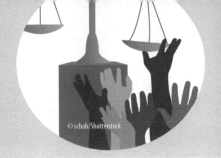

© schab/Shutterstock

Durant's Model for Diversity and Inclusion

APPENDIX VIII-1 Evidence-Based Practices That Work	
Practice	**Description**
1. Scholarships	Develop a financial assistance package that includes sources of financial aid. Offer competitive funding for reducing cost of degree program, including full and partial scholarships.
2. Mentorship	Develop a mentoring program by providing Black faculty with names and email addresses of Black students each semester.
3. Summer bridge	Identify promising sophomores and juniors for summer enrichment programs.
4. Minority faculty/ administrative representative	Develop an Office of Diversity Affairs to serve the needs of Black students. Create paid positions for persons with the responsibility of recruitment. Continue to keep open lines of communication between faculty in reference to recruitment and retention of Black students.
5. Recruitment	Hire a recruiter, plan an annual Minority Career Day, and provide rewards to Black faculty who are engaged in recruitment and retention efforts (e.g., reduce teaching load). Provide faculty with recruitment packages to take to local, state, and national meetings, which they attend.
6. Support groups	Develop an administrative unit for planning, programming, and counseling Black students.

APPENDIX VIII-1 Evidence-Based Practices That Work

Practice	Description
7. Institutional linkages	Institute a "buddy" program for new students from the current student body. Form an alumni network of interested Black graduates of your institution to assist with recruitment.
8. Multimedia advertising	Promote your program and Black students and faculty on social media, with brochures, and in ads.
9. Direct visits	Encourage faculty members to participate in recruiting by visiting Black colleges and universities.
10. Direct visits to the institution	Identify promising sophomores and juniors for summer enrichment programs. Sponsor a reception for Black students.
11. Referrals from alumni	Identify Black alumni faculty at predominantly Black institutions and predominantly White institutions who would be interested in receiving information about the healthcare program at your institution and referring students.
12. Diversity environment	Improve the university's environment so that Black students feel more comfortable. Develop the capacity to monitor the progress disposition and status of Black graduate students. A factual database must be developed from which to establish policy.

Appendix IX

Association of American Medical Colleges (AAMC) Diversity Portfolios

The Association of American Medical Colleges (AAMC) has created diversity portfolios as part of its commitment to diversity, which includes embracing a broader definition of diversity. The AAMC website describes its Human Capital, Organizational Capacity Building, and Public Health Initiatives portfolios as follows.

▶ Human Capital

The Human Capital portfolio involves impact-driven initiatives, research, and professional development aimed at cultivating and enhancing the knowledge, skills, abilities, and behaviors of individuals. It focuses on cultivating the skills of individuals along the medical continuum from aspiring physicians at the premedical stage to practicing physicians, faculty, researchers, and administrators, through initiatives, programs, and research. Topics include the following:

Premedical
- Enrichment Programs on the Web
- Medical Career Fairs
- Medical Minority Applicant Registry (Med-MAR)
- Summer Medical and Dental Education Program (SMDEP)

Medical Students and Faculty
- Herbert W. Nickens Awards
- Grant Writers Coaching Group for NIH Awards
- Minority Faculty Career Development Seminar
- Mid-career Minority Faculty Seminar
- Striving Toward Excellence: Faculty Diversity in Medical Education
- *The Diversity and Faculty Development Digest* (*DiFac*)

▶ Organizational Capacity Building

The Organizational Capacity Building portfolio is aimed at improving an organization's ability to use diversity as a driver of institutional excellence. It focuses on cultivating organizational capacity building through services, reports, and training that strengthen leadership recruitment, retention, and professional development, cultural competence, and climate and culture assessment, and it addresses diversity issues at the institutional level. Topics include the following:

- Group on Diversity and Inclusion (GDI)
- Tool for Assessing Cultural Competence Training (TACCT)
- Healthcare Executive Diversity and Inclusion Certificate Program
- Learning Lab on Unconscious Bias in the Health Professions
- Diversity Engagement Survey
- Diversity in the Physician Workforce: Facts and Figures 2010
- Diversity Research Forum Publications

▶ Public Health Initiatives

The Public Health Initiatives portfolio is intended to improve the integration of public health concepts into medical education and to enhance and expand a diverse and culturally prepared health workforce. Topics include the following:

- AAMC-CDC Cooperative Agreement
- Urban Universities for HEALTH
- AAMC AHEAD
- LGBT Initiatives
- Directory of MD/MPH Educational Opportunities

Appendix X

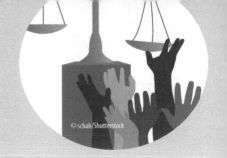
© schab/Shutterstock

Resources: Healthcare Academic Program Accreditation Organizations

Accreditation Review Commission on Education for the Physician Assistant (ARC-PA)
12000 Findley Road, Suite 150, Johns Creek, GA 30097, Phone: 770-476-1224
Accreditation Standards: http://www.arc-pa.org/accreditation/standards-of
-accreditation/

American Veterinary Medicine Association Council on Education
931 North Meacham Road, Suite 100, Schaumburg, IL 60173-4360,
Phone: 800-248-2862
Accreditation Standards: https://www.avma.org/ProfessionalDevelopment
/Education/Accreditation/Colleges/Pages/coe-pp-requirements-of-accredited
-college.aspx
AVMA Diversity Report: https://www.avma.org/KB/Resources/Reports
/Documents/diversity_report.pdf

Commission on Accreditation for Respiratory Care (CoARC)
1248 Harwood Road, Bedford, TX 76021-4244, Phone: 817-283-2835
Accreditation Standards: http://www.coarc.com/

Commission on Accreditation in Physical Therapy Education (CAPTE)
1111 North Fairfax Street, Alexandria, VA 22314, Phone: 703-706-3245
Accreditation Standards: http://www.capteonline.org/AccreditationHandbook/

Commission on Accreditation of Allied Health Education Programs (CAAHEP)
1361 Park Street, Clearwater, FL 33756, Phone: 727-210-2350
Accreditation Standards: http://www.caahep.org/Content.aspx?ID=1

Commission on Collegiate Nursing Education (CCNE)
One Dupont Circle, NW Suite 530, Washington, DC 20036, Phone: 202-463-6930
Accreditation Standards: http://www.aacn.nche.edu/ccne-accreditation
/accredited-programs

Council on Education for Public Health (CEPH)
1010 Wayne Avenue, Suite 220, Silver Springs, MD 20910, Phone: 202-789-1050
Accreditation Standards: http://ceph.org/criteria-procedures/

Joint Review Committee on Education in Radiologic Technology (JRCERT)
20 North Wacker Drive, Suite 2850, Chicago, IL 60606-3182, Phone: 312-704-5300
Accreditation Standards: https://www.jrcert.org/programs-faculty/jrcert-standards/

Liaison Committee on Medical Education (LCME)
330 North Wabash Avenue, Suite 39300, Chicago, IL 60611-5885,
Phone: 312-464-4933
Accreditation Standards: http://lcme.org/
FACTS: Applicants, Matriculants, Enrollment, Graduates, MD-PhD, and Residency
Applicants Data: https://www.aamc.org/data/facts/

National Accrediting Agency for Clinical Laboratory Sciences (NAACLS)
5600 North River Road, Suite 720, Rosemont, IL 60018, Phone: 773-714-8880
Accreditation Standards: http://www.naacls.org/Find-a-Program.aspx

2019 World Population Review, July 11, 2019
http://worldpopulationreview.com/countries/united-states-populationUnited
States Population Projections: 2000 to 2050, United States Census Bureau, March 19,
2018 https://www.census.gov/content/dam/Census/library/working-papers/2009
/demo/us-pop-proj-2000-2050/analytical-document09.pdf

Appendix XI

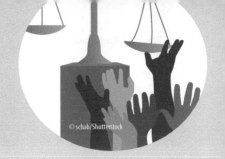

© schab/Shutterstock

University of Mississippi Medical Center (UMMC) Pipeline Into Medical School

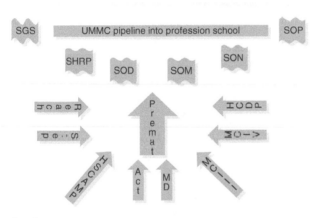

Reach.

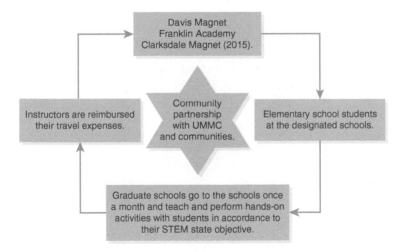

Science training enrichment program (STEP).

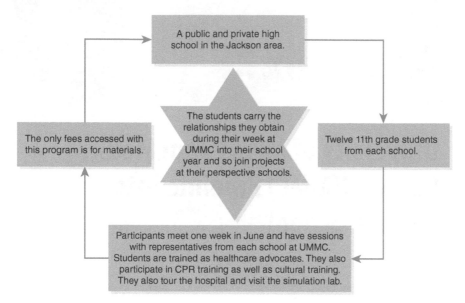

High school healthcare camp.

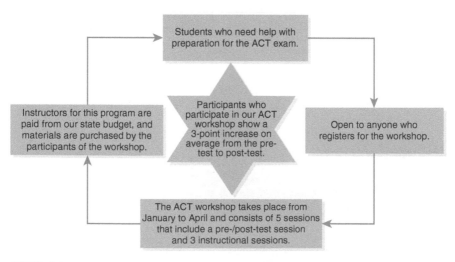

ACT Workshop.

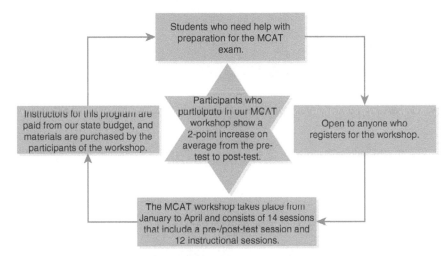

MCAT workshop.

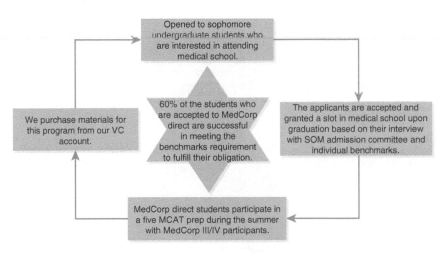

MedCorp Direct.

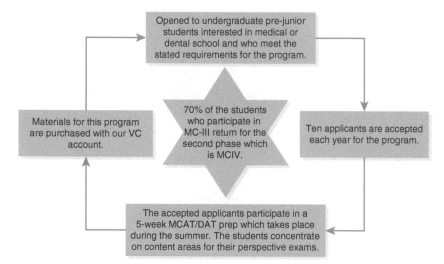

MedCorp III (MC-III).

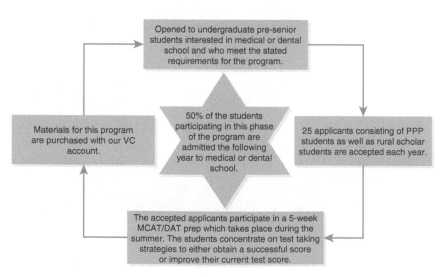

MedCorp IV (MC-IV).

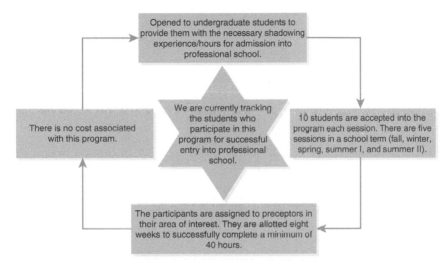

Health careers development program (HCDP).

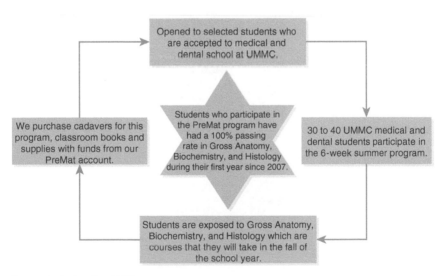

Prematriculation (Pre-MAT).

Reproduced from Office of Health Careers Opportunity. Dr. Gaarmel Funches, Director of Programs, Ms. LaFreda Sias, Program Administrator, Mr. Jonathan Simmons, Administrative Assistant.

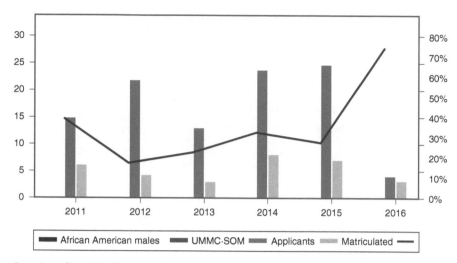

Snapshot of UMMC African American male students.

Reproduced from Office of Health Careers Opportunity. Dr. Gaarmel Funches, Director of Programs, Ms. LaFreda Sias, Program Administrator, Mr. Jonathan Simmons, Administrative Assistant.

Appendix XII

© schab/Shutterstock

Suggested Readings

Bibliography

Anderson, L. M., Scrimshaw, S. C., Fullilove, M. T., Fielding, J. E., & Normand, J. (2003). The tasks force on community preventive services culturally competent health care systems. A systematic review. *American Journal of Preventive Medicine, 24*(3S), 68–79.

Baxter, C. (2001). *Managing diversity and inequality in healthcare*. Oxford, UK: Bialliere Tindall.

Brach, C., & Fraserirector, I. (2000). Can cultural competency reduce racial and ethnic health disparities? A review and conceptual model. *Medical Care Research and Review, 57*(S1), 181–217.

Brondolo, E., Gallo, L. C., & Myers, H. F. (2008). Race, racism and health: Disparities, mechanisms, and interventions. *Journal of Behavioral Medicine, 32*, 1–8.

Brown, C. M., Barner, J. C., & Shepard, M. D. (2003). Issues and barriers related to the provision of pharmaceutical care in community health centers and migrant health centers. *Journal of the American Pharmacists Association, 5*, 1.

Burgess, D., van Ryn, M., Dovidio, J., & Saha, S. (2007). Reducing racial bias among health care providers: Lessons from social-cognitive psychology. *Society of General Internal Medicine, 22*, 882–887.

Byrd, M., & Clayton, L. (2000). *An American health dilemma: A medical history of African Americans and the problems of race: Beginnings to 1900*. New York, NY: Routledge.

Chen, F. M., Fryer, G. E., Phillips, R. L., Wilson, E., & Pathman, D. E. (2005). Patients' beliefs about racism, preferences for physician race, and satisfaction with care. *Annals of Family Medicine, 3*(2), 138–143.

Chettiar, I. (2012). *At America's expense: The mass incarceration of the elderly*. NELLCO Legal Scholarship Repository. New York University Public Law and Legal Theory: New York University school of Law.

Chevannes, M. (2002). Issues in educating health professionals to meet the diverse needs of patients and other service users from ethnic minority groups. *Journal of Advanced Nursing, 39*, 290–298.

Clark, R., Anderson, N. B., Clark, V. R., & Williams, D. R. (1999). Racism as a stressor or African Americans: A biopsychosocial model. *American Psychologist, 54*(10), 805–816.

Dovidio, J. F., Penner, L. A., Albrecht, T. L., Norton, W. E., Gaertner, S. L., & Shelton, J. N. (2008). Disparities and distrust: The implications of psychological processes for understanding racial disparities in health and health care. *Social Science & Medicine, 67*(3), 478–486.

Emery, J., Crump, C., & Bors, P. (2003). Reliability and validity of two instruments designed to assess the walking and bicycling suitability of sidewalks and roads. *American Journal of Health Promotion, 18*(1), 28–46.

Hausmann, L. R. M., Jeong, K., Bost, J. E., & Ibrahim, S. A. (2008). Perceived discrimination in Health care and health status in a racially diverse sample. *Medical Care, 46*(9), 905–914.

Institute of Medicine (IOM). (2004). Health literacy: A prescription to end confusion (Report brief). Retrieved from https://www.nationalacademies.org/hmd/~/media/Files/Report%20Files/2004/Health-Literacy-A-Prescription-to-End-Confusion/healthliteracyfinal.pdf

Jones, D. (2006). The persistence of American Indian health disparities. *American Journal of Public Health, 96*(12), 2122–2134.

Kirsch, I. S., Jungeblut, A., Jenkins, L., & Kolstad, A. (1993). *Adult literacy in America: A first look at the results of the National Adult Literacy Survey (NALS)*. Washington, DC: National Center for Education Statistics, U.S. Department of Education.

Kopp, W. (2011). The newest silver bullet: Providing every child with an effective teacher. *One Day Alumni Magazine*, Spring, Edition XI, 29.

Kuzma, J. (1998). *Basic statistics for the health sciences*. Mountain View, CA: Mayfield.

Ladson-Billings, G., & Tate, W. (1995). Toward a critical race theory of education. *Teachers College Record, 97*(1), 47–68.

Mak, W. W., Poon, C. Y., Pun, L. Y., & Cheung, S. F. (2007). Meta-analysis of stigma and mental health. *Social Science & Medicine, 65*(2), 245–261.

Massey, D. S. & Denton, N. A. (1993). *American apartheid: Segregation and the making of the underclass* (Chps 2 & 3). Cambridge, MA: Harvard University Press.

McKinney, J., & Kurtz-Rossi, S. (2000). *Culture, health, and literacy: A guide to health education materials for adults with limited English skills*. Boston, MA: World Education.

Milner, H. R. (2012). Beyond a test score: Explaining opportunity gaps in educational practice. *Journal of Black Studies, 20*(10), 1–26. doi: 10.1177/0021934712442539

National Center for Education Statistics. (2006). *The health literacy of America's adults: Results from the 2003 National Assessment of Adult Literacy*. Washington, DC: U.S. Department of Education.

Naylor, L. (Ed.). (1997). *Cultural diversity in the United States*. Westport, CT: Bergin and Garvey.

Purnell, L., & Paulunka, B. (1998). *Transcultural healthcare: A culturally competent approach*. Philadelphia, PA: F. A. Davis.

Richard, A. (Ed.). (2007). *Eliminating healthcare disparities in America*. New York, NY: Humana Press.

Ross, C. E., & Wu, C. (1995). The links between education and health. *American Sociological Review, 60*(5), 719–745. doi:10.2307/2096319

Rothstein, R. (2004). *Class and schools: Using social, economic and educational reform to close the Black–White achievement gap*. New York, NY: Teachers College, Columbia University.

Sankar, P., Pyeritz, R. E., Bernhardt, B., & Shea, J. A. (2008). Differences in the patterns of heath care system distrust between Blacks and Whites. *Journal of General Internal Medicine, 23*(6), 827–833.

Scott, M. G. (2002). Cultural competency: How is it measured? Does it make a difference? *Generations, 26*(3), 39–45.

Smedley, B., Stith, A., & Nelson, A. (Eds.). (2003). *Unequal treatment: Confronting racial and ethnic disparities in health care*. Washington, DC: National Academies Press.

Srivastava, R. (2006). *The healthcare professional's guide to cultural competence*. St. Louis, MO: Mosby.

Taylor, S., & Lurie, N. (2004). The role of culturally competent communication in reducing ethnic and racial healthcare disparities. *American Journal of Managed Care, 10*, SP1–SP4.

Torres-Rivera, E., West-Olatunji, C., Conwill, W., Garrett, M. T., & Phan, L. T. (2008). Language as a form of subtle oppression among linguistically different people in the United States. *Social Perspectives, 10*(1), 11–28.

U.S. Department of Health and Human Services. (2001). *National standards for culturally and linguistically appropriate services in health care*. Washington, DC: Office of Minority Health.

U.S. Department of Health and Human Services. (2008). *America's health literacy: Why we need accessible health information*. Washington, DC: Office of Disease Prevention and Health Promotion.

Zimmerman, E., & Woolf, S. H. (2014, June 5). *Understanding the Relationship between Education and Health* [Discussion Paper, Institute of Medicine]. Washington, D.C.

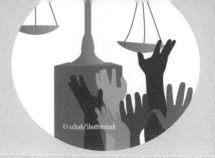

Appendix XIII

Racial and Ethnic Data for Students of Color in Veterinary Medicine

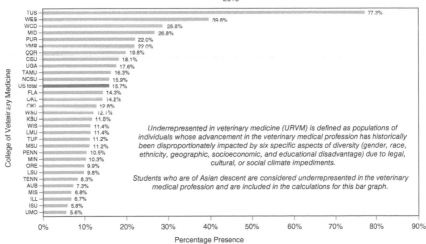

Presence of racially and ethnically underrepresented students at U.S. colleges of veterinary medicine

AAVMC internal reports
2010

College of Veterinary Medicine (y-axis) — Percentage Presence (x-axis)

College	Percentage
TUS	77.3%
WES	39.8%
WCD	28.8%
MID	26.8%
PUR	22.0%
VMR	22.0%
COR	19.8%
CSU	18.1%
UGA	17.6%
TAMU	16.3%
NCSU	15.9%
US total	15.7%
FLA	14.3%
OKL	14.2%
OKI	12.8%
WSU	12.1%
KSU	11.0%
WIS	11.4%
LMU	11.4%
TUF	11.2%
MSU	11.2%
PENN	10.5%
MIN	10.3%
ORE	9.9%
LSU	9.8%
TENN	8.3%
AUB	7.3%
MIS	6.8%
ILL	6.7%
ISU	5.8%
UMO	5.6%

Underrepresented in veterinary medicine (URVM) is defined as populations of individuals whose advancement in the veterinary medical profession has historically been disproportionately impacted by six specific aspects of diversity (gender, race, ethnicity, geographic, socioeconomic, and educational disadvantage) due to legal, cultural, or social climate impediments.

Students who are of Asian descent are considered underrepresented in the veterinary medical profession and are included in the calculations for this bar graph.

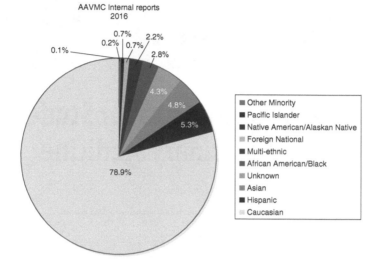

Racial and ethnic demographics of DVM students
at U.S. colleges of veterinary medicine

AAVMC Internal reports
2016

0.7%   2.2%
0.2% 0.7%
0.1%   2.8%

4.3%

4.8%

5.3%

78.9%

- Other Minority
- Pacific Islander
- Native American/Alaskan Native
- Foreign National
- Multi-ethnic
- African American/Black
- Unknown
- Asian
- Hispanic
- Caucasian

Racial Segregation in Veterinary Medicine

Black Enrollments at U.S. Veterinary Schools, 2003

Veterinary School of Medicine	Total Students	Black Students	Percent Black
Tuskegee	228	66	42.1%
Virginia-Maryland Reg. College	360	14	3.9
Cornell University	329	12	3.6
University of Florida	323	9	2.8
University of Wisconsin	317	7	2.2
University of Missouri	253	4	1.6
North Carolina State University	303	4	1.3
University of Illinois	406	5	1.2
Michigan State University	417	5	1.2
University of Georgia	347	4	1.2
Auburn University	363	4	1.1
University of California-Davis	485	5	1.0
Mississippi State University	208	2	1.0
Louisiana State University	320	3	0.9
Purdue University	264	2	0.8
University of Tennessee	268	2	0.7
Tufts University	319	2	0.6
Colorado State University	537	2	0.4
Ohio State University	538	2	0.4
Oklahoma State University	292	1	0.3
Iowa State University	400	1	0.3
Kansas State University	406	1	0.2
University of Pennsylvania	448	1	0.0
Oregon State University	141	0	0.0
Texas A&M University	493	0	0.0
University of Minnesota	311	0	0.0
Washington State University	287	0	0.0

Reproduced from Association of American Veterinary Medical Colleges. (2016). *Annual data report 2015–2016*. Retrieved from http://www.aavmc.org/About-AAVMC/Public-Data.aspx; Morse, E. M. (2008). Minority student perceptions of the veterinary profession: Factors influencing choices of health careers (MA dissertation, Cleveland State University). Retrieved from http://engagedscholarship.csuohio.edu/cgi/viewcontent.cgi?article=1698&context=etdarchive

Appendix XIV

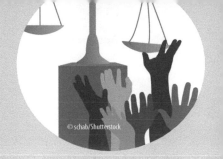
© schab/Shutterstock

First Step Act (H.R. 5682)

MASS INCARCERATION AND CRIMINAL JUSTICE SYSTEM REFORM: FIRST STEP ACT (H.R. 5682)

ACT SECTIONS

1. Creating Evidenced-based Recidivism Reduction Programs
2. Expansion of Good Behavior and Early Release Programs for Federal Inmates
3. Amend Federal Sentencing Laws
4. Miscellaneous Improvements

Proposed Reform Actions	Responsibility for Reform Actions	Timeline for Reform Actions
Develop a Risk & Needs Assessment System ("system") to be applied to each prisoner upon intake and reassessed periodically	Attorney General (AG) in consult with the Directors of the Bureau of Prisons (BOP), Administrative Office of the U.S. Courts, Office of Probation and Pretrial Services, National Institute of Justice, and the National Institute of Corrections	Within 180 days of Enactment (after consultation with the Independent Review Committee created by the Act)
■ Must assess recidivism rate level		
■ An Independent Review Committee shall assist in developing the Risk and Needs assessment system ("system")		Independent Review Committee shall terminate 30 days after the release of the risk and needs assessment system
• Two members with published peer-review scholarship		
• Two corrections practitioners who have developed risk and needs assessment tools	The Bureau of Prisons (BOP) shall list appropriate recidivism reduction programs for each prisoner	Phase-in period of 2 years to give Bureau of Prisons (BOP) time to provide appropriate programming and to develop and validate the risk and assessment system ("system") to be used
• One person with expertise in assessing risk assessment implementation		
■ Assign prisoners to appropriate recidivism rate reduction programs	The Attorney General (AG) shall develop training programs for the Bureau of Prisons (BOP) officers and employees responsible for administering the Risk and Needs Assessment System ("System")	
■ Ensure programs are evidenced-based, effective, and efficient		Initial report due to Congress 2 years after enactment. Subsequent reports due each year for the next 5 years
■ Train Bureau of Prisons (BOP) employees to correctly implement programs		
■ Conduct annual audits of the Bureau of Prisons (BOP) to ensure that the "system" is being used and implemented properly		
■ Congress must receive regular report of results		

The System shall provide incentives and rewards to prisoners in recidivism reduction programs	Attorney General (AG) and Director of Bureau of Prisons (BOP)	Immediately upon law enactment
■ Telephone and visitation rewards (additional time and video conferencing)	Time credits shall be applied toward time in prerelease custody or supervised release	Immediately upon successful completion of recidivism reduction program
■ Transfer to facility closer to prisoners' home residence upon recommendation of warden and if bed is available	Home confinement: 24-hour electronic monitoring; remain in residence except to participate in work, community service, religious/family activities, medical care, or crime victim restoration activities.	Immediately upon law enactment
■ At least two other incentives as follows: increased commissary spending and offerings, enhanced email access, transfer to preferred housing units, and prisoner-solicited incentives		Immediately upon law enactment
■ Time credits for successfully completing a recidivism reduction program (eligible prisoners only)*	Reentry Center: Used when 24-hour electronic monitoring is not feasible.	Immediately upon law enactment
■ Types of prerelease custody include home confinement and residential reentry centers.	Director of Bureau of Prisons (BOP) must ensure sufficient capacity for all eligible prisoners exists within the system	
■ Amends the Second Chance Act to make elderly and terminally ill offenders who are eligible for family reunification through home detention instead of being housed in a federal facility		
■ U.S. Pretrial and Probation Services shall offer assistance to any prisoner not under its supervision during prerelease custody	Director of U.S. Pretrial and Probation Services	
■ All persons released from federal prison must be given their birth certificate and photo identification	Director of Bureau of Prisons (BOP)	

(continues)

Proposed Reform Actions	Responsibility for Reform Actions	Timeline for Reform Actions

Enhanced mandatory minimum sentences for drug felons are reduced
■ The three-strike mandatory penalty is reduced from life imprisonment to 25 years
■ The 20-year mandatory minimum is reduced to 15 years
■ Offenses that trigger these enhanced mandatory minimum sentences are also reformed
  • Qualifying prior convictions must be serious drug felonies (formerly any drug felonies) or other serious violent felonies**
  • Prior felonies must have occurred within the past 15 years**
■ Broadens Existing Safety Valve
■ Application of Fair Sentencing Act (2010)
	Eligibility for Safety Valve sentencing expands the number of criminal history "points" for offenders from one to four
	
	Allows offenders sentenced under prior provisions to petition for reductions in sentence consistent with new crack cocaine sentencing law
		Immediately upon law enactment
		Immediately upon law enactment

Additional improvements for offenders include, but are not limited to, the following: ■ De-escalation Training programs ■ Evidenced-based treatment programs for opioid and heroin abuse ■ Free feminine hygiene products for all female inmates ■ Juvenile solitary confinement adjustment	The Director of Bureau of Prisons (BOP) must include de-escalation training to teach how to de-escalate encounters between law enforcement, Bureau of Prisons (BOP) employees, and a civilian or prisoner. Bureau of Prisons (BOP) must report to Congress it's capacity to treat heroin and opioid abuse through evidenced-based programs. The Director of the Administrative Office of the U.S. Courts must report to Congress a report assessing the availability and capacity for the provision of medication-assisted treatment.	Immediately upon law enactment Not later than 90 days after the date of enactment. Not later than 120 days after the date of enactment. Immediately upon law enactment. Immediately upon law enactment

Director of Bureau of Prisons (BOP)

The Bureau of Prisons (BOP) must restrict the use of juvenile solitary confinement for any reason except as a temporary response to a juvenile's behavior that poses a serious and immediate risk of physical harm. Staff must use the least restrictive means, including "talking it out" and attempting care by a qualified mental health professional.

*Eligibility restricted to prisoners classified as minimum or low risk. Prisoners serving sentence for conviction of certain offenses, including crimes relating to terrorism, murder, sexual exploitation of children, espionage, violent firearms offenses, or those that are organizers, leaders, managers, or supervisors in the fentanyl and heroin drug trade are ineligible to receive these incentives. Deportable prisoners are not eligible for time credits.

**Provision is not retroactive and will not apply to any person sentenced before enactment of this law.

Source: First Step Act Section by Section Summary, December 14, 2018; National Conference of State Legislatures Staff, National Conference of State Legislatures. Retrieved from http://www.ncsl.org/documents/statefed/First_Step_Act _Summary_Dec2018.pdf

Table prepared by Jeffrey A. Rose, B.A., Economics and Political Science, Yale University, 1984.

Appendix XV

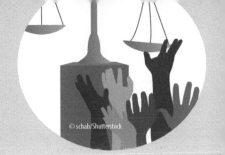

Men's Health

TABLE XV-1 Ten Leading Causes of Death (LCOD) in Black Males in the U.S.	
	Percent of total deaths*
1) Heart disease	23.9
2) Cancer	21.4
3) Unintentional injuries	6.5
4) Stroke	4.9
5) Homicide	4.9
6) Diabetes	4.2
7) Chronic lower respiratory diseases	3.2
8) Kidney disease	2.7
9) Septicemia	1.9
10) Influenza & pneumonia	1.7

*Percent of total deaths in the race category due to the disease indicated. The white, black, American Indian/Alaska Native, and Asian/Pacific Islander race groups include persons of Hispanic and non-Hispanic origin. Persons of Hispanic origin may be of any race. https://www.cdc.gov/healthequity/lcod/men/2015/black/index.htm

Centers for Disease Control and Prevention. Retrieved from https://www.cdc.gov/healthequity/lcod/men/2015/black/index.htm

The CDC reported intentional injuries (ages 1–14) and homicide (ages 15–34) ranked number one as the leading cause of death for Black males. In age group 35–44, heart disease ranked number one as the leading cause of death. However, the CDC reported that Black men ages 45–85+ ranked number one in heart disease and cancer for the leading cause of death.

TABLE XV-2 Ages 1–44 by Age Group—Black Males

Rank	Age 1–4	Age 5–9	Age 10–14	Age 15–19	Age 20–24	Age 25–34	Age 35–44
1	Unintentional injuries 29.4%	Unintentional injuries 31.2%	Unintentional injuries 22.1%	Homicide 49.5%	Homicide 49.7%	Homicide 35.5%	Heart disease 21.0%
2	Homicide 14.9%	Cancer 10.7%	Homicide 15.3%	Unintentional injuries 23.0%	Unintentional injuries 22.3%	Unintentional injuries 22.3%	Unintentional injuries 17.5%
3	Birth defects 8.4%	Chronic lower respiratory diseases 9.5%	Cancer 9.0%	Suicide 8.8%	Suicide 8.5%	Heart disease 8.3%	Homicide 14.2%
4	Cancer 4.6% **(tie rank 4)**	Birth defects 7.3%	Chronic lower respiratory diseases 8.5%	Heart disease 3.0%	Heart disease 3.8%	Suicide 6.8%	Cancer 8.1%
5	Heart disease 4.6% **(tie rank 4)**	Homicide 7.0%	Suicide 8.3%	Cancer 2.7%	Cancer 2.4%	Cancer 3.8%	Suicide 4.2%
6	Perinatal conditions 3.0%	Heart disease 4.6%	Heart disease 4.3% **(tie rank 6)**	Birth defects 1.3%	HIV disease 1.1%	HIV disease 3.0%	HIV disease 3.9%

Rank							
7	Influenza & pneumonia 2.8%	Septicemia 1.5% **(tie rank 7)**	Birth defects 4.3% **(tie rank 6)**	Chronic lower respiratory diseases 1.1%	Chronic lower respiratory diseases 1.1%	Diabetes 1.9%	Diabetes 3.7%
8	Chronic lower respiratory diseases 2.4%	Anemias 1.5% **(tie rank 7)**	Stroke 2.0%	Diabetes 0.8%	Anemias 0.7%	Stroke 1.1%	Stroke 3.5%
9	Stroke 1.9%	Stroke 1.5% **(tie rank 7)**	Diabetes 1.5%	Legal intervention 0.5%	Diabetes 0.7%	Chronic lower respiratory diseases 0.9%	Kidney disease 1.7%
10	Medical & surgical complications 1.3%	Benign neoplasms 1.2% **(tie rank 10)** Influenza & pneumonia 1.2% **(tie rank 10)**	Influenza & pneumonia 1.3%	Anemias 0.4%	Legal intervention 0.6%	Influenza & pneumonia 0.9%	Hypertension 1.5%

Percentages represent total deaths in the age group due to the cause indicated. Rankings are based on number of deaths. Numbers in parentheses indicate tied rankings. The white, black, American Indian/Alaska Native, and Asian/Pacific Islander race groups include persons of Hispanic and non-Hispanic origin. Persons of Hispanic origin may be of any race. Some terms have been shortened from those used in the National Vital Statistics Report. See the next page for a listing of the shortened terms in the table and their full-unabridged equivalents used in the report. To learn more, visit Mortality Tables or Mortality Data (HHS, CDC, NCHS).

Centers for Disease Control and Prevention. Retrieved from https://www.cdc.gov/healthequity/lcod/men/2015/black/index.htm

TABLE XV-3 Ages 45+ by Age Group—Black Males

Rank	Age 45–54	Age 55–64	Age 65+	Age 65–74	Age 75–84	Age 85+	All Ages
1	Heart disease 26.1%	Cancer 27.1%	Heart disease 26.6%	Cancer 29.4%	Heart disease 26.5%	Heart disease 27.4%	Heart disease 23.9%
2	Cancer 18.2%	Heart disease 26.7%	Cancer 25.1%	Heart disease 26.3%	Cancer 24.6%	Cancer 17.7%	Cancer 21.4%
3	Unintentional injuries 10.7%	Unintentional injuries 5.7%	Stroke 6.1%	Stroke 5.6%	Stroke 6.6%	Stroke 6.2%	Unintentional injuries 6.5%
4	Diabetes 4.8%	Stroke 4.9%	Diabetes 4.5%	Diabetes 5.0%	Chronic lower respiratory diseases 4.8%	Alzheimer's disease 5.5%	Stroke 4.9%
5	Stroke 4.5%	Diabetes 4.9%	Chronic lower respiratory diseases 4.5%	Chronic lower respiratory diseases 4.3%	Diabetes 4.7%	Chronic lower respiratory disease 4.3%	Homicide 4.9%
6	Homicide 3.7%	Chronic lower respiratory diseases 2.7%	Kidney disease 3.4%	Kidney disease 3.1%	Kidney disease 3.4%	Kidney disease 3.7%	Diabetes 4.2%

7	HIV disease 3.4%	Kidney disease 2.6%	Alzheimer's disease 2.6%	Unintentional injuries 2.5%	Alzheimer's disease 2.9%	Diabetes 3.4%	Chronic lower respiratory diseases 3.2%
8	Chronic liver disease 2.3%	Chronic liver disease 2.4%	Septicemia 2.3%	Septicemia 2.2%	Influenza & pneumonia 2.3%	Influenza & pneumonia 2.8%	Kidney disease 2.7%
9	Kidney disease 2.3%	HIV disease 2.0%	Influenza & pneumonia 2.1%	Hypertension 1.7%	Septicemia 2.3%	Septicemia 2.3%	Septicemia 1.9%
10	Septicemia 1.8%	Septicemia 1.9%	Unintentional injuries 2.1%	Influenza & pneumonia 1.6%	Hypertension 1.9%	Hypertension 2.3%	Influenza & pneumonia 1.7%

Percentages represent total deaths in the age group due to the cause indicated. Rankings are based on number of deaths. Numbers in parentheses indicate tied rankings. The white, black, American Indian/Alaska Native, and Asian/Pacific Islander race groups include persons of Hispanic and non-Hispanic origin. Persons of Hispanic origin may be of any race. Some terms have been shortened from those used in the National Vital Statistics Report. See the next page for a listing of the shortened terms in the table and their full-unabridged equivalents used in the report. To learn more, visit Mortality Tables or Mortality Data (HHS, CDC, NCHS).

Centers for Disease Control and Prevention. (2015). Leading Causes of Death (LCOD) by Age Group, Black Males—United States, 2015. Retrieved from https://www.cdc.gov/healthequity/lcod/men/2015/black/index.ht

TABLE XV-4 Ages 1–44 by Age Group–All Males

Rank	Age 1–4	Age 5–9	Age 10–14	Age 15–19	Age 20–24	Age 25–34	Age 35–44
1	Unintentional injuries 33.7%	Unintentional injuries 32.0%	Unintentional injuries 28.0%	Unintentional injuries 38.1%	Unintentional injuries 42.3%	Unintentional injuries 41.0%	Unintentional injuries 27.5%
2	Homicide 10.1%	Cancer 17.6%	Suicide 14.1%	Suicide 21.4%	Suicide 18.6%	Suicide 15.4%	Heart disease 15.5%
3	Birth defects 10.0%	Birth defects 7.6%	Cancer 12.8%	Homicide 19.1%	Homicide 18.2%	Homicide 11.5%	Suicide 11.4%
4	Cancer 8.6%	Homicide 6.2%	Homicide 6.1%	Cancer 4.8%	Cancer 3.5%	Heart disease 6.4%	Cancer 10.2%
5	Heart disease 3.4%	Chronic lower respiratory diseases 3.3%	Birth defects 5.0%	Heart disease 2.8%	Heart disease 3.1%	Cancer 5.1%	Homicide 5.1%
6	Influenza & pneumonia 2.1%	Heart disease 3.0%	Heart disease 3.8%	Birth defects 1.5%	Birth defects 0.7%	Chronic liver disease 1.5%	Chronic liver disease 4.0%

7	Perinatal conditions 1.5%	Influenza & pneumonia 1.5%	Chronic lower respiratory diseases 3.3%	Influenza & pneumonia 0.6%	Chronic lower respiratory diseases 0.6%	Diabetes 1.3%	Diabetes 2.7%
8	Chronic lower respiratory diseases 1.2%	Stroke 1.4%	Stroke 1.5%	Chronic lower respiratory diseases 0.5%	Diabetes 0.6%	HIV disease 1.1%	Stroke 2.2%
9	Stroke 1.1%	Benign neoplasms 1.3%	Influenza & pneumonia 1.1%	Stroke 0.4%	Influenza & pneumonia 0.4%	Stroke 0.9%	HIV disease 1.5%
10	Septicemia 1.1%	Septicemia 1.0%	Septicemia 1.1%	Diabetes 0.4%	HIV disease 0.4%	Birth defects 0.7%	Influenza & pneumonia 0.9%

Centers for Disease Control and Prevention. (2015). Leading Causes of Death (LCOD) by Age Group, All Males—United States, 2015. Retrieved from https://www.cdc.gov/healthequity/lcod/men/2015/all-males/index.ht

TABLE XV-5 All Males by Race/Ethnicity—All Males

Rank	All Races	White	Black	American Indian/Alaska Native	Asian/Pacific Islander	Hispanic
1	Heart disease 24.4%	Heart disease 24.6%	Heart disease 23.9%	Heart disease 19.2%	Cancer 26.1%	Heart disease 20.6%
2	Cancer 22.8%	Cancer 23.0%	Cancer 21.4%	Cancer 17.0%	Heart disease 22.8%	Cancer 20.2%
3	Unintentional injuries 6.8%	Unintentional injuries 6.8%	Unintentional injuries 6.5%	Unintentional injuries 13.1%	Stroke 6.4%	Unintentional injuries 10.3%
4	Chronic lower respiratory diseases 5.3%	Chronic lower respiratory diseases 5.6%	Stroke 4.9%	Chronic liver disease 5.7%	Unintentional injuries 5.5%	Stroke 4.6%
5	Stroke 4.2%	Stroke 4.1%	Homicide 4.9%	Diabetes 5.5%	Diabetes 3.9%	Diabetes 4.5%
6	Diabetes 3.1%	Diabetes 2.9%	Diabetes 4.2%	Suicide 4.1%	Influenza & pneumonia 3.3%	Chronic liver disease 4.2%

7	Suicide 2.5%	Alzheimer's disease 2.6%	Chronic lower respiratory diseases 3.2%	Chronic lower respiratory diseases 3.9%	Chronic lower respiratory diseases 3.2%	Chronic lower respiratory diseases 2.7%
8	Alzheimer's disease 2.5%	Suicide 2.6%	Kidney disease 2.7%	Stroke 2.9%	Suicide 2.6%	Suicide 2.6%
9	Influenza & pneumonia 2.0%	Influenza & pneumonia 2.0%	Septicemia 1.5%	Homicide 2.2%	Alzheimer's disease 2.0%	Homicide 2.4%
10	Chronic liver disease 1.9%	Chronic liver disease 1.9%	Influenza & pneumonia 1.7%	Influenza & pneumonia 1.8%	Kidney disease 2.0%	Alzheimer's disease 2.1%

Percentages represent total deaths in the age group due to the cause indicated. Rankings are based on number of deaths. Numbers in parentheses indicate tied rankings. The white, black, American Indian/Alaska Native, and Asian/Pacific Islander race groups include persons of Hispanic and non-Hispanic origin. Persons of Hispanic origin may be of any race. Some terms have been shortened from those used in the National Vital Statistics Report. See the next page for a listing of the shortened terms in the table and their full-unabridged equivalents used in the report. To learn more, visit Mortality Tables or Mortality Data (HHS, CDC, NCHS).

Centers for Disease Control and Prevention. (2015). Leading Causes of Death (LCOD) by Race/Ethnicity, All Males—United States, 2015. Retrieved from https://www.cdc.gov/healthequity/lcod/men/2015/race-ethnicity/index.ht

TABLE XV-6 Ages 45+ by Age Group—All Males

Rank	Age 45–54	Age 55–64	Age 65+	Age 65–74	Age 75–84	Age 85+	All Ages
1	Heart disease 22.6%	Cancer 29.5%	Heart disease 26.7%	Cancer 32.0%	Cancer 25.2%	Heart disease 30.4%	Heart disease 24.4%
2	Cancer 20.1%	Heart disease 24.4%	Cancer 23.8%	Heart disease 24.2%	Heart disease 25.2%	Cancer 15.0%	Cancer 22.8%
3	Unintentional injuries 13.6%	Unintentional injuries 6.2%	Chronic lower respiratory diseases 6.5%	Chronic lower respiratory diseases 6.8%	Chronic lower respiratory diseases 7.3%	Alzheimer's disease 6.1%	Unintentional injuries 6.8%
4	Suicide 6.1%	Chronic liver disease 4.2%	Stroke 5.1%	Diabetes 4.0%	Stroke 5.2%	Stroke 5.8%	Chronic lower respiratory diseases 5.3%
5	Chronic liver disease 5.5%	Chronic lower respiratory diseases 4.1%	Alzheimer's disease 3.6%	Stroke 3.9%	Alzheimer's disease 3.4%	Chronic lower respiratory diseases 5.6%	Stroke 4.2%
6	Diabetes 3.7%	Diabetes 4.0%	Diabetes 3.1%	Unintentional injuries 3.0%	Diabetes 3.2%	Influenza & pneumonia 3.3%	Diabetes 3.1%

7	Stroke 2.7%	Stroke 3.2%	Unintentional injuries 2.8%	Chronic liver disease 1.9%	Unintentional injuries 2.6%	Unintentional injuries 2.9%	Suicide 2.5%
8	Chronic lower respiratory diseases 1.9%	Suicide 2.6%	Influenza & pneumonia 2.4%	Kidney disease 1.9%	Parkinson's disease 2.3%	Kidney disease 2.5%	Alzheimer's disease 2.5%
9	Homicide 1.5%	Kidney disease 1.5%	Kidney disease 2.2%	Septicemia 1.6%	Influenza & pneumonia 2.2%	Diabetes 2.2%	Influenza & pneumonia 2.0%

Percentages represent total deaths in the age group due to the cause indicated. Rankings are based on number of deaths. Numbers in parentheses indicate tied rankings. The white, black, American Indian/Alaska Native, and Asian/Pacific Islander race groups include persons of Hispanic and non-Hispanic origin. Persons of Hispanic origin may be of any race. Some terms have been shortened from those used in the National Vital Statistics Report. See the next page for a listing of the shortened terms in the table and their full-unabridged equivalents used in the report. To learn more, visit *Mortality Tables or Mortality Data* (HHS, CDC, NCHS).

Centers for Disease Control and Prevention. (2015). Leading Causes of Death (LCOD) by Race/Ethnicity, All Males—United States, 2015. Retrieved from https://www.cdc.gov/healthequity/lcod/men/2015/race-ethnicity/index.ht

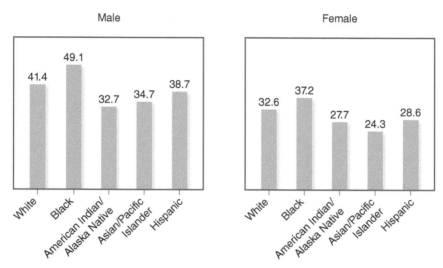

Rate per 100,000 people

FIGURE XV-1 Rate of new cancers by Sex and Race/Ethnicity.

Data from U.S. Cancer Statistics Working Group. U.S. Cancer Statistics Visualization tool, based on November 2018 submission data (1999–2016): U.S. Department of Health and Human Services, Centers for Disease Control and Prevention, and National Cancer Institute. Retrieved June 2019, from https://www.cdc.gov/cancer/dataviz

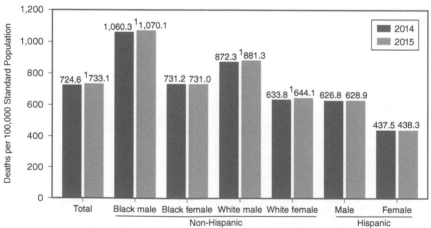

[1]Statistically significant increase in age-adjusted death rate from 2014 to 2015 (*p* < 0.05).

NOTE: Access data table for Figure 2 at: http://www.cdc.gov/nchs/data/databriefs/db267_table.pdf#2.

FIGURE XV-2 Life expectancy at select ages, by sex: United States, 2014 and 2015.

National Vital Statistics System. (2015). Mortality in the United States. Retrieved from https://www.cdc.gov/nchs/data/databriefs/db267.pdf

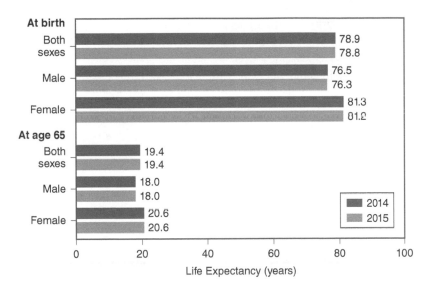

FIGURE XV-3 Age-adjusted death rates for selected populations: United States, 2014 and 2015.

National Vital Statistics System. (2015). Mortality in the United States. Retrieved from https://www.cdc.gov/nchs/data/databriefs/db267.pdf

▶ Resources

Black Men's Health Network
http://www.menshealthnetwork.org/library/Medicaidwelcomephysical.pdf

Black Men's Health Project
http://blackmenshealthproject.org

Men's Health Caucus, American Public Health Association
http://www.menshealthcaucus.net

Association of Black Cardiologists (ABC)
http://abcardio.org

Office of Minority Health
https://www.minorityhealth.hhs.gov

Gerontological Society of America (GSA)
https://www.geron.org

Men's Health Network
http://www.menshealthnetwork.org

National Black Men's Health Network
http://nbmhn.org

Office of Minority Health, AI/AN Male Health
https://minorityhealth.hhs.gov/omh/browse.aspx?lvl=3&lvlid=62

Office of Minority Health, ORISE
https://www.fda.gov/consumers/minority-health-and-health-equity/about
-fda-office-minority-health-and-health-equitys-research-and-collaboration

Prostate Conditions Education Council
https://www.prostateconditions.org

▶ Videos

Harlem Barbershop Serves Up Preventative Medical Care
Andrew Siff NBC New York
Department of Population Health at NYU Langone Medical Center
YouTube: https://www.youtube.com/watch?time_continue=2&v=R05eT8EoEKE

A short video describing the NYU School of Medicine
Department of Population Health, my academic home.
Joseph Ravenell on Public Health Live!
Saving Lives: How New York State is Increasing Colorectal Cancer Screening Rates
https://vimeo.com/157970264
March 2016

▶ Books and Articles

Graham, G., & Gracia, J. N. (2012). Health disparities in boys and men. *American Journal of Public Health, 102 Suppl 2*, S167. doi:10.2105/AJPH.2011.300607

Jack, L., Jr, & Griffith, D. M. (2013). The health of African American men: Implications for research and practice. *American Journal of Men's Health, 7*(4 Suppl), 5S–7S. doi:10.1177/1557988313490190

Parker, L. J., Hunte, H., Ohmit, A., & Thorpe, R. J., Jr. (2017). Factors associated with Black Men's preference for health information. *Health Promotion Practice, 18*(1), 119–126. doi:10.1177/1524839916664488

Ravenell, J. E., Johnson, W. E., Jr., & Whitaker, E. E. (2006). African-American Men's Perceptions of Health: A Focus Group Study. *Journal of the National Medical Association, 98*(4), 544–550.

Ravenell, J. E., Whitaker, E. E., Waldo E. Johnson, W. E., Jr. (2008). According to him: Barriers to Healthcare among African-American Men. *Journal of the National Medical Association, 100*(10), 1153–1160.

Ravenell, J., Thompson, H., Cole, H., Plumhoff, J., Cobb, G. Afolabi, L., & Boutin-Foster, C., et al. (2013). A novel community-based study to address disparities in hypertension and colorectal cancer: a study protocol for a randomized control trial. *Trials, 14*(287).

Victor, R. G., Ravenell, J. E., Freeman, A., Leonard, D., Bhat, D. G., Shafiq, M., & Knowles, P. et al. (2011). Effectiveness of a Barber-Based Intervention for Improving Hypertension Control in Black Men. *JAMA Internal Medicine, 171*(4), 342–350.

Glossary of Important Terms

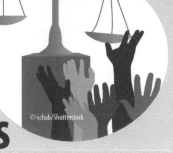

A

American Indian (Native American) or Alaska Native A person whose origins link to any of the original peoples of North America and who maintains a cultural identification through tribal affiliations or community recognition.

Asian/Pacific Islander A person whose origins link to any of the original peoples of the Far East, Southeast Asia, Indian subcontinent, or Pacific Islands. This area includes, for example, China, India, Japan, Korea, the Philippine Islands, and Samoa.

B

Black/African American A person whose origins link to any of the Black racial groups of Africa.

Black Sacred Cosmos A theoretical framework for understanding the religious composition of African Americans.

Black spirituality The notion that Black spirituality is not simply the profession of basic Christian tenets but is a divinely inspired reframing of Christianity that affirms Black existence in the world.

C

cultural competence In conjunction with linguistic competence, a set of congruent behaviors, attitudes, and policies that come together in a system or agency or among professionals to enable effective work in cross-cultural situations. The cultural competence continuum involves ensuring that the needs of diverse patients/clients/customers are met by health service and public health organizations based upon the acquisition of specific skill sets, valuing diversity, and taking concrete steps to ensure efficacy in serving minority populations.

cultural filtration The process by which a person interpreting a situation either includes or removes cultural beliefs or ideas from the interpretation process.

cultural nuance The recognition of subtle differences about a particular culture.

Culturally and Linguistically Appropriate Services (CLAS) Standards designed to address the inequities that exist in the provision of health care and to make services more responsive to the individual needs, on a cultural and linguistic basis, of patients/consumers/clients served.

culture An integrated pattern of learned beliefs and behaviors that can be shared among groups, including thoughts, styles of communicating, ways of interacting, views on roles and relationships, values, practices, and customs.

D

digital divide The notion that in lower socioeconomic status communities, individuals may not have computers.

diversity In regard to health care, the makeup of the workforce of a given healthcare organization. Diversity includes ethnic and racial backgrounds, age, physical and cognitive abilities, family status, sexual orientation, socioeconomic status, religious and spiritual values, and geographic location, and includes all of the dimensions among and all of the differences between people.

E

emerging majorities A term used to describe an inevitable change taking place in U.S. society based on the prediction that by the year 2050, in certain geographic areas in the United States, the majority populations will be Hispanic and Black people and other minorities (combined), and White people will be the minority group.

ethnicity A group's or individual's conception of cultural identity, which includes a wide variety of learned behaviors that a human being uses in his or her natural and social environment to survive, which may result in cultural demarcation between and within societies. In the United States, according to the Office of Management and Budget, there is only one ethnicity, which is Hispanic, based primarily on the commonality of the Spanish language.

F

face validity A review of the items of a survey by individuals who are not trained in the survey development process.

family wage The amount of income for a family to live on, in terms of meeting basic needs.

food desert The absence of supermarkets within poor communities such that individuals cannot get to the stores, and even if they do, they cannot afford the healthy products that are inside of them.

food injustice This disparity/gap in the offering of quality foods in low-income neighborhoods as compared to higher socioeconomic communities.

food mirage The presence of large grocery stores in low-income neighborhoods that include a full selection of products but that are not affordable to the individuals who live in the neighborhood.

freedom Through the lens of Eurocentric normativity, an American pursuit toward individualism; through the lens of the Black Sacred Cosmos, a call to total allegiance to God alone and free reign over one's life to do as God requires.

H

healthcare disparity Differences between groups in health coverage, access to care, and quality of care.

health disparity/health inequality Healthcare inequality or gaps in the quality of health and health care across racial, ethnic, and socioeconomic groups and population-specific differences in the presence of disease, health outcomes, or access to health care.

health literacy The ability to obtain, process, and understand basic health information and services needed to make appropriate health decisions.

Hispanic A person of Mexican, Puerto Rican, Cuban, Central or South American, or other Spanish cultures or origins, regardless of race.

I

inclusion The action or state of including or of being included within a group or structure.

infant mortality rate The number of infant deaths per 1,000 live births.

L

linguistic competence The capacity of an organization and its personnel to communicate effectively and convey information in a manner that is easily understood by diverse audiences, including people of limited English proficiency, people who have low literacy skills or are not literate, and people with disabilities.

low birth weight A weight of less than 2500 grams at birth.

M

mainstream A term often used to describe the "general market" and usually referring to a broad population that is primarily White and middle class.

maternal mortality rate (MMR) The annual number of female deaths per 100,000 from any cause aggravated by pregnancy or its management, excluding accidental or incidental causes.

Medicaid A means-tested (income-based) health insurance program for low-income individuals, including children.

Medicare A health insurance program that originated for people 65 years of age and older, people with long-term disability, and people with end-stage renal disease. It was signed into law by President Lyndon Baines Johnson on July 30, 1965.

middle passage The transport of slaves from Africa to the New World on slave ships across the Atlantic Ocean.

mission (of an organization) A brief statement that attempts to answer the question of why an organization exists and states the purpose of an organization, namely to those in it and to the public.

N

nationality An identity that can be defined by a person's place of legal birth or by a person's associational citizenship status governed by where the individual resides and works, which may defy national boundaries and sovereignty.

P

Patient Protection and Affordable Care Act A federal statute, pertaining to health insurance, that was signed into U.S. law by President Barack Obama on March 23, 2010.

people of color Individuals classified in the emerging majority groups, namely Black or African American, Native American or Alaska Native, Asian and Pacific Islander, and Hispanic or Latino people.

R

race Biologic variation including phenotypical differences in stature, skin color, hair color, facial shape, and other inherited characteristics that may or may not be mutually exclusive in each individual.

religion An integrated set of beliefs, rituals, and institutions through which people give expression about that which is holy or held in highest esteem in their lives.

S

school-to-prison pipeline A system of policies and practices in the United States that send children into the criminal justice system rather than helping them pursue education.

soul food A traditional food preparation style of the South, which emerged from slavery in the United States, still used by some African American people.

spirituality A high-order individual endeavor that facilitates both greater personal expression and enhanced personal benefits and outcomes, a viewpoint that is particularly ardent among those who are estranged from organized religion.

stereotype Exaggerated beliefs or fixed ideas about a person or group of people.

T

Temporary Assistance for Needy Families (TANF) Welfare reform, which emerged in 1995; a state-by-state administered program based on federal grants.

tolerance Respect, acceptance, and appreciation of the rich diversity of our world's cultures, our forms of expression, and ways of being human. It is fostered by knowledge, openness, communication, and freedom of thought, conscience, and belief.

V

visual affirmation The physical surroundings of healthcare organizations, such as artwork and images, that reflect the customers/patients/clients served.

W

White A person whose origins link to any of the original peoples of Europe, North Africa, or the Middle East. (Note that there is great debate regarding North Africa, as it is located in Egypt, which is in Africa, and the people, are largely Arab and African.)

Index

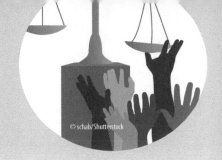

© schab/Shutterstock

Note: Page numbers followed by *f* and *t* refer to figures and tables, respectively.